THE BIRTH OF THE HOSPITAL IN THE BYZANTINE EMPIRE

The Birth of the Hospital in the Byzantine Empire

TIMOTHY S. MILLER

THE JOHNS HOPKINS UNIVERSITY PRESS
Baltimore and London

This Johns Hopkins paperbacks edition was brought to publication
with the generous assistance of the Salisbury State University Foundation, Inc.,
and the Office of the Provost, Salisbury State University.

Johns Hopkins Paperbacks edition, 1997
06 05 04 03 02 01 00 99 98 97   5 4 3 2 1

The Johns Hopkins University Press
2715 North Charles Street
Baltimore, Maryland 21218-4319
The Johns Hopkins Press Ltd., London

Library of Congress Cataloging in Publication Data

Miller, Timothy S.
    The birth of the hospital in the Byzantine Empire.

    (The Henry E. Sigerist supplements to the Bulletin
of the history of medicine; new ser., no. 10)
    Bibliography: p.
    Includes index.
    1. Hospitals, Medieval—Byzantine Empire.   2. Charities—
Byzantine Empire.   3. Public welfare—Byzantine
Empire.   4. Byzantine Empire—History.   I. Title.
II. Series.
RA964.M55   1985   362.1'1'09495   84-26111
ISBN 0-8018-2676-4 (alk. paper)

ISBN 0-8018-5657-4 (pbk.)

A catalog record for this book is available from the British Library

To my father and mother, who helped me board the ship
To Father George Dennis, who set the sails for Byzantium

God works for good with those who love him.

—Romans 8:28

Contents

Introduction to the 1997 Edition

When first published in 1985, *Birth of the Hospital in the Byzantine Empire* represented the first monograph devoted solely to tracing the history of Byzantine hospitals, the philanthropic institutions designed exclusively to treat the physically ill. Byzantine medical texts, imperial laws, monastic rules, saints' biographies, narrative histories, poems, and formal orations all provided information for reconstructing how Byzantine hospitals functioned. The evidence extracted from these sources revealed that Byzantine hospitals (*xenones*) had begun to focus exclusively on caring for and curing the sick as early as the fourth century A.D.; that these philanthropic centers continued to expand their medical services, especially during the reign of the emperor Justinian (527–65); and that by the eleventh and twelfth centuries they had become the principal theaters of the Byzantine medical profession, providing both specialized treatment to hospital patients and walk-in clinical services to the general population. Moreover, by that time these xenones were also providing instruction in the theory and practice of medicine to those who wished to become physicians.

These Byzantine hospitals, tied closely to the medieval Greek medical profession and focused solely on curing their patients, do not fit the image that twentieth-century historians of medicine and medievalists have presented of premodern hospitals—an image of poorly equipped almshouses more concerned with comforting the sick in their distress than providing medical cures. Indeed, since the Enlightenment, intellectuals have ignored the achievements of medieval charitable institutions and have established a wall between enlightened science and the imperatives of Christian morality. As John Locke observed:

> [the study of nature], if rightly directed, may be of greater benefit to mankind than the monuments of exemplary charity that have at so great a charge been raised by the founders of hospitals and almshouses. He that first invented printing, discovered the use of the compass, or made public the virtue and right

use of *kin kina* [quinine], did more for the propagation of knowledge, for the supply and increase of useful commodities, and saved more people from the grave than those who built colleges, workhouses, and hospitals.[1]

The history of Byzantine hospitals, however, clearly reveals that Christian philanthropy and scientific medicine were indeed wed, at least in the Eastern Roman Empire, where a strong medical profession survived throughout the Middle Ages.

Because Byzantine xenones do not fit the accepted notions concerning premodern hospitals, several scholars have rejected some of the evidence presented in *Birth of the Hospital* and questioned its conclusions, especially regarding the kind of treatment xenones provided and their relationship to the medical profession. While many historians have come to hold views similar to those I present in *Birth of the Hospital,* others have raised a series of objections. One critical opinion faulted the book for relying too heavily on evidence regarding a single hospital, the Pantokrator Xenon of twelfth-century Constantinople.[2] A second criticism has been that the book makes assertions without sufficient evidence to support such views.[3] A third assessment, based primarily on currently accepted ideas about the history of hospitals in Northwestern Europe, labeled as absurd the notion that a society before the twentieth century would have organized its provision of medical care around hospitals.[4]

In view of the significance of hospitals in the history of medicine in general and of the lively debate that surrounds the subject of Byzantine xenones, this paperback edition of *Birth of the Hospital* is being issued. In this edition, I have made a number of minor corrections to the original text, especially the footnotes and the bibliography. This new introduction serves in part to restate succinctly the key arguments presented in the book, and also to introduce significant new evidence discovered after its initial publication. Some of this additional material I uncovered myself; other new sources my colleagues found and kindly forwarded to me. In every case, this evidence has confirmed the original conclusions of the book. Some of the new information has been especially valuable in providing a more complete picture of how Byzantine hospitals functioned and how physicians organized their private practice around their xenon duties.

For many years the majority of Byzantinists have maintained that some hospitals in the East Roman Empire were organized to offer the best medical care possible for those afflicted by disease. These scholars based their view on the Pantokrator Typikon, the foundation charter and monastic rule of the twelfth-century monastery of Christ, the Ruler of All.[5] In 1895 a Russian scholar, Aleksei Dmitrievskij, first published the Greek text of this *typikon*, a document which not only regulated the daily routines of the monks but also outlined in detail two philanthropic institutions the monks were to maintain. The first of these was a nursing home for twenty-four aged or infirm men; the second a hospital for fifty patients. The Pantokrator Typikon describes how many physicians and medical assistants were to staff the hospital, how these medical professionals worked in monthly shifts, how much pay they received as compensation for their work, and even how these professional employees advanced to the higher ranks of the medical staff.[6]

Impressed by the hospital regulations of the Pantokrator Typikon and by the similar but less extensive descriptions of Byzantine xenones in the seventh-century *Miracula S. Artemii*, the tenth-century Sampson *Miracula*, the thirteenth-century Lips Typikon, and a variety of other sources, historians such as Georg Schreiber, Alexandre Philipsborn, Herbert Hunger, Hans Georg Beck, and Demetrios Constantelos have recognized the superiority of Byzantine hospitals over any institutional health care available in the Latin West.[7] Recent studies by Paul Magdalino and Armin Hohlweg have reiterated the importance of xenones not only as centers of medical care, but also as institutions that organized and sustained the medical profession, especially through their training of young physicians.[8]

Although historians have recognized the sophistication of Byzantine hospitals and their role in sustaining the medieval Greek medical profession, *Birth of the Hospital* was the first attempt to describe how the xenones actually functioned with respect to the Empire's physicians. In the course of my studies I noticed that the physicians at the Pantokrator hospital received extremely low salaries. Even the *primmikerioi*, the highest-ranking physicians on the staff, received only 11.75 *noumismata* a year, a salary slightly below a living wage in twelfth-century Constantinople (pp. 161–63). More than a century later the Lips Xenon also paid its doctors a remarkably low salary (pp. 201–4). How could hospital physicians survive with so little remuneration?

The Pantokrator Typikon itself and several other sources offered the key to solving this riddle. Since the seventh century A.D., hospital physicians had been working in two shifts. Each month one shift served in the hospital, while the other shift engaged in private practice; the next month the shifts exchanged roles. The rules of the Pantokrator Xenon thus allowed its physicians to pursue a private practice for six months a year, but it restricted this practice to patients who lived within Constantinople. Staff physicians were not to leave the capital to visit patients at their country estates, even if these people held high office or were members of the emperor's personal retinue.[9] These Pantokrator rules imply that the potential private patients of hospital physicians came from the pinnacle of Byzantine society.

Soon after I submitted the final typescript of *Birth of the Hospital* to the Press, Robert Volk published his thorough study of references to philanthropy and medical care in the many surviving Byzantine *typika* (the medieval Greek term for monastic rules). Of course, Volk devoted many pages to analyzing the Pantokrator Xenon, but in addition he called attention to two other twelfth-century typika which also mentioned hospitals, two references I had not included in my reconstruction of how the hospitals functioned.[10]

The first of these two references comes from the typikon prepared for the Mamas Monastery in 1158/59. Although originally founded in the sixth century, the Mamas community became prominent only in the late tenth century, but it continued to have financial problems until George Kappadokes and Athanasios Philanthropinos restored the monastery in the twelfth century and drafted a new typikon for its monks.[11] Chapter Thirty-four of this rule stipulates how the community was to care for sick monks:

> The monks who fall ill with a sudden attack of disease should be allowed to rest in their cells with the knowledge of the superior and to receive there the proper food which fits their sickness. Whoever is commanded by the superior is to serve the sick in all ways: with food, with drink, or with anything else they might need. . . . Moreover, since two *xenones* are close to our monastery, if the monastery should be able—as I hope and pray it will—the superior should make arrangements that one of the physicians nearby visit the sick brothers [the monks] each day, bring them the required medicaments, and consider them worthy of all possible care. On the other hand, if the monastery should not be able to afford this—which I pray will not be the case—then, the superior is to go for assistance to those who work in the *xenones* so that the monk in need of medical treatment can obtain a bed, and lying there [in the hospital], he can receive medical treatment. Provision for his food, however, must be made by the monastery so that the monk might not be constrained in some way and utter evil statements, for what is provided in the *xenon* is not sufficient.[12]

At the Mamas Monastery sick monks were normally to receive in-house care at the hands of their fellow ascetics; if necessary, they also enjoyed the services of a trained physician who visited them daily and prescribed their medicines. The Mamas document, however, contains two additional pieces of information regarding xenones which both confirm and expand the picture of Byzantine health care presented by the Pantokrator Typikon and other earlier sources. First, the physicians hired to visit the ailing monks at the Mamas were attached to the neighboring xenones (the superior of the monastery was to arrange for one of the hospital doctors to visit the sick monks in their cells). Second, the Mamas Monastery would have to pay a considerable sum for these private visits. The authors of the typikon expressed concern that the Mamas community might not always be able to afford the house calls. If the monastery's finances were not sufficient, then the superior was to transfer the sick monks to hospital beds in one of the two neighboring xenones. The Mamas Typikon thus indicates that physicians charged a high fee for visits to residences or monasteries. Usually, private patients would therefore have come from the class of wealthy and powerful laymen or from well-endowed monasteries such as the Mamas.

The second passage appears in the typikon written for the Heliou Bomon Monastery in 1162. The author of this document, a certain Nikephoros Mystikos, copied much of his rule from the Mamas Typikon, including sections of chapter thirty-four, the Mamas' guidelines for the treatment of sick monks.[13] Nikephoros, however, made sufficient alterations in these regulations to prove that he did not simply borrow from his archetype with no thought toward application. He altered precisely those requirements which did not suit his institution and its location—the Monastery of Heliou Bomon did not stand within the walls of Constantinople, as did the Mamas community, but had been built somewhere in Bithynia across the Bosporos from the capital city (its exact location is unknown).[14]

Just as at the Mamas, when a monk fell ill at the Heliou Bomon Monastery, the superior assigned one of his brother monks to care for the patient and to bring him whatever food or drink was suitable for the illness. If the disease proved severe or lasted many days, the superior was to have the patient transferred to one of several xenones for medical treatment. Unfortunately, the typikon provides no information on where these hospitals were located or how far away they were from the monastery. It is possible that they were in Constantinople.[15]

The author of the Heliou Bomon Typikon made one major change in the regulations he had borrowed from the Mamas Monastery: if a monk of Heliou Bomon were seriously ill, he had to go to a hospital because physicians never visited the sick at the monastery. That physicians were not available to attend the sick in this monastery might have been a result of urban hospital rules that prohibited staff physicians from leaving Constantinople to treat private patients in the Thracian or Bithynian countryside. Certainly, such restrictions would have barred the Pantokrator doctors from visiting sick monks at Heliou Bomon (pp. 48 and 162).

The evidence from these three monastic typika—Pantokrator, Mamas, and Heliou Bomon—suggests that Byzantine physicians of the twelfth century charged a high price for private visits. As a result, most people in Constantinople, both the poor and the middle class, came to the hospitals for treatment. The evidence for this I have presented in *Birth of the Hospital*. One passage from the annals of John Kinnamos, however, provides a particularly vivid picture of the central role hospitals played in providing medical services for most twelfth-century Constantinopolitans. Kinnamos had served in the government of the emperor Manuel I (1143–80) and wrote a detailed account of the emperor's reign, which the historian completed shortly after the emperor's death.[16] In a digression illustrating Manuel's skill in the art of medicine, Kinnamos wrote: "And [the emperor Manuel] has contributed many things to the science of the Asklepiads [i.e., the physicians], medicines which had been unknown in every [previous] age. Some of these medicines were to be used as salves, others as potions. For anyone who wishes, it is possible to pick up these medicines from the public *nosokomeia* which are usually called *xenones*."[17] Kinnamos clearly states that citizens of Constantinople visited the city's xenones not only when they were incapacitated, but also when they needed medicines for less serious illnesses. For this they visited infirmaries like the one the Pantokrator Xenon staffed with four novice physicians.

After completing *Birth of the Hospital,* I found, among the published poems of an anonymous twelfth-century poet, a passage which supports Kinnamos's statement. The Mangana Poet, as Byzantinists often refer to him, composed a great number of poems which date from the first half of Manuel I's reign. The Mangana ᵖoet worked for the emperor's brother Andronikos and, after Andronikos's death, for his widow Eirene, the *sebastokratorissa* (a Byzantine title for a high-ranking person).[18] In Poem no. 62, addressed to Andronikos and Eirene, the Mangana Poet complains that he has fallen ill in a province outside Constantinople while working for this august couple. He has become so sick that he has decided to leave his home province and go to the capital, where he would be able to find "both medicines and hospitals."[19] The Mangana Poet did not belong to the very poor or even the struggling artisan class. He had a position of some importance as a manager of Andronikos's estates, and he had also enjoyed the advantages of a good education.[20] Still, he did not mention that he was seeking doctors in private practice at Constantinople but, rather, that he was journeying to the capital because of its hospitals.

Three additional passages concerning hospitals refer not to xenones of the twelfth century but to those of the fourteenth and fifteenth centuries, a period during which Byzantine society was disintegrating. After I discovered these passages, I realized that I would have to revise to some extent the view I expressed in the 1985 edition of *Birth of the Hospital*—namely, that the Byzantine system of hospital care declined noticeably during the difficult Palaeologan period (1261–1453).

The first of these passages appears in the fourteenth-century *Vita Athanasii* written by Theoktistos. Athanasios was a forceful protagonist of Byzantine monasticism who twice ascended the patriarchal throne: for the first time in 1289 and again in 1303. When the emperor Andronikos II deposed him for the second time in 1309, Athanasios withdrew to the Constantinopolitan monastery of Xerolophos.[21] While there, one of his disciples fell ill with a severe infection of the throat. The disciple approached the holy Athanasios and asked the great man "either to send me to the xenon for treatment or heal me yourself—either with physicians' medicines or with the medicine of prayer." After receiving a scolding for his lack of faith, the disciple was reported to have experienced a miraculous cure when he secretly touched the hem of Athanasios' robe in imitation of the woman who was healed by touching Christ's garment (Matt. 9:19–22; Mk. 5:25–34; Lk. 8:42–48).[22]

In this story, Athanasios's disciple considers a stay at a xenon as one of the two usual ways to receive therapy for a serious disease. Apparently, sick monks at the fourteenth-century Xerolophos Monastery had the same opportunities for care available to them as did the brothers at the twelfth-century Mamas community. They could remain in the monastery and be treated by a fellow monk—in this particular case the disciple asked Athanasios to care for him—or they could go to the nearest xenon.

The second passage describing late Byzantine hospitals appears in a sermon delivered by Philotheos Kokkinos, Patriarch of Constantinople from 1354 to 1355 and again from 1364 to 1376. In this homily Philotheos was commenting on Luke 13:10–17, the passage in which the chief rabbi of the synagogue criticizes Jesus for having healed a crippled women on the Sabbath. The patriarch used an extended metaphor to illustrate how selfishly the chief rabbi had responded to the miraculous healing when he demanded that the sick come for such care only on the six days of the week but not on the Lord's day. Philotheos asks what sort of a hospital would a person establish, what medicines would he prepare, what sort of physicians and servants would he hire, and what routine for treating the sick could he devise, only to then order that the sick not seek care on the Sabbath.[23]

Philotheos's image clearly depicts a hospital founded by a wealthy individual who purchases the medicines, hires the staff, and establishes the routines to be observed. From other sources presented in *Birth of the Hospital*, we know that private individuals of the fourteenth and fifteenth centuries opened hospitals during the very period in which the emperors were forced to cut back on their support of imperial philanthropic institutions (pp. 195–99). Philotheos's sermon indicates that such privately endowed xenones were common enough to serve as a metaphor in explicating the Gospel text.

The third passage comes from the writings of the famous Western intellectual and prelate Nicholas of Cusa (1401–64), the learned German theologian who eventually supported Pope Eugenius IV against the Council of Basel. In 1437 Nicholas made a voyage to Constantinople on behalf of Pope Eugenius. While on this embassy he also attempted to find manuscripts containing the Arabic text of the Koran. In searching for these manuscripts, Nicholas met a learned Turk whom he described as *supremus praeerat hospitalibus,* an officer who apparently supervised all the hospitals of Constantinople. This Turkish physician and several Moslem associates had become interested in Christianity and wished to visit the pope with Nicholas serving as their escort. Before the Turkish physician could leave with Nicholas for Rome, however, he had to inspect the hospitals of the Byzantine capital. On his rounds, he caught the plague and died.[24]

Nicholas's strange account indicates that a system of hospitals still functioned in Constantinople as late as 1437. There is no reason to reject this account because Nicholas portrays a Moslem as the supervisor of Christian hospitals. A late fourteenth-century manuscript (*Vaticanus graecus* 299) refers to a Moslem physician named Abram who served as director of the Mangana Xenon (pp. 150 and 205). I have found no references, however, to a general supervisor of all hospitals. Nicholas possibly misunderstood the office his Turkish acquaintance filled; instead of supervising all hospitals, the Turkish physician may have served as director of one of the more prominent hospitals of the capital, perhaps as *aktouarios* (director) of the Mangana Xenon, the post that the Moslem Abram had held.[25] Despite the questions it raises, Nicholas's testimony provides additional evidence that a hospital system still existed in fifteenth-century Byzantium.

In the course of examining how Byzantine xenones functioned, *Birth of the Hospital* addressed the question of finances. Given that these xenones did not demand that patients pay for either medical care or room and board while at the hospital (the Pantokrator Typikon specifically banned any payments or tips for medical services), how did these institutions meet their expenses? My research has shown that support for hospitals came from major sectors of Byzantine society: the imperial government, the church, the monastic movement, wealthy families, and the medical profession itself through many hours of low-paid service in the xenon wards. In addition to large initial grants of land that emperors or wealthy private patrons donated, I supposed that former patients, both rich and poor, often left hospitals legacies or *inter vivos* gifts in place of payment at the time of treatment (p. 209). I have recently found evidence for such gifts.

A sixth- or early-seventh-century papyrus from Egypt (a province of the Byzantine Empire) preserves part of a will designating a woman as the heiress of an estate. The surviving text does not include the name of the testator or the name or relationship of the female heir. The text does mention, however, that the author of the testament had left a substantial legacy to a hospital, and the will refers clearly to Justinian's Novel 1, a law issued in 535 allowing a testator to disinherit his heir if that person failed to carry out the legacy within one year after the testator's death. The author wanted to ensure that the woman he had named as his heir did not fail to deliver the legacy to the hospital he had designated.[26]

A second testament comes from twelfth-century Constantinople. In drafting his will, the testator, a monk, left almost all his property to the Monastery of Saint George Tropaiophoros in the Mangana. He specified particular books for the monastic library, including service books for Holy Week compiled by Theodore Prodromos, the most famous contemporary writer and teacher of the capital. The monk also left twelve gold hyperpyra to the Mangana hospital: eight hyperpyra to purchase sugar and four to buy olive oil for the medicines.[27]

A third donation, this time an *inter vivos* gift, sheds some light on what motivated these donations and legacies to hospitals. The tenth-century version of the *Vita Sancti Sampsonis* added to the text of the saint's life a series of miracle tales recounting how Saint Sampson had cured patients at his hospital.[28] In one of these tales, a *protospatharios* named Eustathios developed a serious eye infection; he sought assistance from his friend Leo, who had just accepted the responsibility of supervising the finances of the Sampson Xenon. Leo persuaded Eustathios to sign a written contract promising to supply the hospital with olive oil. As a result of his promise, Saint Sampson miraculously cured Eustathios's eye infection.[29] Such cures, both natural and supernatural, no doubt moved many people to offer some remuneration in return for the help they had received either in xenon wards or in the outpatient clinics.

Having highlighted some of the most important features of Byzantine hospitals and introduced several new sources that help to illustrate how these institutions treated the sick and financed their philanthropic services, I shall now address the questions that my colleagues have raised regarding *Birth of the Hospital*. The most significant group of critics has maintained that *Birth of the Hospital* and other studies describing Byzantine xenones rely too much on the detailed description of the Pantokrator Xenon, found in the twelfth-century typikon for the Pantokrator Monastery. These critics claim that this remarkably well-organized hospital was an exception, perhaps even a unique institution in the history of the Byzantine Empire. They warn that the Pantokrator Xenon should not be used as an example of hospital care in most Byzantine xenones. According to these scholars, the majority of Byzantine hospitals offered general charitable assistance—food, shelter, and some nursing care—to many categories of needy people.[30] In sum, they believe these xenones differed little from the hospices and hospitals of the medieval West. Some of these critics have even suggested that the Pentokrator Typikon's hospital instructions were never implemented. They were meant to serve, instead, as an example of a perfect hospital—a utopian ideal for hospital planners, not a description of a functioning institution.[31]

In addressing these views, I shall begin by stating emphatically that the Pantokrator Xenon was not unique, nor did it hold the first place in prestige among Constantinopolitan hospitals. A laudatory *vita* of the empress Eirene, the wife of John II Komnenos and cofounder of the Pantokrator Monastery, states explicitly that the Pantokrator Xenon "almost" held the first place among such institutions, outshining most—but not all—of them in beauty, fame, location, and effective organization.[32] Two hospitals which it surely did not surpass were the ancient Sampson and the more recent Mangana, founded in the eleventh century.

Byzantine texts, both legal and literary, always accorded the greatest honor among hospitals to the renowned Sampson Xenon. Opened sometime in the late fourth century, the Sampson was indisputably the oldest philanthropic medical institution in Constantinople. After the Nika fire of A.D. 532

destroyed the original hospital, the emperor Justinian rebuilt it as a multistoried complex of elaborate buildings. Before A.D. 600 the *archiatroi*, the leading physicians of Constantinople, were supervising patient treatment in its wards. In the seventh century, it had specialized rooms for surgery and for patients with eye diseases. Sources from the eighth and ninth century reveal its continuing importance. The Miracle Tales of Saint Sampson, a tenth-century addition to the ancient *vita* of the hospital's founder, reveals that even a leading aristocrat of a patrician family, a courtier of the emperor Romanos II, was assigned a hospital bed by the Sampson Xenon staff.[33] When Constantine Akropolites described the Sampson hospital in the late thirteenth century, he compared it to Justinian's great church of Hagia Sophia.[34] Although two panegyric texts praise the beauty of the Pantokrator Monastery, the hospital, and the gardens which surrounded the complex, neither compared this foundation to the great domed church of Justinian.[35]

Among the more recent philanthropic foundations of Constantinople, the Mangana Xenon also outranked the Pantokrator hospital. The emperor Constantine IX (1042–55) had expanded the old imperial palace of the Mangana into a vast complex of buildings including the Monastery of Saint George Tropaiophoros, a dependent xenon and *gerokomeion* (old-age home), and a renowned law school. Evidence presented in *Birth of the Hospital* links the Mangana Xenon with the imperial physicians who supervised the emperor's health. For example, the *aktouarios*, the highest-ranking physician attached to the imperial court, also served as a key official on the Mangana Xenon staff, probably its director (pp. 149–50). The imperial government restored the Mangana Xenon after Michael VIII regained control of Constantinople from the Latins in 1261 and continued to support this hospital throughout the fourteenth century; such government attention reflects the high status held by this hospital (pp. 183–84 and 195). Meanwhile, there is no evidence that the Byzantine government considered restoring the Pantokrator Xenon after 1261.

Though it is beyond doubt that the Pantokrator Xenon was not a unique institution in Constantinople, one must admit that *Birth of the Hospital*, as well as other studies of Byzantine philanthropic institutions, have relied heavily on the wealth of detailed information supplied by the Pantokrator Typikon. In many areas of ancient and medieval studies, however, historians often must depend on a single source to reconstruct the past. For example, without the *Notitia Dignitatum*, a detailed outline of the late Roman bureaucratic structure ca. A.D. 400, historians would have been unable to reconstruct the complex civil and military bureaucracy of the imperial government after the reorganizations of Diocletian and Constantine.[36] Without the comments of Galen, penned in the second century after Christ, we would understand much less about the development of Greek medicine during the Hellenistic period.[37]

In writing *Birth of the Hospital*, I attempted to use the Pantokrator

Typikon with care. I have never assumed that organizational features of the twelfth-century Pantokrator Xenon were present in earlier hospitals unless I found contemporary evidence to justify such an assumption, nor have I ignored the element of change while tracing the evolution of Byzantine hospitals through the many centuries covered by the book. In the final analysis, it rests with each reader of *Birth of the Hospital* and with future scholars to determine whether I have correctly employed the Pantokrator Typikon in explicating earlier sources describing xenones.

With regard to the most extreme position advanced by these critics—that the Pantokrator Xenon hospital, as described in the typikon, never in fact existed—one should consider several other twelfth-century sources besides the typikon which describe the Pantokrator Xenon as a center of medical care. Robert Volk cited three of these sources in his study of Byzantine typika.[38] A fourth source was recently discovered by Michael Jeffreys among the many unpublished poems of the Mangana Poet, a work Jeffreys has identified as Poem 59. Since this poem remains unpublished, I provide a summary here of its contents relevant to the Pantokrator hospital.[39]

The Mangana Poet addressed Poem 59 to his employer, the *sabastokratorissa* Eirene, widow of Andronikos Komnenos and sister-in-law of the emperor Manuel I (1143–80). In many of his poems, the Mangana Poet begs Eirene for financial support or for assistance in obtaining favors from the emperor Manuel I. In Poem 59, however, the Mangana Poet describes an illness Eirene contracted and the treatment she was receiving for it from the doctors of the Pantokrator Xenon. Two verses make clear that Eirene was occupying a bed reserved for patients of the hospital, a bed the Mangana Poet prays someone else will soon occupy.[40] That a member of the imperial family would seek help at the Pantokrator is an indication of the high-quality medical care available at this hospital. Other sources, however, also prove that Byzantine aristocrats occasionally made use of public hospitals when they were ill. The tenth-century Miracle Tales of Saint Sampson describe a high court official who occupied a hospital bed while receiving treatment at the Sampson Xenon.[41]

Poem 59 mentions at least three physicians assigned to treat Eirene: two younger doctors and a third, older physician who outranked the others. These doctors gave Eirene a pill and sprinkled her with a concoction made from figs. The senior physician also bled her by using a leech, a treatment the Mangana Poet harshly criticizes. The poem also stresses how the younger physicians had mastered the *logos* of medicine and obtained boundless professional experience as well—doubtless a reference to the hospital's training program, which involved studying medical texts under the teacher of physicians and also an extended period of serving as an apprentice physician in the hospital wards (pp. 156–59).

In reviewing Poem 59, the Pantokrator Typikon, and all the other texts describing the Pantokrator Xenon and comparing the findings with what Byzantine sources reveal about other hospitals, one can confidently state that the Pantokrator offered excellent medical care, adequate even for the reigning emperor's sister-in-law. On the other hand, the Pantokrator Xenon operated fully within the tradition of Constantinopolitan hospitals, a tradition stretching back to the reign of Justinian. In the complex rules governing the Pantokrator Xenon, the Typikon does not employ a single novel term or introduce a single new feature of hospital organization. Every term the Typikon has selected, every title ascribed to members of the medical staff, and every detail of daily regime can be documented in sources describing earlier Byzantine xenones.

Some scholars have raised a second objection to *Birth of a Hospital*, namely that it has attempted to explain too much, to derive more information from the extant sources than they in fact contain. On the basis of such an argument, these historians have rejected my conclusion that the emperor Justinian played a key role in the evolution of Byzantine hospitals by transferring the leading physicians of the Empire, the municipal archiatroi, from the payroll of the Empire's cities to the staffs of the Christian xenones (pp. 44–49). These historians have stressed that no specific law survives in the huge corpus of Justinianic legislation and administrative regulations to indicate such a shift. Without primary evidence for the reassignment of archiatroi, these critics have denied that Justinian ever carried out this fundamental change in the classical medical profession.[42]

My argument in support of Justinian's reassigning archiatroi to hospital service relies on three considerations: first, that all references to archiatroi after the mid-sixth century represent these doctors practicing their profession in association with Christian hospitals; second, that during the reign of Justinian other institutions of the classical polis passed under the supervision of the Christian church; and third, that Prokopios, the chronicler of Justinian's reign, makes an oblique reference to the emperor's reform of the archiatroi.

Birth of the Hospital presents the physician Flavius Phoibammon as the first example of an archiatros closely associated with a xenon (p. 48). A lengthy papyrus document dated 570 preserves a testament prepared by Phoibammon, an archiatros of the Egyptian city of Antinoopolis. In addition to other properties listed in the testament, Phoibammon had inherited the supervision of a xenon in Antinoopolis from his father, who had also been an archiatros of the city. The testament does not make clear how Flavius Phoibammon's father came to administer this hospital, but it is significant for our argument that he was supervising this institution in the years prior to 570, the later years of the emperor Justinian (527–65).[43]

After describing this Egyptian case, *Birth of the Hospital* next examines the *Miracula Sancti Artemii*, a seventh-century text that describes the archiatroi working in monthly shifts at the Christodotes Xenon of Constantinople.[44]

After publication of the book, I discovered another source that refers to an archiatros assigned to the Sampson Xenon during the reign of the emperor Maurikios (582–602). According to this story, Maurikios had managed to capture a vicious robber who had terrorized the countryside of Thrace. After the emperor imprisoned him in Constantinople, the robber fell seriously ill and was assigned a bed in the Sampson Xenon. At the moment of the robber's death, the archiatros in charge of the hospital had a dream revealing that God had forgiven the criminal.[45] This detail of the story supports the evidence from the Antinoopolis papyrus that archiatroi were supervising Christian hospitals by the late sixth century.

In addition to this consistent evidence, I also considered relevant Justinian's general policy of realigning polis government around Christian institutions. Completing a program initiated by the emperor Anastasios I (491–518), Justinian transferred the selection of important polis officials such as the *defensor civitatis* and the *sitones* (the official in charge of the city's grain supply) from the old municipal council (*curia*) to a new group of wealthy landowners headed by the local bishop. Recent research has shown that, as a result of Justinian's legislation, the patriarch of Alexandria was supervising that great city's emergency grain stores by the beginning of the seventh century.[46] At Constantinople, the director of the capital's largest Christian philanthropic institution, the Orphanotropheion (orphanage), had assumed responsibility for maintaining emergency grain supplies by the time of the Persian-Avar assault in the early seventh century.[47]

A recent study on the baths of the Byzantine Empire has shown that the great public bathing facilities of the Eastern cities began to experience serious difficulties in the sixth century. In the late fifth century, a monastery replaced a bath and gymnasium built on the island of Chios during the reign of Constantine. Excavations at Aizanai in Asia Minor have revealed that the bath complex at that city was converted into a church and a number of other facilities during the reign of Justinian.

As these ancient baths waned, new Christian institutions called *diakoniai* began to spread throughout the East. Although initially the Monophysites sponsored these philanthropic foundations, orthodox Chalcedonians eventually copied them (pp. 130–32). The main philanthropic service of these *diakoniai* was to provide baths for the poor. Some *diakoniai* built their own bath houses; others rented existing facilities. In addition to these *diakoniai*, monasteries in the sixth century began to build and maintain small bath houses to serve laymen. These smaller Christian baths gradually replaced the vast bathing facilities of the classical *polis*.[48]

The imperial government mandated the transfer of polis government from the ancient city councils to the local bishops and encouraged the concomitant expansion of church responsibility by issuing many constitutions confirming the new powers of Christian officers. The decline of the ancient bathing facilities and their replacement by Christian baths, on the other hand, seems to have occurred spontaneously, perhaps as the result of economic forces or of moral considerations—the cavernous classical baths had been difficult to police, and Christian homilists had attacked them as places of immorality. It is, nevertheless, significant that the transformation of polis institutions, whether government sponsored or spontaneous, took place in the sixth century, the same time period during which the municipal archiatroi began to appear as physicians in the Christian hospitals.

The foregoing considerations would not necessarily indicate that Justinian altered the organization of the city archiatroi. The change from municipal physicians to hospital doctors could have occurred spontaneously, as the transformation of bathing practices did. The historian Prokopios, however, specifically mentions that Justinian altered the method of remunerating archiatroi. In his *Anekdota*, a vicious attack on the character and policies of Justinian and his ministers, Prokopios tries to portray not only Justinian's wicked personal qualities, but also his ill-conceived government programs, which Prokopios believed were destroying the core of ancient society, the classical city-states. As an example of Justinian's ruinous acts regarding the ancient cities, Prokopios states:

> Nay more, he [Justinian] also caused physicians and teachers of freeborn children to be in want of the necessities of life. For the allowance of free maintenance which former Emperors had decreed should be given to men of these professions from the public funds he cancelled entirely. . . . And thereafter neither physicians nor teachers were held in any esteem.[49]

Since the second century, the only physicians who received stipends from the government were called archiatroi (p. 46). In this passage, Prokopios clearly records a major change in the nature of the city archiatroi, the direct heirs of the public physicians of classical Greece. But did Justinian merely cancel the government subsidies to these doctors? In view of Prokopios' love of ancient institutions, his coolness toward the Christian church, and his hatred of Justinian, it is easy to see how he could interpret the reassigning of archiatroi to Christian hospital service as the destruction of the traditional profession of medicine.

Prokopios's statement implies that a reorientation of city archiatroi resulted from a policy decision by Justinian. Since no official law ordering a major revision of how these doctors were paid survives, it is also possible that the movement of archiatroi into Christian xenon service might have occurred spontaneously, just as the changes in bathing facilities had evolved. With their large endowments, xenones might have offered a more dependable source of income than the financially troubled municipal governments. Moreover, as Christianity grew stronger, devout physicians would have seen hospital service as a way of fulfilling the Gospel's command to assist those in need.

Whether as the result of imperial policy, as Prokopios seems to indicate, or of a spontaneous development, there is no doubt that the decades of the sixth century saw the archiatroi assume a leading role in treating the patients of Byzantine hospitals. These archiatroi, in turn, bound the Christian xenones more tightly to the medical profession and helped to ensure that these philanthropic hospitals continued to focus on curing illnesses, not simply on caring for the sick (pp. 156–61).

Some researchers, particularly among the historians of medicine, have developed a third argument against the conclusions reached in *Birth of the Hospital,* an argument based not so much on interpreting Byzantine sources as on experiences in studying how other premodern societies, particularly Western Europe, organized medical care. As one historian of medicine has put it, hospital care in Byzantium "took very much a second place to treatment in the home by privately engaged and self-employed physicians. That is what our literary sources emphasize, and to argue otherwise flies in the face of common sense and of all other parallels for societies before this century."[50] But were there no societies prior to the twentieth century which developed a medical system in which hospitals occupied a central place?

From the ninth century on, Islamic society maintained a medical organization in which hospitals played a primary role, particularly in collecting important manuscripts, promoting translations into Arabic, and educating new physicians.[51] So important did hospitals become to the organization of Islamic medicine that the famous twelfth-century Egyptian physician Ibn Jumay recommended good hospitals as a key step in maintaining a high-quality medical profession because such institutions offered ideal opportunities for the proper training of doctors.[52] No historians of Islamic medicine have yet thoroughly studied the role of these hospitals in providing medical care to the people of Baghdad, Aleppo, or Cairo, but it is possible that such institutions performed services similar to the xenones of Constantinople.

Renaissance Florence offers another example of a society prior to the twentieth century in which hospitals occupied a central position in the treatment of illnesses and the training of young physicians. Katharine Park and John Henderson have focused attention on the Hospital of Santa Maria Nuova, an institution that one fifteenth-century humanist hailed as the first hospital among Christians. The rules of this hospital engaged the services of the six best physicians in Florence and required that they come to the hospital each day and supervise the treatment of the sick. In addition, the hospital supported three young physicians who lived on the premises and received room, board, and an unparalleled opportunity to learn from experience in return for dedicating their full-time service to the hospital patients. In addition to its patient wards, Santa Maria Nuova also maintained an outpatient clinic, and everyone who could not afford private physicians came to this dispensary for medicines and other sorts of treatment.[53]

We have no idea what percentage of Florentines used the hospital compared to those who paid for private treatment, but surviving records of the individual patients at Santa Maria Nuova from the years 1502–14 reveal a discharge rate from the hospital proper of between 86 and 91 percent.[54] In other words, only 9 to 14 percent of the patients admitted during these years died in the hospital's care. These statistics indicate that Santa Maria Nuova was not the death trap that Enlightenment reformers of the eighteenth century imagined philanthropic hospitals to be.

The physicians at Santa Maria Nuova also kept a record of effective remedies that they had devised in the course of their hospital practice, the very same kind of lists which xenon physicians collected in Constantinople.[55] During the sixteenth century the Florentine guild of physicians added hospital experience as a requirement for licensing, and by the end of the same century surgeons had organized formal instruction at the hospital. The medical profession of Renaissance and early modern Florence increasingly came to see hospitals and hospital experience as an essential part of medical practice. In this, they were following the same paths that Byzantine physicians had pursued half a millennium earlier.[56]

In sum, hospital medicine did not always take "a second place to treatment in the home" by self-employed physicians up until the twentieth century. In Islamic cities as well as fifteenth- and sixteenth-century Florence (and perhaps in other Italian cities), physicians integrated hospital practice into the fiber of the medical profession, especially in training new physicians. After one considers these two examples, the Byzantine xenones cease to appear so exceptional, so isolated from developments in the Latin world of the West and from medical institutions in the Moslem society of the East.

To conclude this introduction, I shall briefly outline three paths for further research which promise to yield additional information concerning Byzantine xenones and their development through the centuries. The first path we have just examined—that is, the history of medieval and Renaissance Italian hospitals. Recent research I have conducted on the *Antidotarium magnum,* the major twelfth-century pharmacopoeia used at the medical school of Salerno, demonstrates that this treatise included at least three entries derived from Constantinopolitan xenon treatment lists. There might be many more Byzantine remedies in the Salerno text, but determining how many would require a critical edition of the *Antidotarium magnum,* as well as a careful comparison with the many extant xenon treatment lists. After such careful philological and codicological analysis, it might be possible to gauge to what extent Byzantine hospital medicine influenced the Salerno physicians.[57]

The hospitals of Renaissance Florence and Siena offer another area of fruitful study. Did the Florentine hospital of Santa Maria Nuova, so strikingly similar to Byzantine hospitals, evolve its organizational features independent of any outside influence, or did Byzantine refugees from the Ottoman advance instruct their Italian hosts not only in ancient Greek but also in contemporary Byzantine medical practice? One of the leading Greek immigrant scholars at Florence was John Argyropoulos (Giovanni Argiropulo), who had taught science and medicine at a Constantinopolitan xenon before the Turkish conquest of the Byzantine capital in 1453.[58] So far, historians have found no connection between Argyropoulos and the Florentine hospitals, but the study of these remarkable Tuscan institutions has only just begun.

Archaeology represents the second promising path to future discoveries concerning Byzantine hospitals. Visitors to Hagia Sophia can still see the ruins of the ancient Sampson Xenon to the northeast of the Great Church. One can find there a maze of walls and what appears to be a courtyard. A scientific survey of the aboveground ruins might reveal important information concerning Constantinople's most famous hospital.[59] It might also be rewarding to study more thoroughly the walls and vaults surrounding the Pantokrator monastery churches which still stand today in central Istanbul. All around these domed churches one can see the substructures of what once were the xenon, the *gerokomeion,* and the monastic quarters of the Pantokrator community (p. 12).

Although almost all the documentary evidence presented both in *Birth of the Hospital* and in this introductory essay refer to xenones at Constantinople, evidence exists that some hospitals served other cities such as Thessalonica, Philadelphia, and Nicea (pp. 165, 193, and 197). Moreover, in the preamble to his Novel 19, a law restricting new monastic foundations, the emperor Nikephoros II Phokas stated that the Empire not only had enough monasteries, but also sufficient xenones and *gerokomeia* to serve his subjects' needs. His statement implies that a network of hospitals for the sick and rest homes for the aged and chronically ill existed by the tenth century. Rather than establish new ones, Nikephoros recommended that donors increase the endowment of existing charitable foundations so that these institutions could maintain the facilities they already had.[60]

If such a network of provincial hospitals functioned throughout the Empire, perhaps archaeologists surveying Byzantine sites in Asia Minor or Greece will discover the remains of some of these other xenones. During recent excavations at Corinth, Charles Williams and Orestes Zervos have, in fact, identified the remains of a hospital. This particular structure dates from the years of Frankish occupation (second third of the thirteenth century), but it may contain information applicable to provincial Byzantine xenones of the twelfth century.[61]

Opening the third path to a better understanding of Byzantine hospitals will require painstaking research by philologists and historians of medicine, in order to prepare thorough studies of the many edited and unedited Byzantine medical treatises and treatment lists. In his detailed analysis of the fourteenth-century physician John Zachariah, Armin Hohlweg discovered that Zachariah had made some of his medical observations while working in a xenon. Hohlweg found these references in a work of Zachariah published in the 1840's.[62] Other references may also appear in the extensive unedited writings by this late Byzantine physician.

In addition to the many unpublished works of John Zachariah, Byzantine codices contain a myriad of treatment lists, pharmacopoeias, and epitomes of Classical medical treatises. Careful study of these works and the manuscripts which preserve them may reveal much information on Byzantine hospital practice. Such studies would not only seek to establish the oldest versions of particular treatment lists or pharmacopoeias, but they would also record just as carefully which new therapies physicians added and which they removed as the lists were recopied in later manuscripts. An accurate knowledge of the transformations experienced by these treatment lists and a careful record of the physicians credited with discovering new therapies might unveil much about the practice of hospital physicians.[63]

In Chapter Nine, "Hospitals and Medical Literature," *Birth of the Hospital* only touches on this vast subject, but the wealth of information uncovered simply by examining one xenon treatment list, found in *Vaticanus graecus* 299, folios 368–393[v], demonstrates how fruitful careful philological and codicological research focused on a wider selection of Byzantine medical manuscripts might be in the future.

This introductory essay presents new evidence regarding Byzantine hospitals and attempts to answer some of the objections raised by scholars regarding the history of medical xenones presented in *Birth of the Hospital*. It is perhaps useful to close this discussion by reducing the debate concerning xenones to its simplest terms. Were Byzantine xenones hospitals in the modern sense of the term, medical centers controlled by trained physicians and designed to cure the sick, as *Birth of the Hospital* maintains, or were they facilities established primarily to provide care and comfort to the suffering? A passage from the tenth-century biography of Saint Luke the Stylite should help answer this question. (It is important to notice that the Constantinopolitan xenon described in this hagiographical source is neither the ancient Sampson nor the twelfth-century Pantokrator hospital.)

> [Sergios, having been severely beaten] was found sometime later by those assigned the task [of searching out the sick]. Sergios was lying as though dead, scarcely breathing. Sadly, they lifted Sergios up, and carrying him in a litter, they left him at the hospital called Euboulos. There, those learned in the medical art consulted together and examined his condition carefully from the first day to the seventh, but seeing that the injury was greater than any medical study or therapy, they completely gave up and abandoned hope for his life. Moving on, they left him unattended and urged those in charge of his care to make

preparations because of this. . . . The people who were responsible for taking care of him received this painful news; they picked up the hopeless Sergios in a litter and carried him to a home in a holy house nearby, named after the martyr of God, Nicholas, and located next to the place called the Tyche of the City. Here they placed him to breathe his last according to the situation.[64]

Sergios, however, did not die in the hospice of Saint Nicholas. Having been judged incurable by the physicians and thus removed from the Euboulos hospital, he received divine healing through the prayers of Saint Luke.

Notes

1. John Locke, *An Essay Concerning Human Understanding,* IV.12.12.

2. Recent works which have presented views similar to those expressed in *Birth of the Hospital* are: Paul Magdalino, *The Empire of Manuel I Komnenos, 1143–1180* (Cambridge: Cambridge University Press, 1993), pp. 360–66; Alexander Kazhdan and Ann Wharton Epstein, *Change in Byzantine Culture in the Eleventh and Twelfth Centuries* (Berkeley: University of California Press, 1985), pp. 156–58; Stanley Samuel Harakas, "The Eastern Orthodox Tradition," in *Caring and Curing: Health and Medicine in the Western Religious Traditions,* ed. Ronald L. Numbers and Darrel W. Amundsen (New York: Macmillan, 1986), pp. 146–72; Demetrios Constantelos, *Byzantine Philanthropy and Social Welfare,* 2d ed. (New Rochelle, N.Y.: Caratzas, 1991), pp. 113–39; Evelyne Patlagean, "Les donateurs, les moines et les pauvres dans quelques documents byzantins des XIe–XIIe siècles," in *Horizons Marins, Itinéraires spirituels (V^e–XVIIIe siècles). Vol. 1: Mentalités et Sociétés,* ed. Henri Dublois et al. (Paris: Publications de la Sorbonne, 1987), pp. 223–31; Armin Hohlweg, "La formazione culturale e professionale del medico a Bisanzio," *Koinonia,* 1989, *13.2:* 165–88, esp. pp. 184–87; and Michael Angold, *Church and Society in Byzantium under the Comneni, 1081–1261* (Cambridge: Cambridge University Press, 1995), pp. 308–14.

Among those works which warn against overdependence on the Pantokrator Typikon are the following: Michael W. Dols, "The Origins of the Islamic Hospital," *Bull. Hist. Med.,* 1987, *61:* 367–90, esp. p. 370: "Unfortunately, Miller interprets the long history of the Byzantine hospital in terms of the large, twelfth-century Pantocrator Hospital in Constantinople"; Ewald Kislinger, "Der Pantokrator Xenon, ein trügerisches Ideal?" *Jahrbuch der österreichischen Byzantinistik,* 1987, *37:* 173–79; Review by Gary Ferngren, *Transactions and Studies of the College of Physicians of Philadelphia: Medicine and History,* 1987, *5.9:* 138–41; Review by Angeliki E. Laiou, *The American Historical Review,* 1989, *94:* 426.

3. Vivian Nutton, "Review essay," *Medical History,* 1986, *30:* 218–21; Review by Gary Ferngren, *Transactions and Studies,* p. 140; Review by John Scarborough, *Isis,* 1986, *77:* 372–73.

4. Nutton, "Review essay," p. 221. This also is the assumption of most of the earlier works on medieval hospitals such as Henry Sigerist, "An Outline of the Development of the Hospital," *Bull. Hist. Med.,* 1936, *4:* 579. See the bibliography in *Birth of the Hospital,* p. 218, note 3 for other references. See also Peregrine Horden, "A Discipline of Relevance: The Historiography of the Later Medieval Hospital," *The Society for the Social History of Medicine: Bulletin,* 1988, *40:* 359–74, who offers important considerations for the proper understanding of the history of welfare, but his suggestions cannot be applied to evaluating the role of Byzantine xenones because of their exclusively medical orientation.

5. See Schreiber, "Hospital," pp. 3–80; Philipsborn, "Krankenhauswesen," pp. 338–65; Hunger, *Reich,* pp. 173–80; Constantelos, *Philanthropy,* pp. 152–84 (1968 edition); and Hans

Georg Beck, *Das byzantinische Jahrtausend,* 2d ed. (Munich: Verlag Beck, 1994), pp. 216 and 340–42.

6. Dmitrievskij, *Opisanie,* pp. 656–705. See *PantTyp,* the modern edition edited by Paul Gautier, pp. 1–145. For an analysis of the Typikon, see below, *Birth of the Hospital,* pp. 14–21.

7. For a partial list of these historians see note 5 above. Regarding the *Miracula S. Artemii,* there is now an English translation of this valuable text with extensive commentary and a reprint of the Greek text edited by Athanasios Papadopoulos-Kerameus; for this edition see Vergil S. Crisafulli and John Nesbitt, *The Miracles of St. Artemios* (Leiden: Brill, 1996).

8. Magdalino, *The Empire of Manuel I Komnenos, 1143–1180,* pp. 361–66; Hohlweg, "La formazione culturale e professionale," p. 183.

9. *PantTyp,* p. 87.955–58 (regarding monthly shifts); p. 107.1305–12 (regarding the restrictions on leaving Constantinople).

10. Volk, *Klostertypika,* pp. 134–99 analyzes the Pantokrator Typikon; pp. 215–21 and pp. 222–24 present the two *typika* not discussed in *Birth of the Hospital.*

11. Ibid., pp. 215–21 and Janin, *Eglises,* pp. 314–19.

12. "Τυπικὸν τῆς Μονῆς τοῦ ἁγίου μεγαλομάρτυρος Μάμαντος," ed. Sophronios Eustratiades, *Ellenika,* 1928, *1:* 287–88.

13. Volk, *Klostertypika,* pp. 222–24.

14. Raymond Janin, *Géographie ecclésiastique de l'empire byzantin. Vol. 2. Les églises et les monastères des grands centres byzantins (Bithynie, Hellespont, Latros, Galèsios, Trébizonde, Athènes, Thessalonique)* (Paris: Institut Français d'Études Byzantines, 1975), pp. 142–48.

15. Typikon of Nikephoros Mystikos for the Monastery of the Theotokos tôn Bomon, in Dmitrievskij, *Opisanie,* pp. 748–49.

16. Hunger, *Literatur,* 1:409–15.

17. Kinnamos, 4.21 (p. 190).

18. Magdalino, *The Empire of Manuel I Komnenos, 1143–1180,* p. 348, p. 440, and p. 494. See also the entry "Prodromos, Manganeios" in *The Oxford Dictionary of Byzantium,* ed. Alexander Kazhdan et al. (New York: Oxford University Press, 1991), 3:1726.

19. Poem II, *De Manganis,* ed. Silvius Bernardinello, Studi bizantini e neogreci, 4 (Padua: Liviana editrice, 1972), p. 33. Michael and Elisabeth Jeffreys, who are preparing an edition of all the Mangana Poet's poems, have established a new numbering system for these works. By this system, Bernardinello's Poem II becomes Poem 62. See the list of the Mangana Poet's poems published in Magdalino, *The Empire of Manuel I Kmonenos, 1143–1180,* pp. 494–500.

20. Magdalino, *The Empire of Manuel I Komnenos, 1143–1180,* p. 348.

21. For the biography of Athanasios, see *The Correspondence of Athanasios I, Patriarch of Constantinople: Letters to the Emperor Andronicus II, Members of the Imperial Family, and Officials,* ed. and trans. Alice Mary Talbot, Dumbarton Oaks Texts, 3 (Washington, D.C.: Dumbarton Oaks, 1975), pp. xv–xxviii.

22. *Theoctisti Vita Sancti Athanasii,* ed. A. Papadopoulos-Kerameus, *Zapiski istoriko-filogičeskogo fakulteta Imperatorskogo S.-Peterburgskago Universiteta,* 1905, *7:* 41–42.

23. *Logos 10,* Φιλοθέου Κοκκίνου λόγοι καὶ ὁμίλιες, ed. Basileios Pseutogkas, Thessalonian Byzantine Writers, 2 (Thessalonica: Kentron Byzantinon Ereunon, 1981), pp. 221–22.

24. *Nicolai de Cusa cribratio Alkorani,* ed. Ludovicus Hagemann (Hamburg: Felix Meiner, 1986), pp. 5–6. Dr. Robert Trone of Gettysburg College discovered this reference to late Byzantine hospitals.

25. *Vaticanus graecus,* 299, fol. 374; see *Birth of the Hospital,* p. 249 n. 56.

26. For the text mentioned, see Pap. no. 62, *An Alexandrian Erotic Fragment and Other Greek Papyri Chiefly Ptolemaic,* ed. Bernard Grenfell (Oxford: Clarendon Press, 1896), pp. 102–3; for an excellent commentary, see Mario Amelotti and Livia M. Zingale, *Le costituzioni giustinianee nei papiri e nelle epigrafi,* 2d edition (Milan: Dott. A. Giuffrè editore, 1985), pp. 77–78.

27. Silvio G. Mercati, "Un testament en faveur de Saint-Georges des Manganes," *REB,* 1948, *6:* 46–47.

28. For a description of the various versions of the *Vita Sancti Sampsonis,* see Timothy S. Miller, "The Sampson Hospital of Constantinople," *Byzantinische Forschungen,* 1990, *15:* 101–35, for the Miracle Tales, see pp. 120–21.

29. *Miraculum* VII, PG, 115, col. 301 (sec. 18).

30. Dols, "Origins," p. 371; Peregrine Horden, "The Byzantine Welfare State: Image and Reality," *The Society for the Social History of Medicine: Bulletin,* 1985, *37:* 7–10. See also Carolina Cupane and Ewald Kislinger, "Xenon und Xenodocheion im spätbyzantinischen Roman," *Jahrbuch der österreichischen Byzantinistik,* 1986, *36:* 201–6.

31. Kislinger, "Der Pantokrator-Xenon," pp. 178–79; Horden, "The Byzantine Welfare State," pp. 7–10.

32. See the section of the *Vita imperatoris Irenes* reproduced in Volk, *Klostertypika,* p. 191.

33. The history of the Sampson Xenon is retraced in Miller, "The Sampson Hospital," pp. 101–35.

34. Ibid., pp. 101–2 note 2. The *Vita Sampsonis III* of Constantine Akropolites is still unedited. It is preserved in *Codex Ambrosianus,* H.81 suppl., fols. 152ᵛ–169ᵛ.

35. Volk, *Klostertypika,* pp. 189–92.

36. See Guido Clemente, *La "Notitia Dignitatum"* (Cagliari: Sarda Fossataro, 1968), pp. 63 and 123.

37. Eustace D. Phillips, *Greek Medicine,* Aspects of Greek and Roman Life (London: Thames and Hudson, 1973), pp. 139–60; G. E. R. Lloyd, *Greek Science After Aristotle* (New York: Norton, 1973), pp. 75–90.

38. Volk, *Klostertypika,* pp. 189–92.

39. Poem 59 is described briefly in Magdalino, *The Empire of Manuel I Komnenos, 1143–1180,* p. 497. Michael Jeffreys kindly sent me a copy of lines 147–99 of the poem, the section describing hospital doctors. The paraphrased text presented here is based solely on my own interpretation of the Greek.

40. καὶ πόρρω (the physician) παρασύροι σε καὶ βάψοις ἐς τὴν κοίτην. Εἰς δὲ τὸν τόπον ἕτερος εἰσέλθοι σου καὶ βάψοι.

41. Miller, "The Sampson Hospital," pp. 125–66.

42. Vivian Nutton, "Essay review" *Medical History,* 1986, *30:* 219–20; Ferngren, *Transactions and Studies,* pp. 139–40.

43. *Papyrus* (Maspero), no. 67151. Although Egypt retained many distinctive political and administrative features during the Early Roman Empire, the reforms of Diocletian at the end of the third century set in motion a process whereby Egypt adopted most of the urban and provincial structures seen in the other provinces of the Late Roman Empire. See Leslie B. MacCoull, "Egypt," in Kazhdan et al., ed., *The Oxford Dictionary of Byzantium,* 1: 679–81 and Hunger, *Reich,* p. 149.

44. *Miracula Artemii,* mir. 22, pp. 28 and 30.

45. *Sancti Anastasii oratio in psalmum VI,* PG, 89, col. 1112–13.

46. Jones, *LRE,* 1: 757–59; Jean Durliat, *De la Ville antique à la ville byzantine: Le problème des subsistances,* Collection de l'École Française de Rome, 136 (Rome: École Française de Rome, 1990), pp. 457–84. For the role of the Patriarch John at Alexandria, see pp. 343–49.

47. For some of the evidence that the office of the Orphanotropheion managed an emergency grain supply for Constantinople, see Timothy S. Miller, "Joseph of Egypt and the *orphanotrophoi* of Constantinople," *Abstract of Papers: Sixteenth Annual Byzantine Studies Conference, October 26–28, 1990* (Baltimore: The Walters Art Gallery, 1990), pp. 38–39. For the Orphanotropheion during the early seventh-century siege of Constantinople, see *Chronicon paschale,* p. 721–22.

48. For a study of the transformation of Byzantine baths, see Paul Magdalino, "Church, bath, and *diakonia* in medieval Constantinople," *Church and People in Byzantium,* ed. Rosemary Morris, Twentieth Spring Symposium of Byzantine Studies (Manchester: Center for Byzantine, Ottoman, and Modern Greek Studies, 1986), pp. 165–88. Regarding the transformation of other urban institutions during the sixth century, see Helen Saradi-Mendelovici, "The Demise of the Ancient City and the Emergence of the Medieval City in the Eastern Roman Empire," *Echos du Monde Classique/Classical Views,* 1988, *n.s. 7:* 365–401.

49. Prokopios, *Anecdota,* 26.5, translation by H. B. Dewing, *Procopius,* Loeb Classical Library (Cambridge, Mass.: Harvard University Press, 1960), 6: 303.

50. Vivian Nutton, "Review essay," *Medical History,* 1986, *30:* 221.

51. Dols, "The Origins of the Islamic Hospital" (see note 2 above), pp. 367–90.

52. Ibn Jumay, *Treatise to Salāh ad-Dīn on the Revival of the Art of Medicine,* ed. and trans. Hartmut Fähndrich, Abhandlungen für die Kunde des Morgenlandes, 46.3 (Wiesbaden: Kommissionsverlag Franz Steiner, 1983), p. 28.

53. Katharine Park and John Henderson, "'The First Hospital Among Christians': The Ospedale di Santa Maria Nuova in Early Sixteenth-century Florence," *Medical History,* 1991, *35:* 164–88; Katharine Park, "Healing the Poor: Hospitals and Medical Assistance in Renaissance Florence," *Medicine and Charity before the Welfare State,* ed. Jonathan Barry and Colin Jones (London: Routledge, 1991), pp. 26–45; Katharine Park, *Doctors and Medicine in Early Renaissance Florence* (Princeton: Princeton University Press, 1986).

54. Park and Henderson, "The First Hospital among Christians," pp. 174–75.

55. Ibid., p. 174; cf. *Birth of the Hospital,* pp. 178–80.

56. Park and Henderson, "The First Hospital among Christians," pp. 174–75; cf. *Birth of the Hospital,* pp. 156–63.

57. Alfons Lutz, "Der verschollene frühsalernitanische Antidotarius magnus in einer Basler Handschrift aus dem 12. Jahrhundert und das Antidotarium Nicolai," *Veröffentlichungen der internationalen Gesellschaft für Geschichte der Pharmazie,* 1960, *n.s. 16:* 97–133.

58. For a complete biography of John Argyropoulos, see Giuseppe Cammelli, *I dotti bizantini e le origini dell' umanesimo, II: Giovanni Argiropulo* (Florence: le Monnier, 1941). A fifteenth-century miniature from a manuscript of Aristotelian texts (*Baroccianus,* 87, fol. 34ᵛ) preserves a drawing of Argyropoulos teaching in a Constantinopolitan xenon. This drawing has been reproduced on the cover of this 1997 edition of *Birth of the Hospital.* See also text, *Birth of the Hospital,* p. 206.

59. Miller, "The Sampson Hospital," 104–5.

60. Nov. 19 (Nikephoros II Phokas), *Jus,* 1: 249–52.

61. Charles K. Williams and Orestes H. Zervos, "Frankish Corinth: 1994," *Hesperia: Journal of the American School of Classical Studies at Athens,* 1995, *64:* 1–11; idem, "Frankish Corinth: 1996," *Hesperia,* 1996, *65:* 1–7.

62. Hohlweg, "Aktuarios," pp. 302–21; edition of John Zachariah, *De urinis,* in Ideler, 2: 2–192.

63. Hohlweg, "Formazione culturale" (see note 2), pp. 166–68.

64. *Vita Lucae Stylitae,* p. 218.

Preface to the Original Edition

When Professor Demetrios J. Constantelos completed a study of Byzantine philanthropic institutions in 1968, he helped to focus attention on a subject long neglected in writings on the East Roman Empire. After combing the Greek patristic sources and later Byzantine religious and secular writing, Constantelos presented an impressive picture of the large and complex network of charitable agencies supported by Byzantine society—its church, its government, and its subjects—a network which included orphanages, hostels for the poor, old-age homes, and hospitals for the sick.

Constantelos identified many of the Byzantine charitable institutions and examined some of the religious attitudes that motivated emperors, bishops, and citizens of substance to support them. By limiting research to a single category of charitable foundation, however, one can study more thoroughly both the institutions and the society which sustained them. Orphanages, for example, offer an opportunity to investigate changes in the East Roman legal system, since the directors of these institutions replaced relatives as tutors or curators of the children in the institutions they supervised. These orphanages and the rights of their administrators raise deeper questions about the pattern of family life in the East Roman Empire. Do they indicate that relatives outside the nuclear family were no longer willing to support orphans within the extended family? Building on the research of Constantelos, the present monograph pursues similar avenues of research with regard to hospitals for the sick in the Byzantine Empire. It probes the sources to discover as much as possible about the hospitals themselves—their medical personnel, their administration, their sources of financial support. At the same time it casts its gaze beyond the hospital wall to explore the powerful forces within Byzantine society that helped to shape these institutions.

Surprisingly, the idea of writing on Byzantine hospitals first came to me in a seminar on Western medieval history at Catholic University, a seminar directed by Professor Elizabeth Kennan. She suggested that I write a paper on the Knights of Saint John. As I inquired into the origins of the Knights and especially examined their hospital at Jerusalem, I became aware of the close relationship between the order's famous charitable institution in the Holy City and the vast array of Byzantine philanthropic foundations. After completing an article on the Knights and their hospital, I began to investigate the charities of the East Roman Empire, particularly those which cared for the sick. I would never have succeeded in pursuing this topic without the help of Professor George Dennis of Catholic University, who guided me through the maze of Byzantine primary sources and saved me on many occasions from consulting a superseded edition.

As research proceeded, it became clear that a study of Byzantine hospitals posed many difficult questions. Did medical institutions similar to the Byzantine hospitals exist in the pre-Christian Greek and Roman world? Did the Christian faith, with its tradition of healing miracles, encourage or retard the development of medical centers? Who paid for these hospitals? What effect did the hospitals have on Byzantine physicians and the quality of medical treatment? Each of these questions demanded specialized knowledge; consultations with many colleagues helped in answering them.

Professor Darrel Amundsen read the chapters on hospitals in the ancient world and on Christianity and suggested several significant changes and valuable additions. Professors Rochelle Snee and George Dennis advised me in writing about the fourth century. Professor John Thomas provided valuable insights on the shifting relationships among state, church, and private sources of support for philanthropic agencies in general and hospitals in particular. With regard to the practice of medicine, Professor Lawrence Bliquez advised me of his research on Byzantine surgical instruments, while Professor Alexander Kazhdan directed me to several passages which describe East Roman doctors performing autopsies. With the information from Bliquez and Kazhdan I was able to complete my chapter on Byzantine medicine and propose some intriguing possibilities regarding the nature of medieval Greek medical science. Professor John Scarborough read the entire manuscript and suggested many additions to the bibliography. Finally, by offering an opportunity to talk with many researchers, acquire new information, and sharpen my ideas, the Dumbarton Oaks Symposium on Byzantine Medicine (29 April to 1 May 1983) contributed immeasurably to the final form of this book.

I would also like to thank Mrs. Betty Lou Gutekunst of the Mullen Library, Catholic University, and Dr. Irene Vaslef of Dumbarton Oaks for their assistance in conducting the research for this project; Mrs. Carolyn Moser for her careful editing of the manuscript; and Mrs. Diane Abresch of Blackwell Library, Salisbury State College, for her help in completing the bibliography. I owe special thanks again to Professor Amundsen, who not only corrected the manuscript but also advised me step by step in the process of finding a publisher. I should mention as well Dr. Edmund Pellegrino who as president of Catholic University enthusiastically supported the project.

I would never have completed the necessary research nor finished writing this book without a generous fellowship from the National Humanities Center in North Carolina. With the Center's assistance, I was able to devote the entire academic year 1982–83 to Byzantine hospitals. In addition to financial support, the Center provided me with a spacious office, excellent typing services, library assistance, and lush surroundings. For that year my wife Vicki and I thank everyone on the Center's staff.

Salisbury State College
Salisbury, Maryland

THE BIRTH OF THE HOSPITAL IN THE
BYZANTINE EMPIRE

CHAPTER ONE

Introduction

In 1936 the renowned historian of medicine Henry Sigerist maintained that only in the second half of the nineteenth century did hospitals become anything more than the last refuges of the desperately poor. Although sentiments of Christian philanthropy had given birth to hospitals as early as the fourth century A.D., these institutions had failed to evolve into centers of scientific medical treatment and had remained primarily poor houses providing some nursing care.[1] Developing these ideas in his study of medical institutions in the United States, Paul Starr stated that hospitals and the practice of scientific medicine had moved in separate spheres until the nineteenth century: "From their earliest origins in preindustrial societies, hospitals had been primarily religious and charitable institutions for tending the sick, rather than medical institutions for their cure."[2] In the final analysis, they functioned simply as ersatz homes for the homeless poor. These two views, and many similar ones in a wide range of historical and institutional studies, are correct only with reference to the tradition of philanthropic institutions—hospitals or hospices—in Western Europe. They totally ignore the elaborate medical facilities that appeared in the provinces of the East Roman Empire—what the modern world identifies as the Byzantine Empire.[3]

With their highly specialized medical personnel and their careful rules regarding hygiene, private beds for patients, and proper heating, East Roman hospitals (or *xenones,* as they were often called in Greek) challenge the accepted image of premodern institutions for the sick—an image of cold, overcrowded, unhealthy places providing little or no medical attention for their patients. Moreover, the existence of these East Roman institutions alters the common notion that the quality of health care drastically declined in all regions during the Middle Ages. A study of Byzantine hospitals will force scholars in many fields to reevaluate their assumptions both about medieval health care and about the possibility that philanthropic agencies can provide the best medical treatment society has to offer.[4]

Exploring the birth and development of Byzantine facilities for the sick is all the more important since these institutions were in fact the first to offer hospital care, certainly in the Western tradition if not in the world. Historians of medicine such as Sigerist as well as those interested in the evolution of Christianity and its institutions agree that the ancestors of the modern hospital originated in the Eastern provinces of the Roman Empire during the fourth century.[5] From here these philanthropic foundations were brought westward to Italy and Gaul, where they managed to survive until the eleventh century without any major impact on secular or religious culture.[6] In the twelfth century, the Crusaders reintroduced the hospitals of the East Roman Empire into Western Europe; this time these institutions fired the zeal of a number of new religious orders and have flourished to the present day.[7] The Moslems to the East also received the inspiration for their famous *bimaristan*s (houses of the sick) from the Byzantine Empire; the Nestorian Christians brought the East Roman hospitals to Persia in the sixth century and later introduced them to the Abbasid califs of Bagdad.[8] Thus, the Byzantine xenones represent not only the first public institutions to offer medical care to the sick, but also the mainstream of hospital development through the Middle Ages, from which both the Latin West and the Moslem East adopted their facilities for the ill. To trace the birth and development of centers for the sick in the Byzantine Empire is thus to write the first chapter in the history of the Hospital itself.

At the outset of a study on Byzantine hospitals, it is essential to define two key terms: *hospital* and *Byzantine*. The word hospital has experienced many shifts in meaning and connotation over the centuries, as the remarks of Sigerist and Starr suggest. Fixing a definition requires a comparison of what modern society has defined as a hospital with agencies which bore that name in the premodern Western world. Defining the second term, *Byzantine,* will help to set this discussion in the proper historical, chronological, and geographical framework.

Men and women of the late twentieth century can define a hospital with no difficulty, since most have had some personal experience with such an institution, either as patients themselves or as friends or relatives of patients. Most would readily agree that a hospital is an institution which provides beds, meals, and constant nursing care for its patients while they undergo medical therapy at the hands of professional physicians. In carrying out these services, the hospital is striving to restore its patients to health. Its goal— healing its sick patients—marks it off from institutions for the aged, from convalescent homes, and from nursing homes for the permanently disabled, facilities which also offer some medical care for their residents but not the intensive routine of medical treatment, including major surgery, which distinguishes hospital service. Finally, hospitals accept patients of all classes from the wealthy to the poor. Some hospitals might admit only wealthy patients or those with good insurance coverage, but such distinctions arise from financial considerations, not from the very nature of the institution. Hospitals qua hospitals serve the public; institutions which admit only members of a group—military men or monks of a monastic community, for example—are classed as infirmaries.[9]

Because they have confined their study of medieval and early modern facilities for the sick to those of Western Europe, some researchers have maintained that institutions which tried to aid the sick before the nineteenth century fall outside the boundaries of this modern definition for *hospital* in several ways.[10] First, these medieval houses for the sick did not limit their efforts to curing the ill or injured; they were supposedly general agents of charity where pilgrims, poor persons, the aged, and those who suffered from disease or accident could find food, shelter, and care. One of the earliest hospitals of the Latin West, the modest institution founded by King Childebert in Laon during the sixth century, served both the sick and pilgrims.[11] Theodulf, the ninth-century bishop of Orleans, described the charitable house in his city as a place where the weary received support, the sick medicine, and the sorrowful joy.[12] Behind such general philanthropic institutions the words of Christ on the throne of judgment echoed across the Christian centuries: "In so far as you did this to one of the least of these brothers of Mine, you did it unto Me" (Matt. 26:40; Jerusalem Bible).

Such researchers next emphasize that hospitals before the nineteenth century did not serve the sick from all classes, but only those who were without means. The thirteenth-century statutes of the famous hospital in Paris, the Hôtel-Dieu, refer to the dormitory for patients as the *infirmaria pauperum* (the infirmary of the poor).[13] The contemporary Hospital of the Holy Spirit in Rome was also designed solely for receiving patients who suffered both from poverty and from disease.[14] Moreover, researchers have argued that medieval hospitals did not support a full staff of physicians to treat their patients. With the exception of a seventh-century example in Visigothic Spain, none of the philanthropic institutions of Western Europe seem to have offered the sick access to professional physicians before the twelfth century.[15] Even then, physicians rarely undertook hospital service. Although Norman England experienced a great increase in the number of institutions to care for the sick between 1066 and 1154, no source confirms that doctors treated any of their patients.[16] As late as the thirteenth century, the Hôtel-Dieu at Paris did not maintain a regular medical staff; its statutes refer only to the religious community of lay brothers and sisters who nursed bed-ridden patients. Before the fourteenth century, physicians and surgeons only occasionally treated the sick there.[17] Even after the hospital acquired a permanent medical staff in 1328, it did not have an impact on the teaching and practice of professional medicine as did hospitals of the modern era after the development of clinical medicine in the late eighteenth century.[18]

Finally, researchers have emphasized that hospitals of the medieval West fell so short of modern notions of proper patient care that they cannot be considered true forefathers of twentieth-century medical centers. Thus, the thirteenth-century hospital at Saint-Pol in northern France assigned only six nursing sisters to care for at least sixty sick people. Such a ratio of nurses to patients would be unacceptable in a modern institution.[19] In the late Middle Ages and early modern period, the Hôtel-Dieu of Paris was notorious for its poor conditions. Often two or three patients were assigned to a single bed, even as late as the end of the eighteenth century.[20] Because the meals served the sick did not include sufficient vegetables or fruits to form a balanced diet, frequent outbreaks of scurvy plagued the patients. Heating methods were so poor in the dormitories that during an extreme winter in the sixteenth century, many of the sick suffered frozen noses. Even in 1838, the wards were so badly heated that the temperature fell to three degrees centigrade.[21]

Some medievalists might argue with those who deny emphatically that institutions such as the Hôtel-Dieu of Paris or the Hospital of the Knights of Saint John in Jerusalem were true hospitals. Indeed, medieval institutions for the sick provided their patients with meals, beds, full-time nursing care, and some access to physicians. The Knights of Saint John even staffed their great hospital in the Holy Land with two doctors and two surgeons.[22] Moreover, some of these medieval institutions, like modern medical centers, hoped in some cases to restore patients to health, not simply to house them until their deaths.[23] Still, historians of medicine, physicians, and hospital planners surely have good reason for paying little attention to medieval hospitals, since they were in fact poorly equipped facilities which reflected little careful thought for the comfort, the cleanliness, or, ironically, the health of their patients. It is important to stress, however, that the medieval hospitals of Western Europe had not developed spontaneously from Western institutions. They had been imported from the East Roman Empire but had never taken firm root in Latin Christendom so that they could draw on the support of physicians, pharmacists, the state, and the aristocratic classes. It is revealing that the emperor Frederick II issued a series of regulations for Sicily regarding doctors, pharmacists, and medical licensure without once mentioning an institution even resembling a hospital.[24] Even in the kingdom of Sicily, a society with Byzantine roots, Latin physicians of the thirteenth century usually practiced as individual craftsmen who saw some patients in their private offices and visited others in their homes, entering the dingy wards of the hospitals only rarely, if at all.

Although modern researchers are wrong in claiming that medieval houses for the sick in the West had no relationship with physicians, the sources suggest that their role was indeed limited. The thirteenth-century rules of the Hospital of the Holy Spirit describe the steps taken to find the sick paupers in the city of Rome, their reception into the infirmary, and their twice-weekly sponge baths, but nowhere do they mention a physician or the provision of medicines.[25] So, too, in the many hospice-hospitals of late-medieval Germany, physicians rarely appeared.[26] As late as the eighteenth century, doctors visited the ancient hospital of Saint Bartholomew in London only once a week, even when they were receiving a regular salary from the institution.[27] In Western Christendom, then, hospital practice did not absorb the best efforts of the medical profession until the nineteenth century.

In addition, the great religious movements of the West—the Cluniac and Cistercian reforms with their vast resources in men and property—never accepted the maintenance of hospitals for the sick from outside their monasteries as essential to their religious service. Thus, when Latin Christendom began to build new hospitals for the sick during the twelfth century or convert old hospices into centers of some medical care, the strongest impulse came, not from venerable monastic orders or from episcopal leadership, but from the lay *milites Christi,* the Knights of Saint John.[28] To see hospitals of the Middle Ages in their native environment, in the society which gave them birth, it is necessary to cross the linguistic, cultural, and geographic barrier which has always divided the Mediterranean into two distinct regions, to leave the hospitals of medieval Italy and its Western European hinterland for Greece, Asia Minor, Egypt, and Syria—the ancient provinces of the East Roman Empire.

The term *Byzantine* properly applies to the medieval state ruled from Constantinople, the great city on the shores of the Bosporos. The men and women who lived under the sway of Constantinople, however, never thought of themselves as Byzantines; they claimed to be the true *Romaioi,* Romans. The Byzantine Empire, in fact, never existed; it is a myth which historians have spun to distinguish a phase in the evolution of the Roman Empire, the immense state which had dominated the entire Mediterranean from the birth of Christ to the end of the fourth century (A.D.) and survived for another thousand years as a significant power in the Middle East. Scholars have used the Byzantine myth to underscore a critical turning point in ancient history occasioned by the reign of the emperor Constantine (306–37).

Constantine drastically altered the course of the Roman state by making two decisions of the greatest importance for the subsequent development of world history. First, he became a Christian, a personal act which began the transformation of the ancient world from a pagan to a Christian society. Second, he determined to move the capital of the Roman state from the ancient city of Rome in Latin Italy to a Greek town in the Eastern provinces called Byzantium. He greatly expanded the city of Byzantium, decorated it with new buildings, crowned it with fortifications, and renamed it Constantinople—Constantine's city. Shifting the capital, however, had far greater consequences than simply moving the seat of government from one geographical point to another. The new capital lay, not in the homeland of the ancient Romans nor in the provinces of the West which were in the process of adopting Roman language and culture, but in the Greek-speaking East. After Constantine dedicated his new capital in 330, Greeks rapidly came to dominate the imperial government at Constantinople and gave a strong Hellenic color to Roman society in the East. After 395 the city of Constantinople no longer ruled the Western provinces of the old Roman Empire. It now consolidated its position in the eastern Mediterranean as the capital of a new world, still governed by Roman administration and legal institutions, but predominantly Greek in language and culture, and confessing Christianity as its official religion.

This new East Roman, or "Byzantine," Empire experienced two centuries of prosperity and expansion until the beginning of the seventh century, when Avar, Persian, and Arab invasions radically altered the size and structure of the state. Within new borders and with a reorganized army and civil bureaucracy, the Byzantine Empire withstood these assaults and entered an era of renewed prosperity about 850. At the end of the eleventh century, it suffered another disaster at the hands of the Seljuk Turks, but revived again under the Komnenoi emperors of the twelfth century. In 1203, however, the Latin knights of the Fourth Crusade and the ships of the Venetian state in Italy invaded the empire from the west and managed to capture Constantinople, whose massive fortifications had resisted every siege by barbarian armies or rebellious legions since Constantine first dedicated his new city.

The Byzantine provinces of Asia Minor, however, never fell to the Western conquerors; with these as a base of support, the East Roman government was able to recapture the imperial city in 1261. For almost two hundred years thereafter, the last imperial dynasty, the Palaiologoi, governed the empire and attempted to parry the thrusts of hostile Turks to the east and rapacious Italians, Spaniards, and French to the west. Finally, on 29 May 1453, the ancient capital of the East Roman state—the Second Rome, the new Jerusalem—fell to the Ottoman sultan.[29]

From the dedication of Constantinople in 330 to the Turkish conquest in 1453, the cities of the Byzantine Empire supported organized philanthropic institutions. Even before 330, the Christian church of Antioch and its daughter churches in the Syrian hinterland maintained houses of charity which they called *xenodocheia*. In 332 the emperor Constantine granted a share of the public tax revenue to these agencies of the church, an act which inaugurated the tradition of close cooperation between the Byzantine state and the Christian church in financing charitable institutions.[30] By the reign of Theodosius I (379–95), Constantinople had a number of xenodocheia or xenones.[31] Throughout its long history, the Byzantine capital prided itself on its many philanthropic institutions. In describing the fall of the city in 1453, Andronikos Kallistos lamented the destruction not only of the stoas, palaces, and baths which adorned the capital, but also of the hospitals, old-age homes, and poorhouses.[32]

References to philanthropic institutions within Constantinople occur frequently throughout Byzantine history. Outside the capital, on the other hand, they are more difficult to find, since East Roman society tended to focus its attention on the imperial city, especially after the retrenchment which followed the invasions of the seventh century. Nevertheless, sources reveal that as early as the fourth century, small towns in Egypt had xenodocheia.[33] During the early years of the disastrous seventh century, Germiōn in Asia Minor maintained several houses of charity for the sick and insane which it called xenones.[34] In the eleventh century the port of Raidestos on the Sea of Marmara possessed a house to shelter the homeless poor.[35] Finally, twelfth-century Ainos in Thrace had an old-age home close by to nurse both its aged and its sick.[36] Combing Greek patristic and later Byzantine sources known in the seventeenth century, the famous scholar Charles Du Cange identified thirty-five philanthropic institutions in Constantinople alone.[37] Even Edward Gibbon noticed them, although his preconceptions about the moral decay of Late Roman society prevented his studying them carefully.[38]

Since the day Gibbon finished the *Decline and Fall of the Roman Empire* in 1787, many new sources have come to light: saints' lives, collected letters, speeches, legal sources, and medical treatises. References scattered among these newly edited works have added valuable information regarding the vast network of charities in the East Roman Empire. Moreover, historians now have available a substantial number of monastic *typika,* documents which founders of monasteries issued to regulate their institutions. In such a *typikon,* a founder would spell out in great detail how the monks of his monastery were to live, pray, and govern their community. Some of these typika required the monks to maintain philanthropic institutions for the benefit of the unfortunate from the community beyond the monastery's walls. In their instructions for setting up such services, typika offer the most complete pictures of Byzantine charitable agencies so far available. Two such typika, one from the twelfth century and one from the thirteenth, describe institutions which undoubtedly functioned as hospitals, even in terms of the twentieth-century definition.

The twelfth-century typikon—the constitution of the Pantokrator monastery in Constantinople—regulates its hospital's procedure in sufficient detail to raise the curtain of uncertainty regarding many aspects of Byzantine medical centers. By examining this document carefully and comparing the hospital, or xenon, it established with the much briefer illustrations of philanthropic foundations in earlier hagiographical and narrative sources, we can isolate those facilities that functioned as hospitals and also gain some idea of how they served the sick. Moreover, such comparisons can aid in tracing the evolution of hospital facilities from the birth of the first philanthropic institutions to care solely for the sick to the collapse of these agencies at the hands of the Turks in the fifteenth century. A thorough survey of Byzantine xenones will demonstrate that these were remarkably tenacious institutions which enjoyed the full support of the society they served. Despite the many political, military, and economic upheavals which beset the Byzantine state during its long history, the government, the church, the aristocracy, and even the medical profession never faltered in patronizing hospitals for the citizens of the empire.

A complete study of Byzantine hospitals also must emphasize that such institutions did not exist in a vacuum. Just as East Roman society set up its xenones to perform functions analogous to those of twentieth-century medical centers, so too it allowed them to attain a position at the intersection of many interest groups very similar to the place that modern hospitals occupy. First, Byzantine xenones came to dominate the medical profession. They employed the leading physicians of the empire; they were the theaters in which doctors performed their most impressive feats. They also provided students with the opportunity not only for instruction in the theory of medical science, but most importantly, for careful direction in the practice of the healing art; they promoted a form of clinical teaching. Second, Byzantine hospitals were closely linked to the communities they served. Indeed, they took root in the basic unit of the ancient world—the *polis*. By the sixth century, Byzantine society considered the hospital one of the essential amenities of city life. Third, both the central government and the local city bore responsibility for supporting and regulating xenones so that they were always capable of providing the sick with the best possible care. Fourth, the Christian church both created xenones and nurtured their growth. Not only the bishops of the official church but also the charismatic leaders of Eastern monasticism continually rejuvenated enthusiasm for the support of hospitals. Finally, private persons—the great aristocrats of the empire—occasionally demonstrated their philanthropy by founding and sustaining hospitals.

Although Christian bishops of the East Roman Empire organized the first hospitals amid the struggles of the fourth century, they did not generate them *ex nihilo*. They combined elements of the ancient culture of pagan Hellenism with the traditions of the early Christian church. As one hagiographical source eloquently phrased it, hospital physicians united the commands of Christ with the laws of secular medicine.[39] Thus, a thorough study of Byzantine hospitals requires an analysis of both ancient pagan institutions and attitudes as well as those of the early church to appreciate how elements of both traditions were fused to form the medieval xenones.

In view of the place which hospitals occupied at the intersection of several spheres of influence within Byzantine society, it would be impossible to study them alone, isolated from the currents of the civilization which formed them.

One must look beyond the hospital walls to examine some of the forces in the East Roman state which acted upon the xenones and gave them form and substance. The hospital can thus serve as a kind of prism through which it is possible to view in a new light powerful components of East Roman society and intellectual life. The ancient Hellenic heritage, the city environ-ment, the Christian church, the monastic movement, Roman law, the imperial bureaucracy, and the medical profession all participated in shaping and sus-taining perhaps the most fascinating institutions of the Byzantine Empire— its hospitals.

CHAPTER TWO

The Pantokrator Xenon

On the northeast slope of a prominent ridge in Istanbul, overlooking the narrow harbor of the Golden Horn, rise five domes from a tight cluster of three buildings which the Turks today call the Zeyrek Kilisi Cami (Zeyrek Kilisi Mosque).[1] Since the late fifteenth century these buildings with their graceful cupolas have served Islam, but before the Turkish conquest of Constantinople, they formed the spiritual center of a great Christian institution, the Monastery of Christ Savior Pantokrator (the Ruler of All).[2]

When the emperor John II Komnenos established the Pantokrator Monastery in 1136, he designed it as a splendid home for a cloistered community of ascetics, providing it with buildings to house the monks and with the three churches which still stand as the Zeyrek Kilisi Cami. As part of his foundation, he also included two philanthropic institutions in the immediate vicinity of the domed churches. One of these charitable facilities—the Pantokrator Xenon—the emperor fitted out to heal the sick of Constantinople. According to his design, it provided those who suffered from disease or injury with clean beds, nourishing food, nursing care both day and night, and the careful ministrations of physicians. In short, the emperor founded what a modern English speaker would call a hospital.[3] Indeed, the Pantokrator Xenon so closely resembles the highly organized medical facilities of today that one noted Byzantinist has described this twelfth-century institution as "astoundingly modern."[4]

North, east, and west of the present Zeyrek Kilisi Cami stretches an area of approximately 250 square meters, crisscrossed with great arched cisterns and retaining walls—the substructures, no doubt, of the xenon, but also of the monastic buildings and of the second charitable agency, called a *gerokomeion* (old-age home). So far, archaeology has revealed only that the xenon, the gerokomeion, and the quarters for the monks together with their service buildings formed a complex of structures about the domed churches, a small campus of buildings the size of an American city block.[5] For more detailed information on these twelfth-century buildings one must turn to the written sources, for the painstaking work of the paleographers, not the archaeologists' spade, has so far uncovered the most interesting information regarding the various institutions of the Pantokrator complex. As the result of the work of several paleographers, historians now have at their disposal an excellent edition of the *Typikon of the Imperial Monastery the Pantokrator,* the constitution which John II Komnenos drafted to regulate this monastic community and its philanthropic agencies.[6] A fourth of the *Typikon* discusses the xenon in sufficient detail to convince even the most skeptical modern observer that this institution was designed to function as a hospital.

Indeed, the Pantokrator Xenon has won the praise of every scholar who has analyzed its complicated rules for patient care, staff organization, and infirmary equipment. But very few have attempted to place this institution in the proper historical context. Because it alone of the Byzantine xenones has left a vivid picture of its operations in the surviving sources, most studies discuss it in isolation. In his essay on East Roman hospitals, Alexandre Philipsborn even suggests that the Pantokrator Xenon adopted some of its features, not from earlier Byzantine hospitals, but from the bimaristans (houses for the sick) which the califs and later emirs constructed in Bagdad, Damascus, and other Moslem towns.[7] In his detailed study of Byzantine philanthropic institutions, Demetrios Constantelos, on the other hand, has assumed that the Pantokrator hospital developed from earlier Byzantine hostels or guesthouses without analyzing the evolution of such xenodocheia or xenones into medical treatment centers, or establishing the terms which distinguished these two very different kinds of philanthropic institutions.[8]

Since only the Pantokrator Typikon presents a substantial description of a Byzantine hospital's physical plant, of its professional staff, and of its administration, it must serve as the primary tool in unraveling the many strands in the history of xenones. Thus, the state of the sources requires a careful study of the Pantokrator Xenon to determine what exactly a Byzantine hospital was and how it functioned. Once the principal features of the Pantokrator hospital have been established, the search can proceed for these same traits in the much briefer descriptions of philanthropic agencies in other sources. By this method it should be possible to discover whether or not Byzantine institutions predating the Pantokrator Xenon were organized along similar lines to serve the sick and to determine when such institutions first developed. It is especially important to reevaluate the evidence regarding early facilities, since, in their studies of fourth-century institutions, most historians of Christianity and its charitable activities have been interested in establishing the existence of philanthropic houses resembling the hospitals which later emerged in the Latin West. They were not looking for anything as specialized and sophisticated as the Pantokrator Xenon. A history of Byzantine hospitals thus requires a new survey of the early charitable agencies sponsored by the church in light of the later development of such institutions in East Roman tradition.

In order to understand correctly the early philanthropic agencies of the church and trace their growth into hospitals such as the Pantokrator, it is imperative to examine the Greek terms which writers coined in the fourth and fifth centuries for these new institutions. An imprecise understanding of the many words applied to charitable foundations has obscured their history and thwarted the proper identification of early hospitals for the sick.

THE PANTOKRATOR XENON

In his constitution for his monastic complex, the Pantokrator *Typikon,* the emperor John II marks off a discrete section (lines 904–1346) to discuss the rules of the xenon. Within this section, however, he seems to follow no logical pattern, ranging through several topics and back again. This peculiar order or lack of it appears in various sections of the Pantokrator constitution and in other monastic typika as well. Indeed, a certain disdain for systematic treatment seems to characterize the whole genre of Byzantine typika.[9] As a result, a simple translation of the text would perhaps be more confusing than helpful in forming a clear idea of how the Pantokrator Xenon functioned. One can achieve better results simply by confronting the text with specific questions regarding the hospital's facilities for the sick, its staff, its administration, its methods of treatment, and the class origins of its patients.

The facilities. What facilities did the Pantokrator Xenon make available to its patients? This question will focus primarily on the hospital's sleeping arrangements for the sick and its other provisions for their basic needs. The *Typikon* never mentions private rooms for patients at the xenon. Rather, it mandated fifty beds, one for each sick person, arranged in five *ordinoi,* or sections (literally, *ordinos* means row or rank).[10] It reserved the first ordinos for patients suffering from wounds or fractures—the surgical ward; the second ordinos of eight beds for patients with diseases of the eyes or intestines or other serious problems; the third ordinos of twelve beds for women; and the fourth and fifth ordinoi of ten beds each for male patients afflicted with other kinds of illnesses. Each of the fifty beds was to have a mattress, a pillow, sheets, and a cover, and in winter two blankets of goat's hair. For patients who were extremely weak or incapacitated by pain, the hospital had ready six special beds with perforated mattresses so that the sick person need not rise to use the latrine. Each ordinos also had an extra bed besides the assigned number in case more than fifty patients were admitted, a provision which demonstrates that the Pantokrator Xenon did not assign more than one patient to a bed as did hospitals of the Latin West.[11] Finally, the *Typikon* required that the hospital replace worn bedding and yearly card the wool in the mattresses and pillows.[12]

The Pantokrator hospital also met the other physical needs of the patients. Three hearths—one large one in the main hall and two smaller ones in the surgery and the women's ward—were positioned in such a way as to guarantee the comfort of patients even during the cold spells of winter. The xenon included two latrines, one for men and one for women. These were to be cleaned regularly and were illuminated at night.[13] Patients also had access to a bathing facility maintained by the monastery where each sick person could wash twice a week or as often as their attending physician prescribed. The hospital always kept clean and ready for use basins and pitchers for the bath and towels of various sizes for drying.[14]

The Pantokrator *typikon* also specified the meals which the patients should receive. Every day each of the sick was to be served 850 grams of bread, two vegetable dishes dressed with olive oil, and two onion heads. Also every patient was to receive each day one *noumisma trachy* (¹⁄₄₈ of the standard gold coin, the noumisma) to buy wine and any additional food he or she might want. Although the Pantokrator menu contains no meat, modern nutritionists claim that it represents a well-balanced diet sufficient to prevent the kind of vitamin deficiencies which struck patients in the hospitals of the Latin West.[15]

The staff. Who staffed the Pantokrator hospital? The *Typikon* answers this question in great detail, revealing a large and specialized work force. Two physicians (*iatroi*) attended each of the five sections in the hospital. They were aided in their labors by three ordained medical assistants (*hypourgoi embathmoi*), two extra medical assistants (*hypourgoi perissoi*), and two servants (*hyperetai*) in each of the four sections for men. The categories "ordained" (*embathmos*) and "extra" (*perissos*) designated ranks within the guild of professional medical assistants. The two doctors of the women's ward had the help of one female physician (*iatraina*), four female medical assistants of ordained status (*hypourgissai embathmoi*), two female assistants of extra status (*hypourgissai perissai*), and two female servants (*hyperetriai*). Moreover, the hospital maintained four physicians—two specializing in surgery and two in internal medicine—to staff an outpatient clinic. Four ordained medical assistants and four extra medical assistants assisted these doctors. The *Typikon* assigned two more physicians to treat the monks of the monastery and their servants in a separate infirmary, not part of the hospital.[16]

The Pantokrator *Typikon* established a carefully graded hierarchy among the ward physicians. At the top stood the two doctors assigned to the section for serious diseases, including ocular and intestinal illnesses. These physicians bore the distinctive title of *protomenites* (first of the month). Next came the two surgeons assigned to the ward for wounds and fractures. The four doctors of the two general wards for men ranked after the surgeons, and below these four physicians came the two in charge of the women's section. Following these the *Typikon* placed the doctors assigned to the monastery's infirmary. At the very bottom of the list came the four physicians serving in the outpatient clinic, doctors who ranked as extra physicians or physicians of unordained status (*iatroi perissoi*). The *Typikon* indicates that there were other extra physicians at the hospital besides the outpatient doctors, but it is silent about their role in the institution. The *Typikon* stipulated that promotions would follow the order of precedence; a diligent nonordained physician could move from service in the outpatient clinic to the monastic infirmary, and from the infirmary to the women's ward, and then up the ladder of the professional hierarchy to the highest office of protomenites.[17]

The Pantokrator *Typikon* also provided for two additional physicians, the *primmikerioi,* who outranked even the *protomenitai.* They supervised the entire treatment program of the hospital. When on duty, a primmikerios made daily rounds through the ordinoi, reexamined each patient, monitored their therapies, and received their complaints. He also checked the diagnosis of the outpatient physicians in serious cases. During the liturgical commemorations of the Komnenoi founders, the primmikerioi represented the staff by lighting the great torches for the services.[18]

The hospital's physicians did not all work at the same time. The two primmikerioi alternated every other month in supervising the xenon. So too, all the other physicians of the hospital—the two protomenitai, the doctors assigned to the remaining wards, the two in the monastery infirmary, and those in the outpatient clinic—worked monthly shifts so that each month only one physician in each section (two in the outpatient clinic) was on duty.[19] It is unlikely that the medical assistants (hypourgoi) served in the same manner, since they also had to staff the night shift, a skeleton crew composed of one hypourgos in each ward. If half of the hypourgoi were off each month, that would have meant that the two on-duty assistants would have worked on the night shift every other day—an impossible burden.[20]

The staff physicians on duty had to report to the xenon each day during the month of their service to make their daily examinations, perform operations, and admit new patients. During the dark days of winter, they came to the hospital only once a day, but from 1 May to 14 September they returned to the hospital for a second session after the evening meal.[21] In requiring an evening work period during the summer, the *Typikon* was simply following the practices of the Byzantine government and its bureaus.[22]

Besides the physicians, medical assistants, and servants, the Pantokrator Xenon employed a staff of six pharmacists—a chief, three ordained pharmacists, and two extra (*perissoi*) pharmacists. In addition, it retained one usher (*ostiarios*), five laundresses, one keeper of the kettles (*lebetarios*), two cooks, one groom, one porter, one purser, two priests, two lectors, two bakers, four pallbearers, one priest for funerals, one latrine cleaner, and one miller. The list of staff salaries also includes allotments for a craftsman to keep the surgical tools clean and sharp and for a specialist in hernia surgery—apparently not a full-time position.[23]

The administration. These were the people who did the work at the Pantokrator Xenon, but who managed the hospital as a whole? We have already discussed one level of administration—the primmikerioi. Although they supervised the medical care of all hospital patients, they had no authority over the material resources of the institution. Since the emperor John II did not establish the Pantokrator Xenon as an independent economic unit or a distinct legal entity, but rather as a part of his imperial monastery, the final authority over the hospital's resources rested with the superior of the Pantokrator community, subject of course to the guidelines which the *Typikon* set forth. The superior, in turn, was advised by four monks of the monastery all holding the office of oikonomos (household manager). The superior and his four oikonomoi formed a board of directors which supervised the entire Pantokrator complex—the monastery and its church of the Savior, the public church of the Theotokos (the mother of God), the chapel of St. Michael, the xenon, and the gerokomeion. As a committee, they were legally responsible for the entire organization; they sold estates, leased property, and appointed estate managers and accountants. One of these oikonomoi specialized in the affairs of the xenon and the gerokomeion. He made sure that both philanthropic agencies had the money and raw materials the *Typikon* assigned to them.[24]

Although the superior and his oikonomoi governed the vast estates and rights from which the xenon drew its material support, the *Typikon* granted them no role in the daily affairs of the hospital. An official of the xenon— the *nosokomos*—actually managed the operation of the hospital. He was assisted in his supervisory duties by the *meizoteros.* These two officials were to ensure that the hospital had available the necessary supplies of food, fuel, and medicine and that these were properly used for the benefit of the sick, both those receiving treatment in the xenon wards and those coming to the out-patient clinic.[25] In fulfilling these duties, the *Typikon* freed these officials from any obligation to account to an official of the monastery regarding their conduct of affairs.[26] Moreover, since both the nosokomos and the meizoteros received salaries, it is unlikely that they were monks of the monastery.[27] As a result, the hospital administration enjoyed a great deal of freedom; in many respects the xenon was an independent institution.

In defining the duties of the nosokomos and the meizoteros, the Pantokrator Typikon emphasizes their responsibility for receiving essential supplies. For example, it begins its description of the nosokomos' job with his obligation to accept sixty-six measures of oil for hospital salves and lamps and fifty measures of honey for the medicinal compounds.[28] The meizoteros was to assure the food supplies for the patients' meals.[29] The *Typikon* does not expressly state that the nosokomos had to be a physician, but another source describes the holder of this office as a prominent member of the medical profession.[30] Another example from the twelfth century indicates that by that time hospital directors were normally chosen from among the leading physicians.[31] In this regard, a careful reading of the nosokomos' responsibilities in the *Typikon* does suggest that he was usually concerned with supervising the hospital's medicines. The meizoteros, on the other hand, functioned as a cellarer who carefully monitored the food supplies, although he also was responsible for stocking simple medical ingredients (i.e., herbs, minerals, and animal extracts not in compounds).[32] In addition to maintaining the medical supplies of the xenon, the nosokomos guarded the copper bowls and pitchers for bathing under lock and key.[33]

The Pantokrator Typikon leaves a number of questions regarding the nosokomos unanswered. His relationship to the other physicians, particularly the primmikerioi, is unclear. Moreover, it does not indicate how he was chosen. Had he advanced through the ranks of the ward physicians to his post, or was he hired by the superior of the monastery or perhaps the emperor? A comparison of the Pantokrator Xenon with other Byzantine hospitals will help to clarify the position of the nosokomos to some degree, but it will not answer all of the questions about his office or about hospital administration generally.

Medical treatment. What kind of medical treatment did the patients of the Pantokrator receive? To this question the *Typikon* does not offer an adequate answer, since it is a document concerned primarily with outlining the hospital's bureaucratic organization, the salaries of its staff, and the rules governing the facilities for the patients. The treatment procedures the *Typikon* left to the wisdom of the physicians and the professional treatises they had available for consultation. Nevertheless, it provides a few indications of therapeutic procedures. First, routine baths formed an important element in therapy. Physicians personally escorted to the bathing facilities those patients who required frequent baths as part of their treatment.[34] Second, from the list of supplies which the nosokomos was to keep in stock, one can catch a glimpse of some medicines which the xenon physicians prescribed. They used such preparations as hydrostat, oxymel, and diospolis, all standard compounds available to Greek physicians at least since the time of Oribaseios (fourth century). The nosokomos also had to purchase supplies not only for internal medicines, but also for salves and plasters applied externally.[35] Third, a short passage describing the duties of the tool sharpener lists some surgical instruments which xenon physicians had available. These included knives for phlebotomy, cautery irons, catheters for bladder problems, dental pliers, and instruments which the *Typikon* simply calls those for the head and stomach.[36] Finally, the daily diet itself must have formed part of the therapy. It was unusual in including absolutely no meat or fish. Normally, the patients received well-balanced vegetarian meals which modern researchers estimate contained 3,300 calories daily.[37]

As part of the healing of the body, the *Typikon* also provided for spiritual treatment. Since the age of the Fathers, Eastern Christianity had stressed the close connection between physical and spiritual health. Thus, the xenon included two chapels, one for men and one for women, each with a priest and lector. Patients could attend the divine liturgy in these chapels four days a week—Wednesdays, Fridays, Saturdays, and Sundays—and on great feasts of the Lord.[38] The patriarch of Constantinople licensed one of these two priests to hear the confessions of the patients, in the words of the *Typikon*, "that they might not die a truly ruinous death, a spiritual one, leaving this world . . . without confession."[39]

The hospital not only provided the patients with an opportunity for spiritual growth; it also required them to fulfill certain religious obligations on behalf of the hospital founders who had made such therapeutic services available. The patients were to pray for the emperor John II Komnenos, for his wife Irene, and for other members of his family. On the anniversaries of the founders' deaths, patients who were sufficiently strong were to assemble in the Church of the Theotokos together with the physicians and other staff members to offer prayers for the departed souls of the Komnenoi founders.[40] John II especially wanted the sick to pray for his salvation, for in the introduction of the *Typikon* he identified the hospital patients, worn down by disease, crippled in body, and eaten away by pain, together with all the poor and helpless, as the special friends of Christ. After the patients of the xenon had received every care and had recovered from their maladies, the emperor asked the Lord to receive them as ambassadors seeking pardon for the sins of their imperial benefactor.[41]

The class origins of the patients. The next question to consider concerns the patients themselves. Does the *Typikon* provide any information regarding their social status? Were all of them paupers, as was the case in hospitals of the medieval West, or did some people of higher status seek the assistance of a xenon like the Pantokrator? Certainly, many of the patients at the Pantokrator hospital were penniless. The xenon kept shirts and gowns for those in the greatest poverty. Other patients, however, must have had sufficient means to supply at least their own bed clothes.[42] A second passage in the *Typikon* likewise indicates that some patients were not totally destitute. This section lays down several rules governing the physicians of the hospital. One rule bans them from receiving any extra fees (*soupera*) for their services. This restriction does not forbid private practice, since the very next rule limits such practice to the city of Constantinople. During the six months when hospital physicians were not on duty in the xenon, they could freely visit private patients so long as they did not leave the city in the course of such work.[43] It would seem, then, that the regulation against extra fees applied to the hospital itself. Thus, doctors were not to take tips from patients. If this interpretation is correct, then some of the patients were clearly not paupers. Evidence regarding other Byzantine hospitals will confirm this conclusion.

The answers which the *Typikon* has given to the foregoing questions have revealed the purpose for which John II established his xenon. He designed the hospital to accept patients of any social status, and to extend medical care with the intent of curing them; he did not establish this xenon simply to offer patients food and shelter, or to grant them a comfortable place in which to die. A brief glance at the second philanthropic institution in the Pantokrator complex—the gerokomeion—will demonstrate the sharp distinction which existed between a xenon and a simpler philanthropic agency.

The Pantokrator *Typikon* devotes only 42 lines to the gerokomeion, compared to the 442 required to regulate the xenon's routine. The head of the gerokomeion—the *gerokomos*—was not a professional man or a physician, as were the nosokomos and meizoteros of the xenon. Rather, he belonged to the monastic community and received no salary for his work. Six salaried servants (*hyperetai*) assisted him in caring for the twenty-four residents, all of whom were men. The gerokomeion was to admit those suffering from old age, or so crippled by an earlier disease or injury that they were unable to earn a living on their own.[44] If, by chance, one of the old men fell ill or if one of those crippled developed a disease other than the chronic affliction which had originally incapacitated him, the gerokomos had no medical staff to offer him help. Rather, the nosokomos of the xenon was notified immediately. He then dispatched a doctor or medical assistant to diagnose the problem and to decide whether or not to admit the man to a hospital bed. If admitted, the new patient received the same treatment as the other sick. Once recovered, he had to return to the gerokomeion, for the xenon was not to serve as a nursing home or hospice for the old or chronically ill, but only as a treatment center.[45]

Thus, the Pantokrator Xenon was a hospital, not very different from what we today understand such an institution to be. But was the Pantokrator Xenon a single case of such a hospital in the Byzantine Empire, as some historians have suggested, or had many similar xenones served the subjects of the East Roman emperor? If there had been many such hospitals, when had the first ones opened to admit the sick? To resolve these questions it is necessary to compare some of the institutions the Christian churches developed to meet charitable needs in earlier centuries with the Pantokrator Xenon. If earlier institutions shared many features visible in the organization of this twelfth-century xenon, this would indicate a continuous tradition of hospitals in the Byzantine Empire.

CHARITABLE INSTITUTIONS FROM THE FOURTH CENTURY ON

As late as the third century, Christian communities had not yet established permanent charitable agencies, even in the larger churches such as that of Alexandria. When a deadly pestilence struck the Egyptian capital in the mid-third century, Bishop Dionysios and his flock shouldered the perilous task of caring for the plague victims and of burying the dead with suitable reverence. In describing this effort, the bishop knew of no hospice for the poor maintained by his church, nor of a facility to treat the sick. He did not even mention a physician as part of the Christian relief program.[46] Under the first Christian emperor, Constantine, the churches began to receive tax immunities and government grants to help carry out their charitable activities. In 320 the emperor freed the clergy and employees of the churches from the obligation of performing *munera sordida* and exempted them from the hated *collatio lustralis,* the quinquennial tax on merchants, so that they could amass extra profits for the poor. Constantine's immunities, however, do not provide any evidence that Christian communities had by that time organized permanent institutions for ministering to those in need beyond the simple distribution of food and clothing practiced by the early church or that they had set aside special places for receiving the sick.[47] In 332, Constantine again favored his coreligionists by granting the churches of Syria an allotment from the grain *annona* to relieve the ravages of famine. The emperor stressed that this grain was to nourish the clergy, widows, and the poor in the *xeno-docheia.*[48] Here the emperor mentioned for the first time permanent institutions of some kind at Antioch and her daughter churches, the xenodocheia reserved to house and feed the poor. Although later sources from the fourth and fifth centuries were sometimes to use the term *xenodocheion* to describe a refuge for the sick or even a hospital, there is no indication that this word had any such associations in the 330s.[49]

When in 344 Leontios became bishop of Antioch, he took special interest in maintaining the existing xenodocheia of his church, appointing pious men to supervise their operation. He also constructed a new hostel at Daphne, a fashionable suburb of Antioch. A later source, the *Chronicon paschale,* emphasized that Leontios expected his xenodocheia, or *xenones,* as the chronicle also called them, to provide a place to stay for the homeless poor or for strangers to his city. The sources, however, provide no direct evidence that these xenones of Antioch and Syria took any special steps for the sick.[50]

To the east of Antioch, the Syrian city of Edessa had no organized charities as late as 373. Famine struck that city around 370, while the famous Syrian holy man, Ephrem, was living there. Since the Christians of Edessa had no church official to administer any large-scale relief program, Ephrem volunteered to assume the task. He collected money and food, set up some three hundred beds for refugees to the city from the starving countryside, and treated those who were ill from lack of nourishment. His were emergency measures, however; the Edessan church seems to have had no permanent hostels for migrants and the poor, not to mention specialized centers to treat the ill.[51]

Less than ten years later, however, evidence from Antioch indicates that an institution to care for the sick had been functioning in that metropolis for some time. In 381, while still a deacon in Antioch, John Chrysostom advised his friend Stagyrios to contemplate the many forms of suffering in this world. He recommended that Stagyrios ask the administrator of the xenon to take him inside to observe those lying there, so that he "could see every root of evil, the strange forms of disease, and the many causes of depression." Although Chrysostom did not mention any physicians working in this xenon, it seems to have been an institution solely for the care of the sick—perhaps a true hospital.[52] Shortly after, Placilla, the wife of the emperor Theodosius, gained a reputation for holiness in Constantinople by going to the xenones attached to the capital's churches to visit the bed-ridden and offer them nursing care.[53] Several years later, when John Chrysostom ascended the episcopal throne of Constantinople in 398, he reallocated the bishop's personal fund to support institutions which his biographer Palladios called *nosokomeia* (places to care for the sick). Palladios mentions that these institutions supported staffs of physicians, cooks, and nursing attendants. Among these, only the nursing attendants were volunteers drawn from groups of urban ascetics in the capital city.[54]

The term *nosokomeion* implies that Chrysostom's institutions were designed especially for the sick, but Palladios refers also to travellers (*xenoi*) who rested there. Since he identifies physicians and nurses at these institutions, however, it is possible that they included separate dormitories for the sick where the medical staff could examine and treat patients without disturbing the healthy guests. Perhaps each of Chrysostom's nosokomeia formed a small complex of different philanthropies, one building serving as a place for the sick and another as a lodge for travellers, just as the twelfth-century Pantokrator maintained a xenon to heal the sick and a gerokomeion to house the aged. In any case, these nosokomeia surely were offering the poor sick of fourth-century Constantinople food, shelter, nursing care, and some access to professional physicians; in other words, they were institutions which come very close to fitting our definition of a hospital.

A somewhat younger contemporary of Chrysostom, Neilos of Ankyra, provides even more conclusive evidence that hospitals existed in Eastern cities by the early fifth century. In a letter to his friend Marinos, Neilos portrayed the sick and the paralyzed in a nosokomeion; but he also described the physician examining each of the patients and recommending a variety of medicines, diets, and regimens prescribed specially for the individual cases. The aim of these therapies was to provide exactly what each person needed and thereby restore the body to the balance of good health.[55] For the first time, a hospital physician appears, performing his daily rounds, a tradition still followed eight centuries later by the primmikerioi of the Pantokrator Xenon. Moreover, this doctor was not trying simply to alleviate pain or to extend to patients food and shelter; he was devising his therapies to restore the sick to health.[56]

Although these early nosokomeia surely restricted the medical care they offered to the poor, in all other respects they fit our definition of a hospital. The few sources which describe them, however, do not refer to a hierarchical and specialized staff such as the one we have seen at the Pantokrator Xenon. The first evidence that hospitals had several grades of medical personnel comes from the seventh century in a curious hagiographical work—the *Miracula S. Artemii*—which provides glimpses of two Constantinopolitan xenones, the Sampson and the Christodotes. At the first, it mentions surgeons and a special section for patients with eye problems; at the second, it describes physicians who worked in monthly shifts, and medical assistants (hypourgoi) who kept night watch in the hospital wards.[57] Each morning the chief physician at the Christodotes made the same kind of rounds through the hospital sections which the primmikerioi were required to perform at the Pantokrator.[58] In summary, both the xenones described by the *Miracula Artemii* show so many similarities to the Pantokrator hospital that they must have been essentially the same kind of institution. Thus, from the seventh century, or more likely from the prosperous days of the sixth century when the emperor Justinian reformed the secular medical profession, one can date the opening of elaborate hospitals comparable to the twelfth-century Pantokrator.[59]

In the beginning of the thirteenth century, the Byzantine empire suffered an almost fatal blow from the rampaging knights of the Fourth Crusade. Even after the trauma of the Latin conquest and subsequent occupation, however, hospitals continued to operate, at least in Constantinople itself. As late as the fifteenth century, the Krales Xenon, attached to the monastery of St. John Prodromos in Petra, still maintained a staff of physicians, a library, and a teaching program.[60] It represents the last hospital in the Pantokrator tradition, for in 1453 the Turks ended the history of the East Roman Empire and its hospitals.

AN EXPLORATION OF TERMINOLOGY

A brief survey of descriptive sources indicates that hospitals on the scale of the Pantokrator Xenon had existed in the East Roman Empire certainly from the seventh century and that institutions recognizable as hospitals had opened as early as 400. Do the Greek sources also establish a terminology to distinguish these hospitals from other philanthropic agencies? In the West, where medical centers comparable to the Pantokrator Xenon did not exist before the Enlightenment or even before the nineteenth century, precise terms for different kinds of philanthropic institutions never evolved; *hospital, hospitium,* and *xenodochium* were practically interchangeable expressions.[61] In Byzantine Greek, however, words had developed by the sixth century to identify institutions designed solely to provide medical therapy for the sick—words different from those which described shelters to feed the poor, to house the strangers, or to support the aged.

Greek sources of the Byzantine era employed many words in discussing philanthropic institutions. The list includes *xenon, nosokomeion, gerokomeion, ptocheion* or *ptochotropheion, orphanotropheion, brephotropheion,* and *xenodocheion.*[62] These terms can be divided into two classes: those which derive from words with relatively precise meanings and which therefore refer to a specific kind of institution, and those which come from roots with broad meanings and as a result can denote a larger range of institutions, at least from the etymological perspective.

Among the class of terms with specific meanings was *orphanotropheion,* a word composed of *orphanos* (orphan) and *trepho* (to nourish). Thus, *orphanotropheion* clearly referred to an institution which sheltered and fed orphans—an orphanage in English. Although this word first appears in the legislation of Justinian, the term *orphanotrophos* describing the director of an orphanotropheion can be found in 458.[63] In that year the orphanotrophos almost attained the episcopal throne of Constantinople. Since the administrator of the orphanage held such a prominent post by the mid-fifth century, the institution he supervised and probably the word which described it were considerably older, perhaps as old as the fourth century.[64]

Like *orphanotropheion,* the terms *brephotropheion* and *gerokomeion* describe institutions with specific functions. The roots *brephos* (infant) and *trepho* (nourish) indicate that a brephotropheion was designed to care for infants and very young children—a foundling house. Only the sixth-century legal and canonical sources mention such philanthropic agencies.[65] The roots *geron* (old man) and *komeo* (to care for) restrict the meaning of *gerokomeion* to an institution that housed the aged—an old-age home. Writing in the sixth century, Cyril of Skythopolis employed this word in listing the institutions the empress Eudocia had founded in Palestine in the mid-fifth century.[66] Constantinopolitan traditions associated *gerokomeion* with three separate philanthropies founded in the first half of the fifth century.[67] Thus, the evidence from Palestine and the capital indicates that old-age homes certainly existed as distinct philanthropies from the early fifth century, and it is likely that the term *gerokomeion* is just as old.

In later centuries *gerokomeion* continued to describe institutions that focused on caring for the aged. As we have seen, the Pantokrator Geroko-meion conformed to the twentieth-century definition of an old-age home, offering the necessities of life to those who were unable to support themselves on account of their old age or in some cases because of crippling injury or disease. A twelfth-century gerokomeion in the provincial town of Ainos, however, seems to have served also as a hospital. It admitted thirty-six male patients who suffered not only from debilitating old age, but also from acute diseases. It even hired one physician and ten medical assistants (hypourgoi) to treat the sick among the residents.[68] Those who recovered after treatment could leave the institution. In this regard, this gerokomeion functioned as a hospital, though with a much smaller staff than a hospital such as the Pantokrator would have had. On the other hand, if some patients wished to remain at the gerokomeion in Ainos after they recovered, they were not required to leave as they were at the Pantokrator Xenon.[69] Here, the institution differed from a true hospital. It would seem that in a small provincial town such as Ainos, a gerokomeion had to serve a dual function as both hospital and rest home, as indeed old-age homes sometimes do in rural areas of twentieth-century America.

Like *gerokomeion,* the sense of *nosokomeion* emerges from its roots, *nosos* (disease) and again *komeo* (to care for). The verb *nosokomeo* (to care for the sick) and the abstract noun formed from it, *nosokomia* (the care of the sick), are found in Greek texts of the classical, Hellenistic, and Roman periods. The noun *nosokomeion* in reference to an institution, on the other hand, appears only in the late fourth century.[70] Indeed, Palladios was among the first Greek authors to employ the term when he described the institutions for the sick which John Chrysostom established in Constantinople.[71] By the sixth century, however, *nosokomeion* had become a common word; Justinian often used it in his constitutions.[72] Later in the same century, the jurist Julian provided a Latin definition of the term for law students who understood no Greek. He defined a *nosokomeion* as a place in which the sick received special care.[73] The tenth-century encyclopedia, the *Suda,* narrowed the definition to a place which treated those suffering from acute diseases as opposed to a refuge for those with some chronic problem.[74] Thus, by this time *nosokomeion* meant an institution for treating diseases, an institution such as the Pantokrator Xenon, and in fact, the Pantokrator *Typikon* once refers to its hospital as a nosokomeion.[75]

Greek sources employed *nosokomeion* both to indicate institutions of medical care for the public, such as the Pantokrator hospital, and to categorize those for a limited group. Thus, in his monastic rules, Basil of Caesarea sometimes called the infirmary for the monks of his monastery a nosoko-meion.[76] The famous eleventh-century typikon of the Euergites Monastery described as a nosokomeion the small infirmary of eight beds which it reserved for sick monks.[77] Indeed, most sources of the later Byzantine period seemed to prefer limiting *nosokomeion* to infirmaries for the monks of a given monastery.[78]

It is significant that three of the terms which denoted specialized charities—*orphanotropheion, gerokomeion,* and *nosokomeion*—gained currency at the end of the fourth century or during the fifth. These new words thus appeared at the time that the descriptive passages considered above first refer to philanthropic institutions which provided special facilities and medical care for the sick. The philological evidence seems to support the conclusion that about 400 Christian bishops were opening philanthropic institutions whose efforts focused on alleviating particular forms of human suffering.

New vocabulary for charitable agencies derived from *ptochos* (poor) or *xenos* (stranger or guest) do not have precise meanings, since both *ptochos* and *xenos* were relative words. *Xenos* meant a traveller with respect to a geographical place, but it also marked out a person from outside the community—a foreigner to a Greek *polis,* someone from the world beyond the cloister wall to a monk. So, too, the early Christian writers often used *ptochos* to describe not only the materially poor but also people suffering from any misfortune, including disease.[79] As a result, *ptochotropheion* or *ptocheion* could designate a place designed to shelter and feed the destitute—a poor house, in its literal meaning. On the other hand, Basil of Caesarea called the philanthropic institution he built in Caesarea during the 370s a ptochotropheion. In describing this agency, he mentions that professional physicians (iatroi) worked there.[80] Thus, a section of it, at least, resembled a hospital. So, too, a ptocheion in fifth-century Ephesus might have received principally the sick.[81] In the sixth century, ambiguity still surrounded these two terms. Julian defined a ptochotropheion as a place where both the poor and the sick were fed.[82] After the sixth century, however, neither *ptocheion* nor *ptochotropheion* refers to a house for the sick. In the eleventh century, Michael Attaleiates founded a ptochotropheion at Raidestos to feed and shelter the destitute, but in his typikon Michael made no provision for nursing or treating the sick.[83]

Reflecting the meaning of *xenos* as guest, the term *xenodocheion* originally applied to a commercial inn. In his book on dreams, the second-century Artemidoros described a man fleeing to a xenodocheion and entering one of its rooms. The context demonstrates that this place was a public inn with individual rooms for guests.[84] By the early fourth century, however, *xenodocheion* had come to describe the houses for the poor which the Christian churches of Syria maintained. Probably most of the poor who stayed in these institutions had wandered into Antioch and other towns from the Syrian countryside and hence were *xenoi* to the *poleis,* but also guests at the philanthropic agencies of the churches.[85] On the other hand, Saint Basil used *xenodocheion* to describe an infirmary for sick monks in his monastery; in this case Basil employed *xenodocheion* interchangeably with *nosokomeion.*[86]

Bishop Rabbula of fifth-century Edessa labeled his institution for both healthy travellers and the sick a xenodocheion. Later Syriac sources continued to use a derivative of the Greek *xenodocheion* to designate institutions only for the sick. Thus, the late sixth-century source attributed to Zachariah of Mitylene describes as a xenodocheion the hospital which Shah Khusro I of Persia built for physicians at his court.[87] In the Greek-speaking world, however, *xenodocheion* did not become an accepted term for a hospital. In the sixth century, Julian defined a xenodocheion as a place "in which travellers are received."[88] So, too, the tenth-century *Suda* considered it simply an institution for the reception of guests, omitting any reference to the sick or disabled.[89] At about the same time, the emperor Romanos I (920–44) constructed what he called a xenodocheion and fitted it out with spacious stables for wealthy guests. Here the word refers to a hotel which served people of means who came to Constantinople on legal or governmental business.[90] When in the early thirteenth century the abbot Neilos legislated for his monastery on Cyprus, he called its simple guesthouse for travelers a xenodocheion.[91] By his time the term no longer had any associations with the sick or the practice of medicine.

A second term derived from *xenos—xenon*—developed along much different lines. Indeed, the twelfth-century Pantokrator *Typikon* normally describes its hospital as a xenon. In classical Greek, however, *xenon* had nothing to do with the care of the sick. Euripides referred to the guest rooms in a palace as xenones.[92] The term retained this meaning throughout the classical Greek and Hellenistic age. In the first century A.D. Josephus still chose *xenon* to describe the guest chambers in Herod's palace at Jerusalem.[93] By the third century, however, *xenon* had acquired a new meaning. An inscription from Syria identifies the hospice which the town of Phaena maintained for travelling officials and perhaps for other strangers as a xenon. Here the meaning is synonymous with *xenodocheion.*[94] Under the Christian Roman emperors *xenon* retained this second meaning. Thus, the fifth-century lexicographer Hesychios defined it as an inn.[95] From the same period, the *Vita Porphyrii* demonstrates that *xenon* could also apply to a shelter for the poor, again following the same evolution as *xenodocheion* had.[96] On the other hand, a xenon which Chrysostom saw at Antioch in 381 seems to have housed only the sick, as did the xenones of contemporary Constantinople, where the empress Placilla waited on patients.[97] By the sixth century *xenon* had certainly acquired the meaning of hospital as we have defined the English word, for authors used it to describe the large and well-organized Sampson—an institution with a specialized staff of physicians and trained assistants.[98]

An inscription from fifth-century Palestine, found in the necropolis of Silwan, may help to explain how some hospitals came to be called xenones. It reads: "A memorial to Philetos, deacon of the new xenon and of the nosokomeion in it."[99] Here the local church operated a hospice for the poor and for travellers that included an infirmary section called a nosokomeion. In larger towns such as Antioch and Constantinople some xenones must have enlarged their nosokomeion sections until the infirmary aspect dominated the raison d'être of the institution. Others, such as the Sampson Xenon, developed from houses of charitable physicians. Here the primitive use of the word *xenon* for guest rooms might well have spread from the quarters assigned to the sick to include the whole philanthropic institution, as two historians of ancient medicine have suggested.[100] Whatever the process, hospitals of Justinian's reign were usually called xenones, while the directors of such philanthropic institutions were known as *xenodochoi,* even though they governed institutions much different than simple xenodocheia for travellers or the poor.

Although *xenon* usually applied to a medical center in the sixth century, it could still have its older meaning of hospice or inn. The classicizing Prokopios described the large hotels which Justinian and Theodora built for poor migrants to Constantinople as xenones.[101] As late as the tenth century the scholarly encyclopedia, the *Suda,* listed two possible meanings for *xenon:* first, a hospice for guests and, second, a hospital for patients with acute diseases.[102] Popular usage, however, had long before narrowed the proper use of the term to a hospital. In the early eighth century, the *Vita Andreae* states that hospitals for the sick were commonly called xenones.[103] Even a conservative classicist such as the ninth-century Arethas interpreted the word *xenon* in the *Onomasticon* of Julius Pollux to mean a hospital, although the context clearly shows that here the ancient author was referring to the guest rooms of a private house.[104]

After the eighth century, *xenon* almost replaced *nosokomeion* in identifying hospitals. Most probably, writers preferred to use *xenon,* since it clearly differentiated a public hospital from a monastic infirmary. Such a distinction was important at institutions like the Pantokrator, where the monastery maintained both its own nosokomeion for the monks and a public hospital for the people outside the monastic community—the xenoi.

To summarize the evidence regarding Byzantine vocabulary for hospitals, *nosokomeion* and *xenon* were the two terms which writers ordinarily selected when they wished to indicate an institution for curing the sick. *Nosokomeion* always referred to a medical center. One must check the context to determine whether or not the nosokomeion mentioned served the public or a special group. Having shed its ancient meaning as guest room, *xenon* functioned as a synonym for *xenodocheion* from 200 to 400. After 400 *xenon* came to designate hospitals for the sick, but conservative writers like Prokopios could still employ the word for xenodocheia. After the radical changes in Byzantine society which began in the seventh century, the older hospice definition of *xenon* fell out of use, except in a treasure house of antiquity such as the *Suda*. Thus, whenever a source refers to an institution as a xenon after 610, it is surely discussing a hospital for the sick, different perhaps in its scale from the imperial Pantokrator hospital, but the same in its essential qualities.

Philanthropic institutions, called either xenones or nosokomeia, offered the subjects of the East Roman emperors hospital services—bed, board, nursing care, and access to trained physicians—from the beginning of the fifth century to the very eve of the Turkish conquest. From the seventh century on, some of these hospitals reached the level of sophistication described by the Pantokrator *Typikon*. In shaping these institutions of medical care, Byzantine society did not depend on models in contemporary Persian or Islamic society, as some scholars have suggested. Rather, it drew on its own rich traditions of classical Greek medicine. Although Christian bishops surely organized the first hospitals, they readily turned to the students of Galen and Hippocrates for the expertise to make their nososkomeia effective centers of medical care.

CHAPTER THREE

Hospitals and the Ancient World

Many aspects of medieval culture both in the Greek East and the Latin West had deep roots in the world of classical antiquity. It is not surprising, therefore, that the professional medical men of a Byzantine hospital such as the Pantokrator Xenon owed much to the physicians of the ancient world. An examination of classical medicine and its practitioners will demonstrate that ancient Greco-Roman society provided medieval hospitals with the traditions of a highly motivated medical profession, with basic medical theory, and with many specific therapies. Working in hospital wards Byzantine doctors were themselves conscious of their own close relationship to the classical practitioners of medicine and saw no break in continuity from the ancient to the Christian age. A twelfth-century nosokomos of the Pantokrator Xenon could boast that the pagan Galen was the teacher of his profession.[1] While institutions for the sick such as the Byzantine xenones were unknown before the fourth century A.D., Greek medicine as it had developed from Hippocrates to Galen influenced medieval hospital development in many ways.[2]

A study of the classical contributions to the development of Byzantine hospitals is especially important since prominent historians of medicine and students of classical civilization have not all held that the Christian xenones or nosokomeia of the fourth century were the first such institutions in the Western world. The great majority of researchers do now agree with the conclusion reached in the preceding chapter, namely that Christian churches of the Eastern Mediterranean opened the first centers of medical care sometime after the middle of the fourth century.[3] The Marxist historian Gerhard Harig has recently reemphasized the crucial role of the Christian church in creating hospitals.[4] Sixty-five years ago, however, in a popular essay regarding institutional care for the sick in the ancient world, Theodor Meyer-Steineg claimed that the pre-Christian world of classical antiquity had established hospitals long before the Christian church began building them in the fourth century. This essay subsequently influenced a number of scholars, including the great historian of medicine Karl Sudhoff. Meyer-Steineg began his essay with a frank statement of his purpose, "to refute the ever-resurfacing opinion that the hospital is a specifically Christian institution, and, on the other hand, to furnish positive evidence that Greek and Roman antiquity had available institutions to house the sick."[5] In his eagerness to prove the existence of hospitals in the ancient world, the author sometimes misinterpreted evidence in the literary sources and stretched meager archaeological information far beyond its ability to support conclusions. Although Meyer-Steineg's essay and the many other studies which adopted his arguments are flawed by a desire to exalt classical civilization, they have uncovered some valuable information regarding institutions of medical care in the ancient world. Upon closer scrutiny one will find that these institutions surely did not offer hospital care. Nevertheless, some of them did exert a significant influence upon Byzantine medical practice in general and upon the nosokomeia in particular.

THE GREEKS

The practice of Greek medicine is at least as old as the Homeric age. In the *Iliad* members of certain aristocratic families entered the epic action as experts in the art of healing.[6] The medical knowledge of these families was a practical affair, each generation learning the collected wisdom of its forefathers regarding the healing properties of herbs and minerals, adding to this treasure its own experience, and passing the knowledge on to its offspring. Throughout its long history the Greek medical profession maintained the outward structure of a great family tradition. When in the archaic period the god Asklepios emerged as the deity of the healing art, myth wove him into the chain of knowledge passed from generation to generation. Zeus taught Apollo; Apollo taught Asklepios; the deified Asklepios, in turn, passed the torch of medical knowledge to mortal doctors.[7] By the fifth and fourth centuries B.C., Greek physicians regularly called themselves the Asklepiads or the Sons of Asklepios.[8] This terminology survived the Roman conquest of the Greek East, survived even the triumph of Christianity, and, protected by the iron-clad conventions of Byzantine classicism, flourished up to the last decades of the Eastern Empire.[9]

The myth reflected reality. Not only in the Homeric age was the healing art kept in the same families, but even when medicine developed a scientific and theoretical framework during the classical period, it tended to pass from father to son. Thus, tradition held that in the sixth century B.C. the Coan doctor Nebros had a son who practiced medicine with him.[10] So, too, both the father and the grandfather of the great Hippocrates were supposedly physicians.[11] After the fourth century B.C. inscriptions from the Hellenistic and Roman era of Asia Minor indicate that the custom of keeping the medical profession in the ranks of the same families was common.[12] Even though the most famous of ancient physicians, Galen, was the son not of a doctor but of a mathematician, he believed that when fathers taught the medical arts to their own sons, they produced the best-trained physicians.[13]

After the fourth century A.D. physicians in the eastern Mediterranean continued to train their sons in the art of medicine. Both the fifth-century Iakobos and the sixth-century Alexander of Tralleis were famous physicians whose fathers had also practiced medicine.[14] The tradition of medical families continued throughout the later centuries of the Byzantine Empire. Though Nikephoros Blemmydes (1192–1272) became famous as a monk, a religious writer, and a classical scholar, he had practiced medicine in his father's footsteps before he took up the monastic life.[15] The family tradition of the medical profession left its mark even in Byzantine terminology. Medieval Greek sources regularly refer to medical students as children of the doctors. The Pantokrator *Typikon* itself described the apprentices at the hospital as the children of the xenon physicians.[16]

In the ancient world as in the medieval Byzantine Empire religion and medicine were always closely linked. In spite of attempts by some historians to separate completely Hellenic religious cults and their emphasis on miraculous cures from the rational approach to medicine which developed during the classical age of Greek culture, a study of ancient physicians demonstrates that such a clear separation did not exist. Demokedes, the famous physician of Kroton, was the son of Kalliphon, whom tradition described as a priest of Asklepios, the god of healing.[17] In third-century (B.C.) Athens, the college of public physicians customarily sacrificed to Asklepios twice a year for themselves and their patients.[18] Xenophon, the personal physician of the emperors Claudius and Nero, also served as a priest at the temple of Asklepios on Kos.[19] Inscriptions from Roman Asia Minor prove that doctors often were priests of Asklepios or at least were associated with the god's cult in some way.[20]

During the sixth and fifth centuries B.C., the traditional practice of medicine at Kroton, Rhodes, Knidos, Kos, and a few other Greek cities fell under the influence of pre-Socratic philosophy. Stimulated by the ideas of Demokritos and other thinkers, physicians began the careful study of disease in an attempt to discern underlying, natural causes. This new activity gave birth to what the classical world would later call the *Corpus Hippocraticum*, a collection of medical treatises emanating from several centers of medical study during the fifth and fourth centuries B.C.[21] Some of the works in the *Corpus Hippocraticum* reveal a rational and empirical approach to diseases and their treatment—a true medical science.[22] For example, in the Hippocratic treatise on epilepsy, the author denies that this disease should be classified as supernatural, since it, like all other illnesses, has its own nature and develops from natural causes. These sentiments some modern scholars have interpreted as a denial of a religious dimension in the thought of scientific Greek medicine. Yet the author of the same text continues: "There is no need to put this disease in a special class and to consider it more divine than the others. They are all divine and all human." Thus, he does not deny the sacred aspect of sickness, but rather, that the scope of the divine can be limited to a specific disease. Moreover, he considers all the elements of nature affecting disease—cold, sun, and the changing winds—to be of divine origin.[23] As Ludwig Edelstein has stressed, most of the Greek physicians from the early days of scientific medicine to the time of Galen acknowledged the existence of God and of the supernatural dimension of life. As a result, ancient physicians were able to retain their close link with the Asclepian cult and with its miraculous cures and yet practice medicine on the basis of observed facts and the theories they deduced from their data. Although secular medicine operated in a different medium than did religion, only a few theorists of the healing art denied divine forces or the possibility of spiritual healing.[24]

After the conversion of Constantine the Asclepian cult with its divine cures did not immediately disappear; it flourished through much of the fourth century A.D., collapsing finally under the onslaught of the emperor Theodosius (379–95) against the pagan shrines.[25] Miraculous healing, however, did not vanish with paganism. The new faith of the Roman Empire also recognized the spiritual approach to health and disease. The New Testament described Christ as both the savior of men's souls and the healer of their bodies. In addition, Christians began to mark out certain of their great men as supernatural physicians, doctor-saints who healed the faithful miraculously. According to popular belief, these saints, unlike the doctors of the world, were willing to effect their cures without collecting a fee, a practice which won them the epithet *anargyroi* (without money).[26] By the sixth century, Constantinople and other Byzantine cities had specific churches dedicated to Cosmas and Damian, the most famous of the doctor-saints, and to other anargyroi where the sick sought the gift of health.[27] Usually, these shrines were associated with Byzantine hospitals, staffed by trained physicians.[28] In xenones that were not dedicated to the anargyroi—such as the Panto-krator—Cosmas and Damian still received special honor. Moreover, in all East Roman hospitals, prayer, liturgy, and the confession of sins were considered integral parts of the healing process.[29] As in the ancient world, so too in the Byzantine Empire secular medicine recognized the significance of the supernatural.

At Kos, Knidos, and the other centers of the healing profession, secular medicine continued to develop during the classical Greek age (fifth and fourth centuries B.C.) and came to exert a powerful influence on Hellenic culture as a whole. After Alexander and his Macedonian generals reshaped the Eastern Mediterranean world at the end of the fourth century, the new capital of Alexandria in Egypt emerged as the leading center of Greek science, including medicine. Here scholars collected and edited the works of earlier physicians, gradually creating the *Corpus Hippocraticum;* they attributed most of these works to a single physician of fifth-century Kos named Hippocrates.[30] At Alexandria and perhaps also at Antioch, some physicians made significant new discoveries. During the third century B.C. Herophilos and his younger rival Erasistratos advanced the study of anatomy and what today is called physiology by conducting careful autopsies.[31]

By the late Hellenistic period and early Roman principate, the Greek medical profession had divided into a number of contending schools, each championing a particular medical theory. The dogmatists of Alexandria stressed the importance of theory in understanding diseases and their cures; their opponents, the empiricists, ignored hidden causes and concentrated on collecting data to determine what treatments were in fact effective against illnesses. At Rome the methodists emphasized rhythms of laxity and tension in diseases and sought to break the baneful grip of sickness by employing astringents and laxatives. Influenced by Stoic philosophy, a fourth school, the pneumatists, asserted that a primordial substance called *pneuma* flowed in the arteries of the body and was the source of life. Much of the work these schools produced has disappeared from the Greek tradition save for comments on their writings found in Galen and excerpts from them collected by early Byzantine physicians.[32]

During the first and second centuries A.D., Greek physicians abandoned the strict doctrinal positions of the Hellenistic schools and adopted an eclectic approach. The greatest of these physicians was Galen of Pergamon. During his lifetime (129–99) he produced a huge corpus of medical writing, building principally on the writings attributed to Hippocrates but gathering much also from the schools of the Hellenistic and Roman periods.[33] Galen insisted on a close relationship between body and mind, between medicine and philosophy. He himself wrote philosophical treatises on Plato and Aristotle and studied astronomy and mathematics. His short tract entitled "The Best Doctor Is Also a Philosopher" presented his case succinctly.[34]

Built on careful observation, experiment, and a wide-ranging synthesis of past medical doctrines, Galen's tremendous achievement so impressed the generations which followed that by the time of Oribaseios (mid-fourth century) his works had eclipsed the writings of all the other Greek physicians. Just as History had its Herodotus and Thucydides, Rhetoric its Lysias and Demosthenes, now Medicine had its canonical texts, the works of Galen and Hippocrates. From the fifth to the seventh centuries the medical curriculum at Alexandria was built around these two men. Here students of medicine continued to study Galen and Hippocrates in their original form, but during these years, too, the process of shortening, simplifying, and explaining their works had begun, a process which eventually led to a forest of commentaries and digests of Galen and Hippocrates, both in the Greek world of the Byzantine Empire and in the Islamic lands.[35]

The sixth-century physician of Alexandria, Palladios summed it up: "Hippocrates sowed; Galen reaped."[36] These two authorities remained the pillars of Greek medicine throughout the long history of the East Roman Empire. The seventh-century doctors of Constantinople boasted of Hippocrates and Galen as the luminaries of their profession.[37] In an excess of rhetorical zeal, a twelfth-century nosokomos of the Pantokrator Xenon claimed that Galen had been a contemporary of Christ, apparently in an attempt to give the pagan head of his profession some connection with the Great Physician of the new dispensation.[38] In ridiculing the physicians of his own time, the fifteenth-century satirist Mazaris accused the doctors of knowing no ancient Greek and of comprehending neither Galen nor Hippocrates. How could men so ignorant of these great medical writers save the sick from death?[39]

Byzantine medicine was thus of the same warp and woof as the healing art of the ancient Greco-Roman world. It shared the same great writers, Galen and Hippocrates, the same dominant medical theory. Through epitomes prepared by Byzantine writers of the fourth through the sixth centuries, the East Roman Empire also inherited the medical wisdom of the Hellenistic and Roman schools. Thus, a patient confined to a ward of the Pantokrator Xenon during the twelfth century could expect to receive medical treatment based on the system which Hippocrates and Galen had developed, although experience and new drugs had altered many of the specific therapies.[40]

THE ROMANS

Hippocrates and Galen as well as Soranos, Rufus, and almost all the other renowned physicians of the ancient world were Greeks. Although the Romans subdued the Hellenes and eventually absorbed their civilization, they did not display the same interest or talent in Greek medicine as they did in Hellenic philosophy, rhetoric, history, and the other fields of science and literature. According to tradition, when the first physician arrived in Rome from the Peloponnesos in 219 B.C., the city welcomed him and gave him a *iatreion,* or medical office.[41] As Rome began to expand her control over the Greek world after 199 B.C., more Greek physicians streamed to the great city on the Tiber, along with many other teachers and craftsmen; some came voluntarily, others as slaves.[42] Among Roman conservatives of the second century B.C. anti-Greek sentiments were quick to surface. Marcus Cato, a paragon of Roman conservative virtue, not only developed a deep-seated dislike of Greeks in general, but singled out medical men as the lowest of the Hellenes, specifically forbidding his son to have any contact with physicians.[43]

By the first century B.C. attitudes had mellowed somewhat in a Rome continually penetrated by Greek culture. The great Latin orator Cicero had read Greek philosophical works thoroughly and had studied rhetoric on the

Isle of Rhodes. In spite of his respect for Hellenic culture, however, he did not think medicine a suitable career for a well-born Roman.[44] Writing in the first century of the empire, Pliny the Elder revived the old conservative hostility toward physicians. He did not criticize medical wisdom per se; rather he attacked the servile dependence of noble Romans on the treacherous advice of foreign (i.e., Greek) physicians. Pliny particularly criticized these doctors for collecting fees from their patients. To correct this situation Pliny wanted to provide his fellow citizens with a Latin summary of remedies for various ailments, many of them culled from Greek works. The liberally educated man could easily develop medical expertise so that he did not need to rely on professional doctors, many of whom Pliny believed were actually murderers and corrupters of virtue.[45]

As a result of this pervasive Latin aversion to the medical profession, it is not surprising that native Romans rarely became physicians. During Roman expansion in the East (199–31 B.C.), Greek slaves and freedmen made up the majority of physicians practicing in the Latin West. Although under Julius Caesar and the early emperors physicians rose rapidly in wealth and prestige as a result of imperial favor, Roman aristocrats did not turn to this field as an avenue of advancement. Pliny found some satisfaction in this reluctance of his contemporaries to study medicine professionally.[46] Epigraphy confirms Pliny's claim. At Ostia most inscriptions found to date are in Latin; the few Greek ones include several funerary dedications to physicians.[47] Throughout Gaul, Italy, and Roman Africa, Greek inscriptions from the principate are usually associated with the medical profession.[48] As an exception to the rule some scholars have cited Aulius Cornelius Celsus, who wrote a long medical treatise, *De medicina,* during the reign of Tiberius (A.D. 14–37). Celsus, however, was most probably not a physician but an encyclopedist who, like Pliny, considered an understanding of medical theory and a knowledge of practical cures within the purview of a well-educated Roman.[49] Scribonius Largus, on the other hand, represents a significant deviation from the rule. He seems to have been a native Roman who both wrote about medicine as a science and practiced it as a profession.[50]

Most Romans of the high empire did not share Pliny's intense hatred for the medical profession. They readily admitted Greek physicians to the capital, sought their services, and encouraged their professional writing. After all, Rome had sheltered both the doctors of the methodist school and Galen during his most productive years. Nevertheless, Romans were influenced by men like Pliny insofar as they considered a professional medical career unsuitable for a Roman of distinction. Most pursued medicine only as one of the liberal arts and thus never developed a strong Latin medical tradition. When the two halves of the Roman world began drifting apart in the fourth century, physicians did not retain a prominent place in the cultural life of the West. The eastern, or Byzantine, provinces, on the other hand, inherited not only the structure of the ancient Greek medical profession and its great corpus of scientific literature, but also the enthusiasm of the Hellenes for medicine as a career.[51]

HEALTH-CARE INSTITUTIONS OF THE CLASSICAL WORLD

Although many professional traditions and much of the medical theory of the Byzantines can be traced back through the centuries of Greek culture to the *Corpus Hippocraticum* and even earlier, still, new elements did emerge in treatment procedures. Of the Byzantine innovations in the practice of medicine the greatest was undoubtedly the creation of the hospital. Although Professor Meyer-Steineg and his followers have suggested that Byzantine medical institutions such as the Pantokrator Xenon had parallels in the ancient world, sources of the classical age indicate that hospitals were not part of the regular practice of medicine in antiquity. Neither the writings of Hippocrates nor those of Galen mention any sort of institution where patients were housed while undergoing treatment.[52] Moreover, a number of passages from ancient sources demonstrate that prolonged medical care for the sick in a hospital setting did not exist.

Writing in the fourth century B.C., the Hippocratic author of the *Decorum* provided some advice for his colleagues on the proper care of patients. "When you go to the sick," he warned, "have each item ready at hand for your work so that you are not at a loss with regard to things which should have been prepared beforehand."[53] Moreover, he advised that the doctor visit his patients frequently to ensure that they were following his instructions. Patients, he said, often lie in an attempt to deceive a physician and will then complain bitterly when their health does not improve. The author advised physicians to leave a guard at the sick person's bed to keep a careful watch on his actions.[54] Clearly, this little guidebook knew nothing of hospitals where physicians and their assistants could monitor patients around the clock.

Plutarch, the biographer and popular philosopher (ca. 45–120), provides a revealing summary of ancient medical practice that omits any reference to hospital care. If a person suffers from some minor complaint such as a toothache or a finger wound, he walks to the doctor; if he is stricken with fever and is confined to bed, he calls the doctor to his house; and if he is violently ill with melancholia or some other form of insanity, he flees the doctor's approach.[55] Here only patients with minor problems visit the physician. Even as late as the fifth century, at a time when xenones and nosokomeia were receiving patients in some cities, a Christian preacher described the doctor's arduous visits to the sick and his careful preparation beforehand of the towels and instruments necessary for surgery.[56] How different this procedure was from that of seventh-century Constantinople, where a deacon, suffering from a severe infection of the groin, committed himself to a hospital bed for surgery and recuperation, or from twelfth-century Thessalonica, where patients facing death sought out the hospitals for medical treatment.[57]

These passages and others show that normally the ancient physician treated patients with serious problems in their own homes. Still, the records of Greek and Roman civilization do mention institutions which provided some sort of treatment for the sick in a central location and thus approximate Byzantine xenones. Whether or not these ancient treatment centers were true hospitals, some of them certainly helped to shape the medieval xenones. It will therefore be useful to study them in depth. Collating the arguments of a number of researchers yields four institutions of the pagan world which in some ways resembled the hospitals of the Byzantine period: the Roman *valetudinaria* for slaves, the legionary *valetudinaria,* the temples of Asklepios, and the doctors' offices, or surgeries (*iatreia*). A fifth institution, the committee of public physicians (*demosieuontes iatroi*) which the typical Greco-Roman city maintained for its citizens, was by the fifth century A.D. providing medical services closely paralleling those of the Christian hospitals.[58]

VALETUDINARIA

The Roman slave *valetudinaria* and the military infirmaries resembled Byzantine xenones in that they also offered a central location where patients received treatment, food, and care under supervision. On the other hand, they cannot be classified as hospitals as I have defined them, since the valetudinaria were designed to serve only restricted groups—the slaves of a particular estate or the troops of a given unit.[59] Moreover, the slave infirmaries did not offer high-quality care at the hands of professional physicians, trained in the skills of secular medicine. Although the Roman aristocrat Columella speaks favorably of slave valetudinaria, Cornelius Celsus paints a negative picture of them, comparing the overseers of such places to veterinarians and doctors in barbarian lands.[60] It is likely, too, that the great military infirmaries of the second century declined rapidly in the chaotic third century. Thus, Alexander Severus (222–35) allowed soldiers who were seriously ill to retire to a city and convalesce with some family of the town.[61] In any case, when the public hospitals of the Greek East arrived in Italy at the very beginning of the fifth century, Saint Jerome, a master of the Latin language, rejected the term *valetudinarium* to describe what he considered new institutions and chose to retain the Greek word *nosokomeion.*[62]

ASKLEPIEIA

Some scholars have seen in the temples of Asklepios, the god of medicine, the origin of hospital care.[63] Although the Asclepian cult had originated in Hellas proper during the archaic age, cities throughout the Mediterranean world had adopted it by the Roman imperial period. *Asklepieia,* the shrines of the god, were everywhere.[64] Men and women stricken with disease fled to the most famous of these in search of relief from their suffering. Since from their earliest days physicians had had close ties with the asklepieia, Meyer-Steineg has claimed that these temples offered some form of hospital care to the sick. Many classicists and historians have accepted this view because of the clear relationship of the medical profession to the Asclepian cult.[65] Even a brief survey of the sources describing asklepieia, however, will prove that they by no means provided hospital care and that they could not have inspired the organization of Byzantine nosokomeia such as the Pantokrator Xenon.

The evidence collected from literary sources and inscriptions indicates that asklepieia did not normally provide their suppliants with a place to sleep, with food, or with nursing care. In his many speeches and essays, the famous orator of the second sophistic, Aelius Aristides, frequently alludes to the famous temple of the healing god at Pergamon. Since Aristides was either a very sick man or an incurable hypochondriac, he made many visits to this asklepieion, but he never mentions that he took up residence in a hospice belonging to the shrine itself. He went to the temple for the all-important incubation, but he actually lived outside the sacred precinct.[66] On a typical visit, both he and his doctor Theodotos roomed at a private house belonging to the temple warden.[67] On the other hand, Pausanias' description of the great asklepieion at Epidauros does refer to a specific building close to the temple where the suppliants slept. Moreover, he mentions that men about to die and women ready to give birth could not remain in the shelter within the temple precinct, implying that other suppliants had some form of housing at the shrine.[68]

Nowhere, however, do the many descriptions of asklepieia throughout the provinces of the Roman Empire mention explicitly that the temples offered any nursing care or food to the sick. In writing of the asklepieion in Phocis, Pausanias provides the only detail which could be interpreted as a reference to attendants to assist the sick. Pausanias states that the sacred precinct included the temple together with dwellings for both the sick and the servants of the god. Perhaps some of these servants ministered to the suppliants staying close by them.[69] It is possible, then, that the asklepieion at Phocis not only sheltered suppliants but organized some kind of care for them. The evidence for this, however, is meager even here. Among the passages describing asklepieia that Edelstein has collected, I have found no other reference to any hospital services for the sick.[70] Even if the temples did house and care for suppliants, they surely fell outside the boundaries of our hospital definition, since they extended to the sick not the secular medicine of the physician, but the supernatural therapy of the god.

Although it is difficult to determine exactly what the practices were, information from archaeological excavations and from the works of Aelius

Aristides have provided an outline of the basic procedures at the large asklepieion at Pergamon, a major center of the cult.[71] When a suffering person
arrived in the town, he usually had to find some kind of lodging on his own.
Then, he walked or was carried to the sacred shrine and entered the temple
precinct. There, he made some sacrifice to Asklepios and withdrew to a
section of the temple area where he could sleep.[72] This was the famous
incubation. Often the suppliant simply found a comfortable spot or brought
along a mat to lay on the floor. But some temples, such as the ones at
Epidauros and Phocis, maintained special buildings where the sick could
sleep. While the suppliants slept, Asklepios worked his wondrous miracles
in one of three ways. The god might simply cure the suppliant in his slumber
so that he awoke in perfect health. Or, he might appear in a dream and
instruct the sufferer to perform a specific action, often of a bizarre nature.
Finally, he might recommend an accepted medical remedy.[73]

In addition to the central rite of incubation, there were also other ceremonies at the temple, including ritual washing, choral chanting, and don-
ning special white robes.[74] A methodical examination by a physician, treatment with specific drugs or dietary regimen, or skilled surgery by a human
hand played no role in the temple procedure. If the god recommended an
established medical treatment, it was not the nature of the cure prescribed
but the obedient response to the divine command which restored health.

In his *Sacred Tales* Aristides several times juxtaposed the uselessness of
the medical arts to the efficacious remedies of Asklepios. In one instance a
doctor recommended that Aristides undergo surgery or chemical cauterizing,
while the god forbade such treatment. The patient followed the divine command and was healed.[75] In another case, Asklepios ordered poor Aristides
to bathe in a nearby river in the middle of winter. The physicians urgently
warned against such drastic treatment. Aristides ignored them, plunged into
the icy waters, and regained his health.[76] In general, Aristides and other
devotees of Asklepios advised against going to physicians and recommended
instead recourse to the healing god. If it was right to recover, Asklepios
would grant it; if not, it was time to die.[77]

Although the medical profession had close ties with the Asclepian cult,
it clearly operated on an entirely different plane. As a result, physicians did
not always understand or accept as proper therapy what some suppliants
claimed to be divine revelation. When Aristides asked for an enema treatment
as the god commanded him, the physicians at first refused, until the orator
forced them to carry out what they considered a harmful procedure.[78] Galen
himself alluded to the extremely austere regimens that some of the god's
suppliants were willing to follow.[79] At the same time many physicians were
closely connected with the asklepieia; some even served as priests. To a
modern reader the position of ancient physicians with regard to the cult of
Asklepios might seem an intolerable contradiction, but one need only visit

a small Greek island or a village in the Italian countryside to see trained physicians willing to practice their craft in conjunction with miraculous springs and healing shrines without too much concern about contradictions.[80]

The sources prove that the Asclepian temples themselves were not centers for the practice of medicine, nor did they regularly provide suppliants with food and nursing care. They were, therefore, not true hospitals and could not have served in any way as models for institutions such as the Pantokrator Xenon. Asklepios and his temples, however, were immensely popular in the ancient world; in the fourth century the emperor Julian placed Asklepios among the greatest of gods, calling him begotten of Zeus and savior of men.[81] The great asklepieion at Pergamon attained such fame among men of late antiquity that it entered the ranks of the wonders of the world.[82] Even in the twelfth century, Byzantine Greeks kept alive the memory of the Pergamon temple as a marvel of antiquity.[83] Christianity succeeded in stamping out the asklepieia despite their popularity, but not by substituting the Christian hospitals for the healing services of the ancient temples. To aid in overthrowing the asklepieia, the church fostered the cult of the anargyroi, those saints who healed the sick as a manifestation of the power Christ had given them. The anargyroi performed their miracles in exactly the same way as Asklepios had. The sick person retired this time to a special church where the holy man's relics had been deposited. Here the sufferer slept through the night. During his sleep the saint would usually appear in a dream and recommend treatment, sometimes sensible, sometimes bizarre or even comic. The cults of the anargyroi are extremely complex phenomena; surely the doctor-saints represent more than the god Asklepios in Christian dress. Nevertheless, the similarity in treatment cannot be denied, and the existence of such doctor-saints—spiritual healers who performed miracles just as Asklepios had—no doubt helped to redirect the habits of pious folk toward shrines and symbols within a Christian context.[84]

IATREIA

Meyer-Steineg and his supporters have built their strongest case for the existence of ancient hospitals on the *iatreion,* the office and surgery of the physician. As early as the time of the *Corpus Hippocraticum* some doctors maintained offices or shops which were specially fitted out for surgical procedures. Casual references found in classical Greek authors reveal that ancient physicians also instructed their apprentices at these iatreia.[85] Since the *De officinis* of Hippocrates and later archaeological evidence from Roman Pompeii indicated that iatreia were primarily surgeries, Meyer-Steineg infers that they must have included recovery rooms where patients could recuperate after enduring the knife or cauterizing iron. The doctor's iatreion resembled other Greek homes and, like them, must have encompassed xenones, rooms for guests according to the classical meaning of the word. Physicians simply followed normal Greek custom, assigning their guests, in this case their recuperating patients, to these xenones. From sheltering surgery patients it was only a step to permitting persons suffering from disease to stay in the iatreion's guest rooms so that the physician could administer treatment under controlled circumstances.[86] In fact, in Plautus' comic play the *Menaechmi,* a doctor tries to force the reluctant hero to spend twenty days in his house, undergoing treatment with hellebore.[87] Although Plautus' plays were written for Italians of the second century B.C., they probably reflected conditions of late fourth- or third-century Hellenistic society. Meyer-Steineg thus supposes that the term *xenon* for the guest rooms of the iatreion gradually came to be applied to the whole institution. The first such example he finds in an order of the emperor Claudius (A.D. 41–54). According to Meyer-Steineg, *xenon* supplanted *iatreion* by the Byzantine era and became the standard name for hospitals.[88]

Meyer-Steineg's account is logical, but most ancient sources argue against his thesis. First, the Hippocratic essay on the iatreion laid down instructions regarding the preparation of instruments, the presence of assistants, the positioning of the patient on the operating table, and proper light, but it did not once mention any provisions for housing recuperating patients.[89] The same is true of Galen's lengthy commentary on this Hippocratic text.[90] Nowhere in this commentary or in any of his many other works did Galen ever mention an iatreion as a place where surgery patients or those being treated for diseases were given room and board. In fact, Galen himself never once described a iatreion of his own, but always pictured himself as visiting his patients in their homes.[91] Only in the case of his friend Protas did Galen refer to his own house as the place of his medical ministrations.[92] Moreover, according to Plutarch, the iatreion was a dispensary for patients not confined to bed; the seriously ill the physician treated in their homes.[93]

Greek Christian writings from the fourth and fifth centuries provide some of the best portraits of the traditional iatreia. John Chrysostom mentioned how the patient who entered the doctor's office was usually amazed by the array of surgical instruments and bandages.[94] In a sermon delivered in Constantinople, he referred to separate rooms in the iatreia for eye operations.[95] Finally, in a commentary on John 5:17, Chrysostom compared the Pool of Bethesda in Jerusalem to the physician's office, where patients suffering from eye injuries or crippled limbs sat together awaiting the doctor's visit.[96] Here and in other such *topoi,* there are no references to beds or any accommodations for the sick in the iatreia even though some of the patients are pictured as suffering from rather serious ailments or injuries. In yet another speech, the archbishop described how people congregated in Constantinople in the marketplaces, in the iatreia, and in other parts of the city to discuss controversial subjects.[97] Here the iatreia seem to be simply shops where people could gather, some waiting for treatment, others just there to pass the time. Such a public environment would have been ill suited for recuperating patients.

One final example should suffice both to demonstrate that the ancient iatreia never developed into hospitals during the pagan period and to illustrate how some of them were indeed transformed into public infirmaries, but only after the beginning of the Christian empire. According to one hagiographical tradition, a holy man by the name of Sampson came to Constantinople from the ancient capital of Rome, where he had studied medicine. Once in the new city on the Bosporos, Sampson opened up his iatreion in a humble house to treat those burdened with illnesses. A version of the *Vita Sampsonis* describes how Sampson not only considered his patients worthy of the care prescribed by the rules of his profession, but also shared food with them and provided them beds in accordance with Christ's laws.[98] Sampson, in fact, turned his office into a hospital where patients received bed, board, and medical attention. The story implies that the typical iatreion, conforming to the established laws of the medical profession, did not include food and housing for patients.

When Sampson came to Constantinople and opened his hospital is not known. Though his *vita* claims that he was a contemporary of the emperor Justinian, the reliable historian Prokopios states that Sampson had died some time before 532, the year in which his xenon was destroyed by fire.[99] One can argue from the evidence that Sampson worked in Constantinople as early as the reign of the emperor Constantius (337–61); certainly he had founded his hospital before the accession of Justinian (526).[100] Thus, his xenon opened sometime between about 350 and 526, during the years when other Christians—bishops, state officials, and laymen—were founding all kinds of new charitable institutions.

The *Vita Sampsonis* and the other passages gleaned from both ancient and early Byzantine sources indicate that the usual iatreion of the classical world, adhering to the norms of the medical profession, did not provide food and sleeping quarters for its patients. As is clear from the *De officiniis* of Hippocrates and the descriptions of John Chrysostom, the doctor's office was a surgery and a walk-in clinic, but not a hospital. On the other hand, the *Vita Sampsonis* also shows that the *iatreion* could easily be changed into a hospital under the proper stimulus. The Gospel norm of *agápe* or *philanthropia* motivated some physicians to carry out such a transformation sometime after the conversion of Constantine.

In association with Christian hospitals the term *iatreion* survived into the later Byzantine centuries. During the ninth century, the bishop Theophylakt erected a two-story hospital in his city of Nikomedeia, an institution which the hagiographer called a *iatreion*.[101] The Pantokrator *Typikon* also uses the term several times, though here it has a variety of meanings: in one passage it refers to the women's ward, in another to the medical staff, and in still a different context to the xenon's hours of operation.[102]

PUBLIC PHYSICIANS

The committees of public physicians (*demosieuontes iatroi*) or chief physicians (*archiatroi*), as they were called by the second century A.D., represent the last of the ancient institutions which some historians have linked to the existence of hospitals in the classical world. One of the standard works on these doctors is still the dissertation of Rudolf Pohl, published in 1905. Pohl carefully traces the history of public physicians from their origins at the end of the sixth century B.C. through their golden age in Roman Asia Minor to the early Byzantine period, when, he maintains, the iatreia of the public physicians simply received a new name, *nosokomeion,* and became the Christian hospitals.[103]

As with many other aspects of ancient medicine the public physicians as an institution did indeed survive the Christianizing of classical civilization and, of even greater significance, were closely linked with Byzantine hospitals. Doctors with the title of *archiatros,* chief physician, were practicing in several hospitals of Constantinople by the beginning of the seventh century. Moreover, as late as the fourteenth century, physicians with the title *archiatros* were still working in the city's xenones.[104] The transformation from a physician who was paid a salary by a city government to a doctor on the staff of a Christian hospital, however, was not accomplished simply by changing the name of the public doctor's office from *iatreion* to *nosokomeion.* It required substantial changes in the institution of public physicians and in the nature and strength of local *polis* government.

The public physicians appeared as early as the end of the sixth century B.C. Herodotos describes how Aegina, Athens, and Samos bid for the services of Demokedes of Kroton, each city offering him a salary and equipment for his art.[105] By the time of Aristophanes' *Acharnenses,* public physicians were well-known characters in Athenian society.[106] Aristophanes paints a picture of the *demosieuōn iatros* Pittalos treating both a poor farmer and a wealthy soldier of Athens.[107] In return for their salaries, paid by the citizens of the polis, public physicians were expected to offer a city competent medical services. In the fourth century Xenophon states that Greek cities generally expected their public physicians to promote the health of all their citizens.[108] In some cases these doctors took a special interest in treating the disadvantaged of the community. In 70 B.C., the Peloponnesian town of Gytheion praised its public physician for treating all—the poor, the rich, the slaves, and the free—with the same care.[109]

On the basis of a few passages in the literary sources and from inscriptions such as the one found at Gytheion, some historians have maintained that the public physicians represented a corps of doctors retained by the cities of Greece to ensure medical care for needy citizens. There is no evidence, however, that such was the case before the late fourth century A.D..[110] As Louis Cohn-Haft has pointed out in his study of public physicians, the inscriptions from the classical, Hellenistic, and Roman days cannot demonstrate that public doctors regularly treated patients without charging a fee or attended to poor patients with the same diligence they devoted to the care of the wealthy. Indeed, when Gytheion praised its *demosieuōn iatros* for treating patients from all classes without distinction, the polis surely did not assume that such philanthropy was expected from any physician who held the job.[111]

Although it was considered praiseworthy for public physicians to offer the poor the same care that they did the rich, the cities did not hire these doctors to provide free health care to the needy. In the case of a smaller polis, the government retained a public physician simply to guarantee that a trained medical man would reside in the city. In bigger cities, selecting public physicians represented a method of identifying practitioners of quality.[112] At Athens in the fourth century B.C., the candidates had to undergo some sort of public scrutiny and were ultimately chosen by a vote of the assembly. A similar system existed at Kos and probably in other cities as well.[113] Though each city had its own method for selecting public physicians, they all tried in some fashion to examine the candidates' education and their professional records in an attempt to evaluate their medical expertise.[114] Under the Roman imperial administration the governors of the provinces were specifically excluded from choosing the public physicians; by that time the choice rested entirely with aristocratic city councils.[115]

Since *demosieuontes iatroi* were the only doctors of the ancient world with some proof of their ability, patients especially sought them out. If the patients were wealthy, they were willing to pay more for the superior skills of these physicians. By the end of the fourth century B.C. some men were ready to accept positions as public doctors without a salary, for they realized that their private practice would improve once they obtained this exalted title.[116] Since the populace respected the public physicians and the rich especially desired their ministrations, it is probable that the poor and the outcasts received little attention from them. Only in the fourth century A.D. does evidence surface that public physicians had an obligation to treat the poor. In return for their salaries from the state treasury—the *annona* allotments—the emperor Valentinian I required that those of Rome provide the poor with medical care on a par with that offered the wealthy.[117]

Physicians good enough to serve as public doctors were relatively rare in the classical Greek and early Hellenistic age. Such men worked as *demosieuontes iatroi* only for short periods; then they would move on to other cities, attracted by higher salaries and, increasingly, by civic privileges such as guest status (*proxenia*) or even citizenship as well as by the promise of special positions in official processions or in seating at the theater. By Roman times, however, most towns had native Asklepiad families who ordinarily kept the office of public physician within their ranks. Since these native doctors had by birthright many of the honors formerly offered to wandering physicians, the cities began to vote their public physicians new privileges in the form of immunities—exemptions from taxes and from city liturgies.[118] In A.D. 74 the emperor Vespasian even granted to the public physicians of the province of Asia exemption from all tribute and freed them from the obligation of quartering Roman troops.[119] Later, Hadrian applied this rule to the whole empire.[120]

By the second century the number of public physicians in many of the cities of the Greek provinces of the empire had increased greatly. At the same time city finances were deteriorating—a problem which was to plague ancient society until the reign of Justinian. In an attempt to relieve the strain on local treasuries, the emperor Antoninus Pius (138–61) decided to restrict the number of public physicians in Greek cities who could claim the immunities. He ordered that small poleis could have only five such doctors, provincial capitals seven, and great cities ten.[121] In the decades after Antoninus Pius released his new regulations, inscriptions from the cities of Asia Minor began referring to the members of this restricted group of public physicians as *archiatroi* (chief physicians), a title borrowed from the courts of the Hellenistic kings.[122]

After Antoninus Pius, two groups of physicians shared the exalted rank of chief physician. The personal physicians of the emperor had borne the title in the Greek East since the days of the Julian House; now the restricted *collegia* of public physicians could also claim it as a mark of their excellence.[123] A chief physician of either category was considered a leader of the medical profession. Origen recounted how a city was smitten by a disease so severe that none of the ordinary physicians could master it. Then, a certain archiatros of great renown arrived and was able to cure the citizens. The other doctors, however, were not jealous, since they recognized the superior skills of a chief physician.[124]

As with other aspects of the medical profession, the Latin West lagged behind the East in developing the colleges of public physicians. Alexander Severus (233–36) seems to have been the first to establish such doctors in Rome.[125] More than a hundred years later, in 369, the emperor Valentinian issued a detailed order establishing fourteen archiatroi in the Western capital. The emperor allotted a salary from the annona levy to each of Rome's fourteen chief physicians, requiring in return that every one of them "serve the poor honorably, not the rich shamefully." The law allowed them to take payment once a sick person was restored to health, but they were not to accept promises made by patients still in danger of death. Finally, the college of archiatroi at Rome was to renew its numbers upon a vacancy by coopting a qualified physician, its choice subject to the emperor's approval.[126] Valentinian also established a salary scale for the members of the college with the newest archiatros receiving the least.[127]

Most probably Constantinople adopted the same system for its public physicians as that at Rome, though no legal record of this has survived. In one of his sermons, delivered at the end of the fourth century to the people of the Eastern capital, John Chrysostom mentions that the doctors of the city treated the same disease in return for different fees. From the rich they took a hundred *solidi*, from others fifty, from still others less, and from the poor they took nothing at all.[128] Since Chrysostom does not identify these physicians as archiatroi, it is not certain whether this practice of sliding-scale fees was followed by all doctors of the capital or only by the public physicians. Of greater interest regarding the chief physicians in the early Byzantine period is a scholion to Aristophanes' *Acharnenses* written in fifth-century Constantinople and reflecting contemporary conditions. The scholiast defines the public physicians (i.e., archiatroi) as those who offered their services for free.[129]

By the fifth century, then, the archiatroi of Greco-Roman cities were providing philanthropic medical care for poor men and women, a service in some ways similar to the charitable medicine practiced in the Christian hospitals. One cannot, however, accept Pohl's suggestion that the shops of the public physicians had always been hospitals and that the Christian nosokomeia were simply the old iatreia of the archiatroi under a new name. To be sure, from their earliest days public physicians must have had iatreia, just as other physicians did. During the late fifth century B.C., the public doctor Pittalos saw patients at his shop in Athens.[130] A papyrus document from Roman Egypt (A.D. 130) refers to the iatreion belonging to a public physician of a small town.[131] During the Antonine age, some cities apparently provided their *demosieuontes iatroi* with offices. In outlining the requirements for proper lighting during surgical operations, Galen mentions these well-equipped iatreia, with spacious windows, torches, and lamps.[132] Although there is abundant evidence that the public physicians had iatreia, the sources do not indicate that these offices or shops differed essentially from those of other physicians. Thus, the arguments that the iatreia of ordinary physicians before the end of the fourth century A.D. did not include hospital services apply equally well to those of archiatroi. In the final analysis, no inscriptions, references in the literary sources, or archaeological finds can offset the claim of the *Vita Sampsonis* that this Christian physician of the early Byzantine period broke with the ancient customs of his profession when he allowed his patients to reside with him and to share his food until they regained their health.[133]

In the fifth century A.D. the city archiatroi and the Christian hospitals still represented different institutions, though they both practiced philanthropic medicine. After the mid-sixth century, however, chief physicians are always found in close association with Christian nosokomeia and xenones. According to the will of the archiatros Flavius, dated 14 November 570, this physician administered a xenon in the Egyptian city of Antinoopolis which provided patients with medical care, food, and housing. Before him, his father, also an archiatros, had supervised this same institution.[134] When in the seventh century the head of the Christodotes Xenon found a poor man suffering from a severe infection of the chest, he entrusted him to the chief physicians of his hospital for medical treatment.[135] In the ninth century, the fabous abbot Theodore the Stoudite described the typical hospital staff as consisting of the head physicians, followed by chief physicians (archiatroi), regular physicians, and assistants.[136] During the same century, court ceremonial required that when the emperor celebrated the tenth day of the Christmas observance, he entertain the hospital administrators of Constantinople accompanied by the archiatroi on their staffs.[137] Moreover, the manuscript tradition of a popular medical treatise emanating from xenon practice always attributes this work to an archiatros named John.[138] Finally, the Pantokrator Typikon itself reveals the vestiges of the archiatroi in hospital service in the twelfth century, although it does not use the term. By requiring that staff physicians of the xenon never practice medicine outside of the city of Constantinople, the *Typikon* reflects the municipal orientation of the pre-Christian public doctors.[139]

Although the old public physicians and chief physicians of the cities had been organized in colleges, they had practiced medicine as individual doctors, each in his own iatreion with his own students, collecting his fees along with the stipend paid all archiatroi by the city governments. The archiatroi mentioned in the sources after Justinian's accession, on the other hand, appear as physicians in Christian xenones. Here they represent the top rank of a hospital bureaucracy which includes several grades of medical personnel. Moreover, they are no longer subject to any magistrate of the local polis, but rather, to the xenodochos of their hospital—a local cleric with the rank of priest or deacon. Although individual Christian archiatroi, moved by the Gospel commands to charity, may have followed the example of Sampson and converted their iatreia into xenones, such voluntary steps would explain only occasional references to archiatroi in Christian hospitals, not the total restructuring of the institution which the sources reflect. One must look, instead, for some sweeping administrative change by the city governments or by the imperial administration to account for the new system one finds after about 532. The emperor Justinian, in fact, did initiate such a sweeping program during his reign, changing the nature of the public physicians throughout the empire. In his *Anecdota,* Prokopios states that the emperor cancelled the annona payments both to the public physicians and to the professors of the liberal arts.[140] Commenting on this passage, Vivian Nutton states that the emperor probably did not abolish archiatroi, but simply re-organized the institution.[141] Indeed, this survey of later sources has proven that Justinian did just that. Terminating the role of the ancient polis govern-ment in supporting archiatroi, he assigned these doctors to the growing Christian hospitals. Justinian thereby succeeded in welding the expertise of the best practitioners of secular Greek medicine to the xenon staff. His reform had a profound effect on the subsequent development of Byzantine hospitals and led to their becoming the nodal points of the medical profes-sion from about 550 to the Latin conquest of Constantinople in 1204.

This brief survey has illustrated again the continuity from classical Greek civilization to the medieval world of the Byzantine Empire. Although East Roman physicians added new therapies to the treatments of Hippocrates and Galen, they continued to study the theories of the great Greek physicians and to employ some of their procedures. Medieval doctors altered the tra-ditions of their professional ancestors most significantly when they began to practice medicine in hospitals, centers where they could treat a number of patients at the same time and could monitor diets and medication closely. Even in the case of the hospitals, however, East Roman physicians borrowed from the classical world. The valetudinaria for slaves and those for soldiers as well as the asklepieia had no relationship to Byzantine hospitals and their kind of treatment, but both the ancient iatreia and the public physicians did help to shape the development of Byzantine nosokomeia after the Christian-ization of the Empire.

Although the pagan world of Greek antiquity had spawned rational med-icine, the Christian church came to consider it as legitimate for believers and even elevated it to a position of great respect among the sciences. In the Byzantine Empire, the church became a patron of physicians, particularly through its hospitals. Nevertheless, this marriage of Christianity and Hellenic medicine took place gradually. It is time now to analyze the process by which the people of the New Israel accepted the medical wisdom of the pagans, a process closely linked to the development of xenones.

CHAPTER FOUR

Eastern Christianity

Christianity created the hospitals of the Byzantine Empire. Not only were the earliest nosokomeia of Constantinople and the cities of Asia Minor Christian institutions, but even the sophisticated xenones of Justinian's reign as well as the Pantokrator and Krales hospitals of later centuries were governed by men of the church. Thus, the opinions Christians held both about the practice of medicine and about its relationship to the virtue of charity played an essential part in the history of Byzantine hospitals.

Early Christians agreed that charity was the supreme virtue and that caring for the sick was one of the manifestations of this love, but they did not all agree that they should use secular medicine in their efforts to serve the suffering. Before the church could contemplate patronizing medical hospitals, it had first to accept the science of healing as compatible with God's will. Thus, to understand early hospitals and their relation to the church, one must examine the stages by which Christians came to view medicine—and even the medical tradition of the pagan Greeks—as a treasured gift from God. As part of such a study, one must, first, consider the early Christian attitude toward charity in general and the tendency for this *agápe*, as Paul called it, to express itself especially in caring for the sick. Second, it is useful to explore the doubts that some Christian writers expressed about the legitimacy of medicine for believers and the arguments which orthodox Christians advanced for accepting it. Third, one must focus on concepts which the Greek Fathers emphasized, concepts which shifted Christian opinion from simply accepting the science of healing to praising its practice as the very epitome of active charity. Finally, one must return to the hospitals themselves to study their close relationship to Greek Christian attitudes concerning physicians and their art.

CHRISTIAN CHARITY

The early Christians stressed agápe as the central virtue of their new faith. Jesus himself had declared that the norms contained in the Law and the Prophets flowed from the love of God and the love of one's neighbor (Matt. 22:37–40). Paul, too, emphasized the primacy of charity: "In short, there are three things that last: faith, hope, and love; and the greatest of these is love" (1 Cor. 13:13). During their earliest days in Jerusalem, the Christians had constructed an ideal community based on love, each one contributing the fruits of his labor to the needs of his brothers and sisters in the faith (Acts 2:42–46).

Along with his general admonitions to love one's neighbor, Christ indicated both by word and example some specific forms of charity, including care for the sick. In his terrifying image of the Last Judgment, Jesus reminded his listeners that God expected his people to visit the sick (Matt. 25:31–46), while in the miracle stories from all four Gospel narratives, Christ demonstrated his deep sympathy for those who suffered from disease. In caring for the sick, however, Jesus never relied on medical remedies, neither the simple herbal treatments of Jewish folk medicine nor the alien wisdom of the Hellenes.[1]

Although during his ministry on earth Christ firmly established the ideal of charity, of love for one's neighbor expressed in aiding people in need— the poor, the homeless, the orphan, the sick—he had not provided practical guidelines for organizing charitable programs. With regard to the sick he did not specify how Christians were to alleviate their suffering beyond visiting them in their distress and praying over them. Before Christian communities could foster the development of hospitals, they had, first, to establish some methods and institutions for carrying out the great commandment to love one's neighbor, and second, to accept the practice of medicine as a valid expression of that love. The early Christians in Jerusalem at first obeyed Christ's commands to love their neighbors by spontaneous giving. As the community expanded, however, its growth demanded some form of administration to assist more people in need. When the Hellenized Jews of the new faith began to quarrel with the converts from among the Jews of Jerusalem concerning the support of widows, the apostles had to appoint officers, the seven deacons, to supervise the community's charitable activities (Acts 6:1–6). As Christian communities sprang up throughout the Greco-Roman world, they adopted the institutions at Jerusalem. Thus, the *Apostolic Constitutions,* a collection of rules reflecting practice in churches from Syria to Rome, indicate that during the second and third centuries the bishop and his deacons directed the local church's charitable functions, collecting from the richer Christians and distributing to the poorer. The *Apostolic Constitutions* also mention that the early bishops were to look after the sick among their flock in fulfillment of Christ's command.[2] The apostle John's student, Bishop Polykarp of Smyrna, also listed the care of the sick among the primary responsibilities of church elders in the early second century.[3] Rules emanating from Rome about 215 obliged the bishop to seek out the sick in their own houses.[4] None of these early guidebooks for Christian conduct, however, mention medicine as part of caring for the sick.

By the third century Christians in large cities had organized to aid the poor and needy on a wide scale. They performed some of their most impressive charitable operations on behalf of the sick. When a plague ravaged Alexandria during the reign of the emperor Gallienus (259–68), Bishop Dionysios directed an extensive relief operation, urging his flock, one of the largest in the empire, to remember Christ's command to visit the sick. In the face of virulent pestilence, the Christians of Alexandria carried out their mission of tending to the plague victims and nursing some back to health. They also fulfilled their obligations toward those slain by the disease, washing and anointing the bodies and burying them in a proper fashion. In his description of the relief effort, Dionysios opposed the behavior of Christians to that of the pagans, who expelled their sick relatives from their homes and left the victims of the plague unburied in the roads because they feared contagion.[5] Even if Dionysios exaggerated the virtue of his own flock and the cowardice of the pagans, still his account provides several valuable comments on the practice of Christian charity in the second half of the third century. First, by that time, a large church such as Alexandria could organize a massive relief effort which offered help to a large number of people in need. Second, the bishop and deacons alone could not have carried out such a task. Under Dionysios' direction, laymen assisted in performing the corporal works of mercy, for the churches had not yet established permanent charitable services with professional staffs. Finally, Christian leaders such as Bishop Dionysios considered the care of the sick the best example of agápe — an activity which clearly distinguished the Christian from the pagan.

Although the early Christians were totally committed to charity, experience soon taught them that some would take advantage of unlimited generosity. Even Paul, the great hymnist of charity, cautioned the Thessalonican Christians to be wary of those who refused to work (2 Thess. 3:6–10). The Syrian *Didache* prescribed that the churches maintain strangers for two or three days only, if they were not willing to work, and added that some pseudoprophets begged bread of the churches as a profession, preferring to barter Christ rather than to work.[6] As a result, Christian communities often required that strangers claiming membership in distant churches present episcopal letters to verify their status before they could receive support.[7] But the church regarded with less suspicion orphans, widows, and the sick, people who clearly needed help. The pious Christian soldier Seleukos, who was martyred under Diocletian, emulated the saints by aiding abandoned children, helpless widows, and those oppressed by disease.[8]

During the fourth century the Greek Fathers especially exalted the care of the sick. In his two sermons on the necessity of loving the poor, Gregory of Nyssa quickly narrowed the argument to a consideration of the sick. Since these people had been robbed of their power by disease and could not help themselves, Christians should especially open their hearts to them.[9] He portrayed in vivid detail the wretched conditions of those who suffered from disfiguring disease.[10] To love and nurse them were indeed taxing duties, but Christ had not offered an easy road to salvation.[11] Gregory elevated the care of the sick to a central position in Christian conduct. By shouldering this difficult task, a Christian fulfilled all that Christ commanded; he assumed the yoke of the Lord.[12] In his sermon on *philanthropia,* Gregory of Nazianz also emphasized mercy toward the sick. Disease attacked persons from all ranks of society. When the wealthy fell ill, they suffered the sharpest pain, for suddenly disease reduced them to wretchedness.[13] When sickness struck the poor, it robbed them of their bodily strength, their only hope of supporting themselves and their families.[14] What sincere Christian, sharing in the spiritual and temporal bounty of God, could turn away such unfortunate men and women?[15] So, too, Saint Basil, bishop of Caesarea, taught the need to care for the ill by example, by ministering to the sick in imitation of Christ.[16]

RATIONAL MEDICINE

Although few Christians disagreed with the sentiments expressed so vividly by these three Cappadocian Fathers, not all of them believed that they should employ medicines and the medical arts as part of this love of the sick. The New Testament demanded charity toward the ill, but nowhere did it sanction the use of medicine. Christ and his apostles had cured through miraculous power, not through medicines. In the story of the hemorrhaging woman, the Gospel of Mark (5:25–34) compares the efficacious power of Jesus to the ineffective efforts of the doctors who had treated the poor woman for twelve years and succeeded only in aggravating her condition.

Since the New Testament did not specifically recommend the use of medicine as a means to care for the sick, Christians felt free to hold differing opinions on this ancient art. Moreover, since medicine was based on knowledge of material things and, in its most developed form, on the works of pagan Greek thinkers, some Christians of the first three centuries attacked it as an evil. Tatian, a Syrian convert to the new faith, had come to Rome during the second century to study under the great Christian philosopher Justin Martyr. Tatian, however, did not share Justin's enthusiasm for some aspects of pagan Greco-Roman civilization, and as a result, broke with him and returned to his native Syria.[17] In his treatise *Adversus Graecos,* Tatian attacked all manifestations of Hellenic culture including medicine, declaring that it was sinful to put one's trust in any form of matter including medicines. One ought to depend solely on the power of God for health. Poisons and medicine both sprang from evil matter.[18] If a Christian still relied on medicine, then according to Tatian, he had not yet freed himself from the snares of the world.[19]

In the Latin province of Africa, the late-third-century convert Arnobius of

Sicca also fulminated against medicine as a manifestation of pagan culture.[20] Arnobius claimed that medicine was wrong on two counts. First, it offered no certain cure; rather, each physician vacillated in his diagnosis. Second, medicine was centered on human knowledge and not on the divine power of God, who needed no herbs or unguents to cure the ill.[21] From Jerusalem, too, came exhortations to seek divine help alone against sickness of the body. The fourth-century Bishop Cyril told his catechumens that the Christian of strong faith sought healing from diseases exclusively in Christ Jesus.[22]

By stressing faith in Christ as the proper medicine for disease, Cyril of Jerusalem implied that recourse to human doctors was a failing, if not a sin. In the case of both Tatian and Arnobius, antipagan sentiments sharpened their hostility toward physicians and the art of medicine. Such considerations continued to color Christian attitudes in the Greek East toward doctors and their craft, especially in ascetic circles. Anonymous treatises which later circulated under the name of the famous Egyptian monk Makarios contained passages hostile to medicine.[23] Although God in his mercy had provided the fallen men of this world with herbs and the skills of physicians to ease the suffering of life, the new man, born again into the Kingdom, ought to have a strong faith in God and turn to Christ alone for health in body and soul.[24] The popular writings attributed to Isaiah, a fifth-century monk of Gaza, echoed Cyril of Jerusalem in advising Christians who strove for perfection to seek Jesus only as a cure for their bodily ailments.[25]

Although some of the literature condemning medicine had a wide circulation among the orthodox, much of it emanated from heretical circles. Despite his early association with the orthodox Justin, Tatian eventually joined a gnostic sect.[26] The writings of Pseudo-Makarios originated in a Messalian community, while the fifth-century abbot Isaiah seems to have been a Monophysite.[27] All of these writers leaned toward dualism; their distrust of medicine with its dependence on human knowledge and material remedies flowed naturally from their condemnation of the visible world. Mainstream Greek Christianity, as it was so elegantly formulated by the Fathers of the fourth century, wholeheartedly rejected a radical dualism and as a corollary accepted the use of secular medicine as proper for Christians.

CHRISTIAN THEOLOGY'S ACCEPTANCE OF MEDICINE

Even before the fourth century, Eastern theologians were laying the foundations for the eventual marriage of Christianity and secular medicine. As part of this work, the Alexandrian theologian Origen presented an impressive defence of both the use of medicine and the physician's craft. Since God knows the weaknesses of the human body, how it suffers from diseases and can be so easily injured, he has provided from the earth the remedies to alleviate the pains of physical suffering, and through his gift of the *logos* (the knowing power of men), he has given us the knowledge of how to use these herbs—the discipline of medicine.[28] On the other hand, Origen stopped short of endorsing medicine for all believers. In his *Contra Celsum,* he argues that ordinary Christians could seek the aid of physicians just as they could marry, but that those who strove for the highest life should avoid both marriage and the use of medicine. For healing they should rather turn to God in faith.[29]

THE GREEK FATHERS

Relying heavily on Origen's work, the Greek Fathers of the fourth century forged an enduring alliance between Christianity and classical culture. To achieve this, they avoided, on the one hand, a blanket rejection of all things pagan, and on the other hand, they proceeded with more caution than Origen had in accepting Platonic concepts into a Christian system.[30] All of them, however, emphasized Origen's more positive attitude toward the science of medicine and developed his position even further. Gregory of Nyssa emphasized the role of experience and cooperation in the medical craft. By observation doctors had discovered over the centuries which plants and minerals were beneficial and which harmful. They had assembled a vast fund of information so that the present generation benefited from the experience of its forefathers.[31] Gregory appealed to the history of medicine as an example of what God allowed men to do when they worked in harmony with him and with one another.[32]

In opposition to dualist notions, Basil of Caesarea stressed the goodness of God's creation despite appearances by elaborating on Origen's image of curative plants. The natural world reflects the unfathomable wisdom of God. Can a mere man find fault with God because he has created poisonous plants? In God's scheme such apparently evil creations have a good purpose. They might nourish certain animals, or, transformed by the physicians' skills, they might provide the proper additive to restore the imbalance of disease to the equilibrium of health. Thus, even apparently destructive elements of the visible world are beneficial when they are used properly by the good physician.[33] In his *Long Rules,* a guide for the ideal Christian life, Basil posed the question directly concerning the healing craft: "Is the use of medicine in conformity with piety?" He answered yes.[34] To those Christians who maintained that one ought only to rely on the supernatural powers of God to banish diseases, Basil responded that the Creator worked just as much through the visible world as he did through the unseen. Thus, God's grace was as evident in the healing power of medicine and its practitioners as it was in miraculous cures. In fact, such natural cures could lead to a greater awareness of God's all-present power.[35] Medicine was in perfect accord with Christian virtue so long as one never lost sight of pleasing God and placing one's spiritual health on the highest plane.[36]

Gregory of Nyssa emphasized sharing among generations in the development of human knowledge and of medicine in particular. John Chrysostom, bishop of Constantinople (398–404), on the other hand, stressed sharing among the people of the same generation in creating a loving, Christian community—the pinnacle of civilization.[37] Each member of the community possessed a special gift—an ability to excel in architecture or medicine, for example—which he ought to use for the welfare of others. Since no one person was capable of mastering all the fields of civilized life, each one needed the others and thereby came to love his fellows. In this exchange physicians had a prominent role. Because God had given them a special talent to save others from pain and sometimes death, they had an urgent responsibility to share their talents.[38] Such political theories and occasional references in his letters indicate how important Chrysostom considered medicine to be in the mosaic of the Christian city. When he was forced into exile from Constantinople, Chrysostom sorely missed the services of the city's physicians and rejoiced when finally he reached Caesarea and its doctors.[39]

Although orthodox writers considered medicine a gift from God and sanctioned its use for Christians, still they occasionally expressed some reservations. Origen had advised the most ardent Christians to depend on prayer for health.[40] Even Basil believed that in some cases a Christian should endure his bodily ailments without the doctor's assistance.[41] Nevertheless, the fourth-century Fathers emphasized the image of medical practice as the most suitable example of love in action—philanthropia, as Clement of Alexandria had called it. Medicine and its practice, thus, came to symbolize the central Christian virtue for Greek Christians. The learned theologian Gregory of Nyssa told his friend, the doctor Eustathios, that the highest Christian virtue of charity belonged especially to the physicians.[42] Because of this, Gregory judged their profession superior to all the others. Popular hagiographical writing readily wove this image into the fabric of its stories. One version of the *Vita Sampsonis* referred to the medical discipline as the practice of philanthropy.[43] Throughout later centuries Byzantine writers continued to associate medicine and charity. The twelfth-century cleric George Tornikes described the doctors' hands and even their cautery irons as "charitable."[44] In his eulogy of the princess Anna Komnena, he praised her study of medicine as an exercise in wisdom and philanthropia.[45] The thirteenth-century archbishop Michael Choniates considered the physician's craft the pinnacle of charity.[46] Once Greek theologians, hagiographers, and other clerical writers came to see the physicians' profession as a paragon of the highest Christian virtue, medicine was assured of the greatest respect in the Eastern Church.

CHRISTIAN PHYSICIANS

That medicine came to symbolize charity in action for Greek Christians is not surprising when one considers how many physicians played prominent roles in the annals of Hellenic Christianity. From its earliest days, when the new faith was still predominantly Greek, come a number of stories regarding Christian physicians. According to an old tradition the evangelist Luke practiced medicine while a companion of Paul.[47] A physician from Asia Minor had died heroically for the faith in Lyons under the emperor Marcus Aurelius (161–180).[48] Greek Christian inscriptions from around the empire indicate that it was not uncommon for priests and deacons to practice medicine. Thus, at Rome during the third century, when Greek Christians still dominated the church there, a priest named Dionysios served also as a physician.[49] In the early fourth century, an illustrious priest of the Sidon church by the name of Zenobios won renown as a doctor.[50] In 305 the Christian physician Theodotos came to the episcopal throne of Laodicea in Syria.[51] At least one source describes as a doctor Basil, bishop of Ankyra, a key figure in ecclesiastical politics during the fourth century.[52]

These doctor-clerics seem to have won great popularity with the faithful in eastern churches. Though only a priest, Zenobios of Sidon was persecuted together with other leaders of the Eastern Church.[53] At the close of the fourth century a Greek physician by the name of Gerantios was consecrated bishop of Nikomedeia. His unselfish practice of medicine while holding the episcopal office won him such popularity among the people of his flock that they fiercely defended him against the attempts of Bishop Nektarios of Constantinople to depose him.[54]

Although the three Cappadocian Fathers did not themselves practice medicine professionally, they all had close ties to physicians and the medical discipline. Gregory of Nazianz had a younger brother, Kaisarios, who had studied medicine at Alexandria and had become a professional physician. After Kaisarios had moved to Constantinople during the reign of Constantius (337–61), his great skill won him a position among the leading physicians of the city (probably the archiatroi of the capital) and eventually brought him to the post of court doctor.[55] Basil himself had excelled in medicine during his student days at Athens, where he pursued the field in a systematic fashion. He later used his medical training to treat his own illnesses and to aid the poor sick of his flock in Caesarea.[56] Gregory of Nyssa, Basil's brother, maintained a close friendship and theological alliance with the physician Eustathios.[57] That the Fathers had among their close relatives and friends prominent physicians should come as no surprise, since they were very much products of the Greek aristocracy in Asia Minor. Unlike the great families of the West, which on the whole rejected medicine as an acceptable career, nobles of the East considered it a worthy field of endeavor. When in the third century many leading families in the East became Christian, they brought the attitudes of their class with them. Gregory of Nazianz, Gregory of Nyssa, and Basil, aristocrats of the East as they were, no doubt considered the medical profession a suitable career for Christian men of their standing, an option not far below an ecclesiastical career.[58]

This close relationship between leading ecclesiastics of the Greek church and the practice of medicine continued throughout Byzantine history. Thus, one of the greatest patriarchs of Constantinople, Photios, took a special interest in medicine, occasionally prescribing remedies for friends as though he were a professional practitioner.[59] The twelfth-century bishop John of Prisdrianai seems to have composed a number of professional medical treatises.[60] After the patriarch Lukas Chrysoberges (1157–70) forbad clerics to join the physician's guild, bishops, priests, and deacons could no longer openly function as doctors.[61] Still, many of them had studied or even practiced medicine before they were ordained, while others dispensed medical advice informally as part of their ministry. Thus, in the fourteenth century, when Matthew of Ephesus arrived in the small Thracian town of Brysis to serve as its bishop, the people naturally flocked to him for medical aid.[62]

THE GREAT PHYSICIAN: CHRISTIAN METAPHOR

Not only did Greek ecclesiastics frequently practice medicine or have friends who did, but Greek theologians also often used metaphors derived from medicine to express many spiritual realities, a practice which further established medicine as a keystone in the Orthodox world view. As early as the third century Origen had employed the image of Christ the Great Physician to express Jesus' philanthropia and power. Christ was the archiatros who could heal every infirmity of the body and soul.[63] Eusebios of Caesarea even borrowed word for word the description of the toiling physician found in the Hippocratic treatise *De flatibus* to embellish his image of Jesus' redemptive suffering.[64] The Cappadocian Fathers readily adopted the figure of Christ the archiatros administering the healing medicine of his Word to those sick with sin. In his commentary on the Our Father, Gregory of Nyssa called Christ "the true doctor of the soul's suffering" who desires to restore spiritual health—openness to the Father's will.[65] One finds the image of Christ the physician in all forms of Eastern Christian literature. Thus, the popular hagiographical text of the early seventh century, the *Vita S. Theodori Sykeon,* refers to the saint as the student of Christ the archiatros.[66]

Although Latin authors such as Augustine also spoke of Christ the physician, this image was not nearly so popular in the West as it was among the Greek Christian writers.[67] That Eastern Christians often represented Christ as a physician was due first to the high regard which the Hellenic world had felt for doctors since the days of Hippocrates. Since Greek society considered good doctors the most charitable of men, it was fitting for Greek Christians to see Christ as the paramount physician. It is also possible that Christians of the Greek-speaking provinces retained a fondness for Christ the physician because their pagan fathers had held Asklepios, the god of the healing arts, in such high regard.

The cult of Asklepios had always been Greek. It had first appeared in the Hellenic homeland some years before 500 B.C. During the Hellenistic and Roman periods the cult had spread rapidly to encompass the whole Mediterranean world. Still, the most famous Asclepian shrines remained in the Greek provinces.[68] Although the Romans had accepted Asklepios as early as 291 B.C. and maintained his cult in Italy through the Principate, the god had practically vanished as a powerful figure there by the fourth century A.D.[69] In a tirade against numerous pagan cults addressed to the sons of Constantine, the Latin Christian writer Firmicus Maternus mentions Asklepios only once in a passage which demonstrates the author's ignorance of the Asclepian legend.[70] At the same time in the East, the cult of the healing god had retained its popularity with pagans. Raised in Eastern pagan circles, the emperor Julian especially revered him.[71]

Since Asklepios had always held a central place in the Greek religious world and continued to claim the affections of a sizable number of Easterners through the fourth century, one would expect that his cult influenced Greek Christians. Moreover, from among all the Hellenic deities and heroes Asklepios most resembled the Christ of the Sacred Scriptures. He, like Christ, had been born of a mortal woman by the power of a god; he had dedicated his life to aiding others; finally, he had been raised to heaven for his virtue. These similarities had made Asklepios seem especially dangerous to early Christian apologists of both East and West.[72] After the year 300 writers in the East continued to worry about him as a deceiver of the faithful, while at the same time borrowing images from the Asclepian cult to embellish Christian truths.[73] It is thus likely that the strength of the *Christus medicus* metaphor among the Greek Fathers and its continued popularity in the centuries which followed owed something to the deeply rooted cult of Asklepios in the Eastern provinces.

Christian theologians of the East employed the physician metaphor to describe not only Christ but also the ministers of his church. According to Origen, all men of God were spiritual physicians. Thus, the apostles Peter and Paul as well as the prophets of old had practiced the therapy of the soul. God also made physicians of souls those to whom he had entrusted his *ecclesia,* the bishops.[74] Along with the image of Christ the physician, the Cappadocian Fathers eagerly received and developed Origen's concept of the bishop as a healer of souls. Gregory of Nazianz compared Basil's work as bishop of Caesarea to that of a doctor. Basil would apply soothing or harsh words as needed to cure sinful souls, just as the physicians employed sweet and bitter medicines in their therapies. According to Gregory, Basil's knowledge of medical principles not only aided him in treating the physically ill of his flock, but served as a model for him in approaching his pastoral work.[75]

By the fifth century the image of the bishop as a spiritual physician had become common throughout the East. In his letter to Bishop Lampetios, the Egyptian monk and abbot Isidore of Pelusium advised him to persevere in cauterizing with burning words Zosimos, whose impiety was indeed hard to cure.[76] The vita of the seventh-century patriarch of Alexandria, John the Alms-giver, pictured the good bishop applying the salve of encouragement and the burning iron of criticism to cure his sinful nephew.[77]

The fifth and sixth centuries saw the introduction of liturgical symbols that strengthened the image of the bishop as a physician of souls. During these years the bishops of both the Latin and the Greek spheres of the old Roman Empire began regularly to carry staffs as symbols of their office. At first, Christians interpreted the episcopal staff in many ways. Writing in the Latin West, Isidore of Seville saw it as a token of the bishop's ruling authority, of his power of correction, and of his duty to support the sick.[78] In the Byzantine Empire, however, the bishop's staff, his *rabdos,* came to symbolize his duty to heal the spiritual ills of his flock and to support them in their weakness.[79] Again it seems likely that the Greek Christians borrowed a symbol from the Asclepian cult, where the god's *rabdos* had early on come to represent the deity's care for and support of the sick.[80] Thus, the standard Byzantine interpretation of the bishop's staff suggests how much the Eastern church emphasized the local leader's role as a spiritual healer—a physician of souls—and as a benefactor of the physically sick. Holding one of the ancient signs of the Greek medical arts, the Christian pastor with his staff also reflected the acceptance by Byzantine Christianity of classical Greek medicine.

Byzantine authors not only used the image of the spiritual physician with respect to the bishops; they also applied the metaphor to monastic leaders. The biographer of Euthymios described the fifth-century founder of the fa-mous Lavra monastery in Palestine as a physician of souls.[81] The seventh-century monk Theodore of Sykeon was "the best physician and a disciple of the true archiatros, Christ our God."[82] In an appeal to his fellow superiors, one of the most influential monastic writers, John Klimax, did not simply ask them to become spiritual physicians for their monks; he employed an extended metaphor listing the plasters, salves, potions, sponges, lances, knives, and cautery irons which a good abbot should have at his command for operating on the spiritual ills of his monks. John's metaphor is so com-plete that it provides a good example of standard medical equipment in the seventh century.[83] The habit of comparing monastic leaders to spiritual phy-sicians lasted into the late Byzantine period. The emperor Theodore II Las-karis (1254–58) addressed as a physician of the soul his friend and advisor, the superior Nikephoros Blemmydes, who, incidentally, had been a prac-ticing physician of the body before he became a monk.[84]

Byzantine writers used the image of the physician and the regimen of medical care to describe every kind of Christian activity. When the fifth-century Theodoretos, bishop of Kyrrhos in Syria, wrote a tract to win over pagans to Christianity, he called it a "therapy for pagan ills."[85] The tenth-century patriarch Nicholas Mystikos spoke of certain therapies which the Greek Fathers employed to cure souls of fornication.[86] He also referred to penances imposed by the Orthodox church as remedies for spiritual disease.[87]

In summary, the Orthodox Christians of the East not only accepted Greek medicine: they moved it to a central place in their theological system. First, they came to see the medical profession as a symbol of charity in action, the cornerstone of Christian morality. Second, they frequently illustrated spiritual truths through medical analogies. Thus, they often conceived of Christ as the Great Physician of bodies and souls—the *archiatros* without equal. Finally, although only some of their religious leaders had practiced medicine or studied it thoroughly, all of them spoke of themselves as physicians of the souls in their care.

CHRISTIAN HOSPITALS

As Christian thinkers were developing their views on scientific medicine and its practice, Christian pastors of the Eastern churches—the bishops and their clergy—were opening the first permanent charitable institutions to include hospital facilities. During the fourth century the ideas of Origen regarding Hellenic medicine had taken firm root in the writings of the Greek fathers—Basil, Gregory of Nyssa, Gregory of Nazianz, and John Chrysostom. In the same milieu in which these men wrote, the first hospitals appeared. In fact, two of the Greek fathers, Basil and John Chrysostom, played significant roles in the early years of Christian hospitals, as we shall see.[88] As the orthodox church came to exalt the medical profession as the epitome of philanthropia, it in turn felt obliged to make this philanthropia available to all—especially the poor—by sponsoring hospitals. Since most Greek church leaders continued to esteem medicine as one of the best expressions of Christian love until the final days of the East Roman Empire, so too they did not falter in supporting nosokomeia. As late as the 1440s the monastery of John Prodromos in Petra still maintained a public hospital.[89]

From their origins in the fourth century until 1453 Byzantine hospitals were conceived as expressions of Christian charity. They carried out in the real world the orthodox doctrine regarding philanthropic medicine. When Basil the Great opened his extensive charitable institution—his *ptochotropheion*—outside Caesarea, he saw its medical services as the deepest possible expression of philanthropia. As Gregory of Nazianz phrased it, one could see there love put to the test in the treatment of disease.[90] John Chrysostom built his hospitals in Constantinople "for the glory of Christ" and staffed them with ascetics who viewed their service to the sick as a religious duty.[91] Sampson, the legendary physician of the Eastern capital, founded his hospital on the principles of the physicians' profession and on the divine laws which Christ laid down.[92] Even after Justinian introduced the archiatroi of the ancient pagan profession into the Christian xenones, a step which encouraged lay professionals to enter hospital service at all levels on the staff, the religious mission of the nosokomeion was never forgotten. When, about 800, Theodore Stoudites described a large nosokomeion with a complex staff of physicians and nurses, he emphasized that all the doctors from the chief physicians to the practical nurses strove to follow the divine plan of philanthropia.[93] When John II Komnenos established the Pantokrator Xenon in the twelfth century, he prayed that it would always be a fount of mercy, a refuge for men and women, a pure offering to the Lord. Moreover, John hoped that the philanthropia which he displayed in founding this hospital would attain for him the forgiveness of his many sins.[94] The emperor also reminded the physicians, medical assistants (hypourgoi), and servants of the Pantokrator that they should never neglect the patients, since Christ, the Creator of All, considered these sick his beloved brethren.[95] Thus, John wanted the monks and the lay staff of the Pantokrator complex to care not only for the buildings he had built—the lifeless temples—but especially for the patients of the hospital—the living temples of God.[96]

As late as the fifteenth century, the doctrine of the Orthodox church regarding medicine and the care of the sick was still bearing fruit. George Goudeles, both a politician and a merchant, remodelled one of his palaces in Constantinople to serve as a nosokomeion. His friend John Chortasmenos praised him for having pursued the highest of virtues—philanthropia toward the sick. The Lord does not require fasting, virginity, nor mortifications of the flesh, but he does demand love and mercy. Chortasmenos ranked Goudeles' hospital as the golden crown of his works.[97] Finally, he described Goudeles' foundation in the words Gregory of Nazianz had used to praise Basil's *ptochotropheion* at Caesarea, thereby linking this fifteenth-century xenon with the earliest hospitals of the Byzantine tradition. Here "disease is studied, suffering made blest, and sympathy put to the test."[98]

AMBIVALENCE TOWARD MEDICINE: THE ANARGYROI CULTS

Though the leaders of the Orthodox church enthusiastically embraced medicine as the embodiment of philanthropic action and wholeheartedly supported hospitals as dispensers of God's love and mercy, certain elements of the Byzantine world did not share this majority view. We have already considered a few critics of medicine from among Christian writers of the fourth and fifth centuries, but these hailed from heretical circles which either were forced underground by the dominant orthodoxy, as the dualists were, or eventually opted out of the Byzantine synthesis of Christian and classical Greek culture, as the Monophysites did. Some tendencies in orthodox Byzantine monasticism, however, were also opposed to physicians and their medicine. The sixth-century monk Dorotheos felt uneasy about studying secular medicine and wished instead to depend on God's divine grace alone, but Dorotheos' spiritual father, a man named Barsanouphios, advised him not to abandon medicine and even suggested that he consult with lay doctors. The reason Barsanouphios desired his spiritual son to continue in medicine reflects the important influence hospitals had in maintaining Christian enthusiasm for medical science in general. Barsanouphios advised Dorotheos to persevere in his medical training so that he could better supervise a hospital, a task which Barsanouphios saw as essential to his Christian life.[99]

In subsequent centuries monasticism continued to support the study of medicine and the maintenance of hospitals. Ascetic movements such as the Stoudite reform of the ninth century and the Athonite movement of the tenth century sponsored the care of the sick through the agency of hospitals staffed by professional physicians.[100] Even in the fourteenth century, when some ascetics had adopted a radically mystical life, the monk Niphon actively promoted xenones in Constantinople.[101]

Greater hostility to the practice of medicine and even to hospitals themselves surfaced in connection with the anargyroi cults. Among the miracle stories of the most famous anargyroi, the doctor-saints Cosmas and Damian, which were recorded at their great church in Constantinople, several emphasized the helplessness of physicians against disease.[102] One hagiographer of the anargyros Sampson stressed that, although the saint had excelled in medical studies, he actually had put little faith in medicine during his lifetime; rather, he had trusted in the grace of God.[103] Moreover, in describing Sampson's treatment of Justinian, this same hagiographer wrote that ordinary physicians had been totally powerless to cure the emperor. They had tried to mask their failure, as physicians usually did, by crediting their lack of success to the patient's refusal to obey their directives. When Sampson finally succeeded in curing Justinian, he used medicine only out of humility to mask his miracle.[104] The tales of the anargyros Saint Artemios contain some of the most vicious attacks against physicians. One recounts how a poor woman sought out the saint's church for her ailing child because the physicians she had consulted previously had demanded fees far beyond her meager means.[105] Another closes with a tirade against the followers of Hippocrates and Galen, sham physicians whose complicated procedures are totally unnecessary when one trusts God and his servant Artemios.[106]

Although some of the anargyroi literature reflected intense hostility toward physicians, one must not forget that the anargyroi tradition intimately linked these saints to the medical profession. Cosmas, Damian, and Sampson had all practiced medicine; though a military man in this life, Artemios assumed the form of a physician after his martyrdom.[107] Moreover, the monks who served the Kosmidion monastery of Cosmas and Damian and the men and women associated with the shrines of Sampson and Artemios all stressed that their patrons were anargyroi—doctor-saints.[108] Nevertheless, writers from these circles produced miracle tales containing some of the empire's harshest judgments on the medical profession, judgments which echo the negative statements about physicians expressed by Aelius Aristides, the fervent devotee of Asklepios, in the second century. Since the anargyroi cults had borrowed so many of their treatment procedures—incubation, special vigils, even the practice of recording miraculous cures—from the temples of Asklepios, they no doubt also inherited the ambivalence of the Asclepian cult toward the medical profession: a close link with the practice of medicine, yet a disdain for its human weakness.[109] Just as Asklepios had been the patron god of pagan physicians, so Cosmas and Damian (and, to a lesser extent, the other anargyroi) were the patron saints of Christian medicine. Just as the divine physician Asklepios possessed such great power that human doctors seemed helpless by comparison, so too the anargyroi had received such grace from Christ that no wise man ought to prefer the treatments of frail physicians of this world to the doctor-saints of God. These parallels demonstrate again the extent to which the old Asclepian worship influenced Greek Christian traditions. They also demonstrate that some of the hostility toward medicine which survived into the Byzantine centuries emanated not only from Christian roots, but also from ancient Greek religion.

Although the antimedical rhetoric one finds in the anargyroi miracle tales owes much to Asclepian traditions, it is possible that one ought to look for the immediate stimulus for such hostile feelings much closer to hand—in fact, to the Christian hospitals themselves. By the sixth century, when the anargyroi cults appear fully developed in the sources, they all have close ties with hospitals. The cult of Saint Sampson had grown up in association with the most illustrious of sixth-century Constantinopolitan hospitals, the Sampson Xenon.[110] The Kosmidion Church of Cosmas and Damian had a xenon next door, probably under the same administration.[111] So too a hospital stood close to the Church of Saint John Prodromos in Oxeia, which housed the relics of Saint Artemios. Since Artemios' suppliants could retire to this xenon for rest, again it is likely that these two institutions—church and hospital—formed part of a single ecclesiastical foundation.[112] The Constantinopolitan church dedicated to Saint Panteleemon, another anargyros, adjoined a hospital of the same name.[113] The Euboulos Xenon was associated with the cult of the doctor-saint Tryphon.[114] Outside of the capital, one finds the same association. When Bishop Theophylakt built and dedicated a church to Cosmas and Damian in ninth-century Nikomedeia, he added a hospital to it.[115] Even xenones like the Pantokrator, which the founders did not dedicate to anargyroi, usually included a chapel or a special celebration in honor of

Cosmas and Damian.[116] Thus the anargyroi churches and the clergy, monks, and laymen who served them always seem to have had close ties with hospitals.

The relationship between hospitals and anargyroi shrines was so close that the miracle-tale writers often pictured the doctor-saints as though they were xenon physicians. Cosmas and Damian would appear in the dreams of the faithful dressed in physicians' raiments. They would then go from suppliant to suppliant inside the church, just as the chief physicians made their morning rounds in sixth-century hospitals.[117] Miracle Six of the Artemios cycle states explicitly that many suppliants saw the saint making his rounds "just as in the xenon."[118] Moreover, the Artemios miracles describe the saint's female assistant as a *hypourgos*—a term which, as we have seen, referred to professional medical assistants working in hospitals.[119] Finally, although the anargyroi sometimes cured simply by touch, they often employed medicines, plasters, or surgical procedures—the kinds of treatments used next door in the xenon.[120] On the other hand, where healing cults were not so closely linked to hospitals and their physicians—as at St. Thekla's in Isauria—there was no tradition that their saints had recourse to sophisticated medicines in working their miracles.[121]

In view of the intimate relationship between anargyroi cults and the Christian hospitals of the sixth century and later, whence came the fierce hostility which some of the miracle tales display toward scientific medicine? A possible answer might be from a spirit of rivalry between the clerical, monastic, and lay staffs who tended the anargyroi shrines and the professional medical men working in the xenones. The authors of the anargyroi literature wanted to demonstrate the inferiority of the hospitals and the scientific medicine they offered to the divine grace which the saints could mediate. Thus, in the twenty-first tale of the *Miracula S. Artemii,* when Deacon Stephen realized that he had an infection of the groin, he asked the surgeons of the Sampson Xenon to operate on him. After three days of cold cautery treatments, Stephen underwent excruciating pains on the operating table, such pains that he abandoned any hope of living. This torture at first seemed to have worked. Stephen joyfully returned home only to see the infection reappear a short time later. Now he went to the relics of Saint Artemios instead of to the hospital and its surgeons. At the grave, the power of the saint truly healed Stephen, and without the pain of the knife or the cautery iron. Here, clearly, the author wished to stress the pointless suffering of xenon treatment compared to the swift, painless, and lasting cures of Artemios.[122] In another tale, the saint successfullly opened a serious infection through supernatural surgery where the hospital archiatroi had been unable to affect a cure.[123] Finally, Artemios restored the health of a young boy whose father—a xenon physician—had been powerless to help.[124]

It is likely too that the people associated with the anargyroi shrines felt deeper resentment against the hospitals and their personnel after Justinian transferred the archiatroi to these institutions. Suddenly the chief representatives of the most popular pagan science were working within the bosom of the church. Even in the sixth century many Christians still feared and hated the ancient pagan heritage of science and philosophy. To appreciate the depth of such sentiments one need only consider the joy with which Romanos the Melode celebrated the closing of the Athenian Academy in 529.[125] Unlike the philosophers, the physicians had not suffered such a dissolution. Rather, the emperor was providing them with new resources, now channelled through the Christian charitable foundations. Many monks, clerics, and ascetic laymen no doubt viewed the Christian confession of such physicians as a mere ruse to obtain government support, since these doctors continued to exalt the teachings of their pagan forefathers, Hippocrates and Galen. The indefatigable champion of Christianity John of Ephesus confirmed such fears when he uncovered a large number of crypto-pagans among the scholars and physicians of Constantinople as late as 546.[126]

Hospitals thus lay behind some of the resentment which Byzantine Christians still voiced against medicine during the sixth century within the context of the anargyroi cults. On the other hand, some aspects of the same anargyroi legends exalted hospitals and their physicians. Two of the doctor-saints, Sampson and Thallelaios, supposedly founded and administered hospitals during their lives. Hagiography depicted these men as they worked tirelessly on behalf of their patients. It canonized them as models and patrons of hospital physicians.[127] Thus, in the twelfth century, the poet Theodore Prodromos counted a kindly hospital doctor among the anargyroi saints—the patrons of Christian medicine.[128]

Hospitals also placed the practice of medicine in a thoroughly Christian environment. According to the oldest version of his *vita,* Saint Sampson ruled his hospital and its physicians according to the norms of the Gospel so that the entire institution functioned in virtuous rhythm.[129] In such a Christian atmosphere, the Greek doctors gradually lost their associations with paganism. After the sixth century, even professional medical literature reflects the values of Christianity.[130] Hospitals thereby helped to eliminate the last major objection on the part of Christians to secular medicine—its pagan ancestry.

Both the Alexandrian theologians of the third century and the Greek Fathers of the fourth century had given their blessing to medicine as a proof of God's philanthropia and of the goodness of creation. Once purged of certain dualist views, Christianity not only accepted medicine, but gradually enshrined it as a paragon of charity in action. The success of such views among leaders of the Eastern churches no doubt encouraged the development of hospitals and certainly aided in sustaining the Greek church's medical centers through the many centuries of the Byzantine era. Hospitals, in turn, helped to secure respect for physicians and their craft by placing the practice of medicine in a Christian context. It would be incorrect, however, to see the hospital as an institution which emerged solely as the result of theological views and of images employed in religious thought. Although the leaders of the Greek churches needed such concepts ready to hand before they could have considered sponsoring institutions which furthered secular medicine, it is doubtful that doctrine alone stimulated these bishops to action. Rather, forces outside the scope of early theological speculation—social, economic, and demographic—provided the immediate stimulus. They forced bishops of the fourth century to address new problems within their Christian flocks and in society as a whole, problems which demanded charitable activity on a larger scale than ever before, problems which required institutions to dispense philanthropia on a continuous basis. Practical demands, not Christian views on secular medicine and its physicians, actually brought the first hospitals into existence.

CHAPTER FIVE

The Fourth Century

None of the references to Christian philanthropic activities in the surviving sources mention any special facilities for treating the sick before the end of the fourth century.[1] By the beginning of the fifth century, however, Neilos of Ankyra portrayed the physician of a nosokomeion examining hospital patients as a familiar figure to Christians of the Greek-speaking world.[2] The decades of the fourth century, then, witnessed the birth of the hospital. So, too, the social, religious, and political forces at work during these years surely influenced Christian leaders of the Eastern provinces in developing new institutions especially for the sick.

The fourth century was a time of change and innovation, a century which began with the most ferocious persecution of Christians since the birth of the new faith in Jerusalem and ended with orders issued by a Christian emperor to close all pagan temples. During this century, too, Christian churches suffered serious internal strife. The theological views of an Alexandrian priest named Areios aroused an unprecedented dispute among Christians concerning the relationship of God the Father and God the Son. As the theological battle broadened, ecclesiastical parties crystallized around the various formulas which Christians advanced to describe this divine mystery. But more than religious change and theological conflict rocked the Eastern Mediterranean provinces of the fourth century; demographic shifts which are just now coming to light altered the basic unit of Greco-Roman society, the *polis*. Population growth and migration to urban centers combined with the rapid Christianization of the leading provincial aristocrats to hasten the death of the ancient pagan city and usher in a new urban constitution centered on the Christian bishop and his clergy.[3] All of these dynamic movements, including the Arian controversy, acted principally upon the urban communities of the Roman Empire. As a result, both the general philanthropic institutions of the first half of the fourth century and the specialized charities at the close of the 300s developed first in cities to assist the urban poor.[4]

These forces pressing on the cities of the empire—demographic growth, rapid Christianization, and theological turmoil—all affected the Greek-speaking provinces; the regions of the Latin West experienced an altogether different set of problems after 300. In fact, with the opening of the fourth century, the society of the Greek East began to evolve along radically different lines from that of the Latin West.[5] First, many among the leading classes of the Eastern provinces had become Christians by the end of the fourth century, while in the West most of the aristocrats remained pagan until the next century.[6] Second, many more among the common people of the cities had accepted Christianity in the East than had in the West.[7] Third, recent research points to a population increase in the villages of Syria, Palestine, and Asia Minor while many provinces of the West were experiencing population decline.[8] Fourth, populations in many Eastern poleis were growing rapidly while those of most Western cities either shrank or showed no growth.[9] Fifth, although the ancient forms of city life in both the East and the West were breaking down, the Christian bishops of the East, with the encouragement of the government, were more successful in their efforts to preserve much of ancient polis life under the wing of the church.[10] Finally, the Arian dispute splintered the Christian communities in Eastern cities, while it disturbed only a few Western congregations. Once one considers carefully these differences between the East and the West, it will no longer seem surprising that the first evidence of hospitals appears in Antioch, Constantinople, and Caesarea, not in Rome, Carthage, or Arles.

The study which follows will not be able to isolate any one of the major upheavals of fourth-century Eastern society as alone responsible for creating hospitals. Rather, it will explore a combination of social, political, and theological problems that gave rise to a new urban environment for Greek-speaking Christians and their leaders. The altered world of the fourth century forced bishops to address social problems and physical suffering on a grand scale. In attempting to meet these needs, bishops and their advisors developed the panoply of philanthropic institutions including the hospitals which emerged by the end of the century.

DEMOGRAPHIC CHANGE IN THE EAST AND CHRISTIAN CHARITY

During the early days of the church, the local Christian communities in both Eastern and Western towns were small enough that they could provide for the needs of their less fortunate members by using the simple system of deacons outlined in Acts 6:1–6 and the later manuals of Christian discipline.[11] In the West as late as the third century Bishop Cyprian of Carthage still managed to know many individuals in his flock personally.[12] To provide housing and shelter for occasional visitors from other churches a bishop either kept a room free in his residence or had a small guesthouse nearby.[13] In smaller towns of the Greek East, such as Rhinokorousa in Egypt, the simple episcopal guesthouse for visitors still sufficed to meet the needs of charity even in the fourth century.[14] In the larger cities of Syria and Asia Minor, however, conditions began to change radically at the beginning of the fourth century. In many Greek cities, the Christian population had been increasing steadily during the second and third centuries, a process that accelerated with the end of persecution and the conversion of Constantine. By the time of the Council of Nicaea some cities of the East had strong Christian communities, the largest of which comprised all ranks of society from the very rich to the wretches of the streets.[15]

The number of Christians in larger cities increased not only because of many conversions, but also because of major demographic changes.[16] Throughout the literature of late antiquity (fourth to sixth centuries) one finds references to masses of homeless people migrating into the cities of the East. Libanius disdained these rootless folk who streamed into Antioch during the fourth century.[17] In the sixth century Justinian, on the one hand, took steps to provide for migrants to Jerusalem but, on the other, tried by force to exclude such people from Constantinople.[18] Most of these newcomers had been simple peasants; with no skills with which to make a living in their new urban homes, they soon sank into desperate poverty. Many were forced to live in wretched deprivation, sleeping in alleys or under porticos without adequate food or clothing. Sermons delivered by bishops of the fourth century frequently described in lurid detail the suffering of the new urban masses.[19]

Historians in the past credited the widespread poverty in the Eastern cities to the general decline of the Roman Empire and its economy brought about by rapid escalation in the costs of government, corresponding increases in taxation, the spread of tax-exempt private estates, and a decline in population.[20] Recent studies, however, indicate that the causes of economic and social disruption in the East were much different from those in the West. Archaeological evidence is accumulating that late antiquity ushered in a period of relative stability and general demographic growth for the East.[21] In Syria and Palestine the population was steadily increasing in the rural areas. Given the static economy of the ancient world, such population increases created grave strains. Younger sons were often forced out of their old villages for lack of land. Some chose to cultivate new land; some joined monasteries; many others sought their fortunes in the cities. Without skills for the limited opportunities of ancient industry and commerce, these men turned to the Christian bishops for help. The church shouldered this heavy task both in response to Christ's commands and as a result of the impotence of local polis governments in responding to the new conditions.[22]

The poleis of the Roman world had been chronically ill even in the halcyon days of the Antonine emperors. Although the catastrophes of the third century ultimately helped to strengthen the imperial government, they hastened the decay of local city councils (*curiae*). Under Diocletian and his successors, the city aristocracies and their councils lost almost all their political power; these curiae now functioned primarily as corporations which assumed responsibility for the payment of the annona tax.[23]

The decline of the curiae, combined with a great many other currents in Late Roman society, eroded the *esprit* of municipal government. Members of prominent families either were unable or reluctant to build careers in service to their polis and looked rather to posts in the imperial bureaucracy for advancement and, if they were successful, enrollment in the senatorial order of the empire. By pursuing such a *cursus honorum,* they deprived their cities of their talents and their financial resources. If they were able to attain the senatorial order, they and their descendants were exempt from financial duties toward their native polis. As wealthy members of the curiae succeeded in fleeing their local responsibilities, they left the city governments impoverished.[24]

The mobility which the *pax romana* of Augustus and his successors had promoted also contributed to the decline of the ancient polis. The classical Greek city-state had rested on the concept of citizenship—hereditary membership in the body politic. Under the Hellenistic kings, the citizens of most cities gradually separated into two classes: a wealthy aristocracy which dominated the council and magistracies and the ordinary people—the *demos.* Both the classical and Hellenistic poleis had permitted outsiders to enter the community only in limited numbers.[25] While the Greek cities were independent, the notion of restricted citizenship flowed naturally from the larger political reality. After Roman conquest had limited the political independence of individual cities, a new era of easy migration from city to city dawned for the Greek world, an era which gradually diminished the significance of local polis citizenship.

The Greek cities, nevertheless, remained the focus of political, social, and economic life for provincials in the Eastern provinces under the principate of Augustus and his successors. As late as the second century, Plutarch, a man famous throughout the empire, still centered his life on his native city of Chaironeia. But Plutarch was extremely conservative in his local patriotism. Some Greek aristocrats of his generation had already become Roman citizens and were moving in circles which carried them far from their *patrides.*[26] In the next century, the Severan emperors further weakened the status of Greek cities by granting Roman citizenship to all free men of the empire.[27] Finally, in the fourth century, when great numbers of rural people began to flow into the Eastern cities, they obliterated totally the significance of ancient citizenship. Although these people had Roman citizenship—membership in the universal empire—they had no status in the local community; they possessed neither rights nor duties in their adopted communities.[28] They created a new kind of demos without the organization or the constitutional rights of the old assemblies of the ancient city-state. Writers of the fourth century came to use *demos* simply to describe the mass of lesser people ranging from the small artisans who worked out of booths along the city streets to the desperately poor who had no source of income nor even a place to lay their heads.[29] The traditional curial governments of the cities, having no desire to assist the new demos nor, indeed, the financial means, willingly allowed the bishops and their clergy to assume this critical task. While still a priest at Antioch, John Chrysostom recognized this demos of the poor and rural migrants. He realized the powerlessness of these men inside the old city government and as a Christian leader felt called to defend these inhabitants who had no vote and no support in the curia.[30] Basil of Caesarea openly acknowledged a novel role for church officials when he included protecting the demos among the duties of a bishop.[31]

The conversion of Constantine also encouraged the bishops, priests, and deacons to assume a greater share of the responsibility in local government. After the emperor had become a Christian, church leaders acquired tremendous prestige in their communities and, as a result, even represented their cities before the emperor or his officials. As a priest and later a bishop, Gregory of Nazianz appeared several times on behalf of his city before the provincial governor, a task formerly reserved for leading curial figures.[32] At the death of Bishop Basil, all the citizens of Caesarea, including the pagans and the Jews, mourned the loss of one of the city's great benefactors.[33] Many bishops of the post-Constantinian age, often drawn from the same aristocratic families which had served on the curial councils, inherited the enthusiasm of the ancient pagans for their cities. For example, Gregory, born of a curial family in Nazianz, displayed fierce pride in his native *patris* and boasted of his father's benefactions on behalf of the city—a behavior with its roots in the classical polis, not in New Testament humility.[34] During the fourth century bishops frequently built churches to adorn their cities, but by the fifth century some bishops, such as Theodoretos of Kyrrhos had taken over responsibility for constructing and maintaining such secular structures as bridges, baths, and aqueducts.[35] John Chrysostom, a leading spokesman of Eastern Christianity, managed to combine both classical and Christian notions of society. He always had before him the old classical ideal of the smoothly functioning polis with all classes and professions working together for the commonwealth. Chrysostom's new polis, however, was bound together not by the ancient customs and distinctions of his pagan forefathers, but rather by Christian philanthropy, which did not distinguish citizen from noncitizen, but only the person in need from the one who could help.[36]

Although these bishops adopted much of the fervor for their cities which their pagan ancestors had formerly displayed, they usually expressed their patriotism in different forms. Whereas the ancient benefactors had provided monuments and services such as baths, libraries, statues, theaters, and gymnasia to enhance the quality of ancient urban life, the Christian bishops applied their own personal resources and those of their congregations first to constructing adequate houses of worship and then to meeting the basic needs of the urban poor.[37]

In the days before Constantine's conversion, the number of Christians who needed economic assistance remained low enough that the bishop and his deacons could carry out redistribution of goods among church members within the traditional organization of the congregation. Meeting the new responsibilities of feeding and housing a large number of poor men and women, however, required specialized institutions with a stable income. Collections at the Sunday services were no longer sufficient. Thus, the churches began to establish permanent machinery to distribute food daily to the poor and to maintain institutions to provide emergency shelter. The first evidence regarding such new foundations comes from Antioch and indicates that the churches of Syria were organizing their philanthropic programs around *xenodocheia,* hostels reserved for the poor.[38] By the reign of Julian (361–63), Christian communities throughout the East had established xenodocheia, xenones, and katagogia (lodges) to house and feed the poor.[39]

Christian charitable activities, which centered in most cities around the xenodocheia, gained popularity for the church among the growing urban masses and no doubt played a significant part in the triumph of the new faith in almost all of the urban centers of the Eastern provinces. When the emperor Julian tried to revive paganism, he was well aware that the xenodocheia had aided considerably in winning the hearts of the people for Christianity. In order to gain back the lower classes to paganism, Julian tried to establish a network of charitable institutions just like those of the Christians. In the words of a Christian critic, "Julian thought that he could deceive the people by trying to imitate the good works of the Christians; thus he ordered that *xenones* and *ptocheia* [poor houses] be organized."[40]

Charitable work also won for individual ecclesiastical leaders tremendous support from the people. While working as the bishop's assistant in charge of charities at Caesarea, Basil established a shining reputation among the inhabitants. As a result of his famine relief program and other successful activities on behalf of the demos, he gained election to the episcopal throne upon the death of Bishop Eusebios (370).[41] In the episcopal office Basil's dedication to expanding the church's philanthropic institutions enkindled such devotion among some elements of the population that when a hostile Arian governor attempted to disgrace him, these people defied imperial authority and threatened to lynch the official.[42] In the same fashion, John Chrysostom achieved such a reputation for philanthropy in Constantinople that the people rioted when the imperial government tried to remove him from the episcopal throne.[43]

A visible role in the local church's charitable operations easily gained for a cleric an instant following among the Christianized demos. When bishops began to appoint assistants (*xenodochoi* or *ptochotrophoi*) to supervise the charitable institutions, these officials became so popular among the people that they often threatened episcopal authority. While serving the poor at Caesarea before his elevation to the episcopal dignity, Basil himself quarreled with his superior, Bishop Eusebios.[44] After Basil's death, his successor as bishop was embroiled in a struggle with Sakerdos, the administrator of the huge ptochotropheion just outside the city.[45] In Alexandria Bishop Theophilos fought bitterly with his xenodochos, Isidore.[46] The ecclesiastical records from the late fourth and fifth centuries are full of such conflicts.[47]

In founding, maintaining, or expanding philanthropic services, ecclesiastical officials were in many cases earnestly striving to observe Christ's command to love others as the good Samaritan had done (Luke 10:30). Even the most spiritual pastors, however, were no doubt aware of the political implications of successful charitable operations. For a man like Basil, a reputation as a philanthropic shepherd gained popularity and support among his flock, support strong enough to translate into political power with which a bishop could defy even the imperial administration. Winning the allegiance of a city's demos was even more important for church leaders during the fourth century because of the Arian controversy, which splintered many local churches into several groups vying for control of the episcopal office.

THE ARIAN CONFLICT

The Arian controversy ushered in an era of both theological conflict and political maneuvering in many Eastern churches of the empire. In the years after the Council of Nicaea (325), theological fighting widened into a power struggle among the various Arian factions, the supporters of the Nicaean Council, and scattered schismatic groups to control congregations and dominate the universal church. In such a contest for control, conspicuous philanthropic activities played an important role in gaining support for a particular faction both from the common people and from the imperial government. Two hundred years later, during the late sixth century, when the Monophysites began in earnest to organize a separate church, their patriarch, Paul of Antioch, established new charitable institutions called *diakoniai* in Constantinople and other major cities to help meet the basic needs of the poor, the weary, and the sick.[48] Doubtless, the Monophysites used these popular institutions as part of a campaign directed against the Orthodox church.[49] In a similar fashion, as I shall show, the various parties in the fourth-century Arian dispute experimented with new forms of philanthropic organizations, a process which, when combined with the demographic pressures we have discussed, accelerated the development of specialized charitable foundations. Since the Arian dispute played a central role in stimulating the foundation of philanthropic institutions, it is useful to consider for a moment how this struggle affected local Christian congregations.

Areios' ideas stirred up much more confusion in the Greek provinces than they did in the Latin West. Although the Council of Nicaea had condemned Arianism, the Nicaean doctrine—the consubstantiality of the Father with the Son (*homoousion* creed)—did not find wide support in the East, and Arian views of various shades resurfaced among the Eastern bishops soon after the council.[50] Disputes over episcopal elections or simple personal rivalries often helped to outline more distinctly theological differences that had initially been quite vague. A prime example of the complex situation which developed in many Eastern sees is the church of Constantinople.

Problems arose in the capital in about 337 with the death of the old bishop Alexander, a man who had ascended the episcopal throne of Byzantium before Constantine had chosen this city for his new capital. Alexander designated as his successor Paul, a man of conservative ecclesiological views. Other elements of the local clergy, more alive to the horizons opening for their church now that Byzantium was the imperial capital, supported a different candidate, Makedonios—a man of greater secular knowledge and political acumen. The two parties contended for two years, until the emperor Constantius interevened by deposing both candidates and selecting his personal chaplain, Eusebios of Nikomedeia.[51]

Each of these three men—Paul, Makedonios, and Eusebios—represented a political party, an interest group within the church of Constantinople: Paul led a theologically conservative party which opposed imperial intervention in the church, Makedonios headed a more political group, and Eusebios represented the clerical circles with close ties to the imperial court. With time each of these parties identified with a specific theological position vis-à-vis the Council of Nicaea, some members from strong personal conviction, but most of them out of a desire to link their local party with a wider faction represented throughout the Christian world. Thus, Paul's party adopted the Nicaean position, the formula *homoousion* (of the same substance), and found support in the West. Makedonios, who eventually succeeded in gaining the episcopal throne after 342, adopted a semi-Arian formula, *homoiousion* (of similar substance), a position close to, but not identified with, the Nicaean creed. As a result, he drew strong support from the bishops of Anatolia. The court party, which won the episcopacy in 360, was composed of moderate Arians who adopted the vague formula *homoion* (similar) in alliance with some powerful bishops of Syria and the East.[52]

A fourth party of extreme Arians had first formed in Antioch, but during the 350s had spread to Constantinople. By the next decade its leaders designated a bishop to head their congregation in the capital. These extremists, who used the formula *anomoion* (dissimilar) to describe the relationship of the Father to the Son, were the only Arians who had a strong moral commitment to their particular creed.[53] Thus, by the time of Bishop Demophilos (370–80), himself a member of the court party, Constantinople had three Arian factions—the moderates of the official court party, the semi-

Arian followers of Makedonios, and the extremist Anomoians—as well as a tiny Nicaean congregation and two schismatic groups, the Novatians and the Apollinarians.[54] All contended with one another for supporters in the court circles and in the ranks of the demos of Constantinople.

Throughout many of the major Eastern cities similar patterns emerged. In attempting to win control of the local church bureaucracy and in struggling to retain a dominant position, factions were pitted against one another in a constant battle to gain favor with the people and support from the imperial authorities. As part of their efforts to win popularity among the demos, factions promoted conspicuous charitable activities, much as the Monophysites were to do two centuries later with their *diakoniai.* So, when the Arian George of Cappadocia was appointed bishop of Alexandria by Constantius II in 357, he constructed a network of xenodocheia for the poor immigrants to the Egyptian capital and organized a free burial service for the poor of the city as part of a campaign to win the affections of the Alexandrian demos away from the arch-Nicaean Athanasios.[55] Unfortunately, there is no surviving source which explicitly states that conspicuous philanthropic projects formed part of an Arian campaign, as the writings of John of Ephesus have so identified the Monophysite program of the late sixth century.[56] Nevertheless, examining a wide range of sources concerning the turbulent years of the Arian schism will illumine new aspects of the struggle for popular support among the various church factions, a struggle which encouraged other bishops besides George of Cappadocia to expand the range and diversity of their charitable projects. The results of such a process were more xenodocheia for the poor and specialized shelters for orphans, foundlings, the aged, and the sick.

ARIAN CHARITIES

When the emperor Julian described Christian charitable foundations during his reign (361–63), he did not mention any facilities designed solely for the sick, but after the Arian dispute had run its course, hospitals were apparently familiar institutions.[57] The chronology of hospital development alone suggests that the Arian controversy played a part in creating philanthropic agencies for the sick. And careful study of each Arian party provides more substantial evidence that the competing ecclesiastical factions in Eastern cities did in fact extend the services of simple hospices to include specialized care for the sick.

The Anomoians (extreme Arians), based in Antioch, seem to have preceded all other factions in stressing free medical care for the poor as part of an organized philanthropic program. Aetios, the founder of the sect, initiated their efforts in philanthropic medicine. Born in Coele-Syria, the son of a low-ranking bureaucrat, Aetios began his higher studies under Paulinos, bishop of Tyre, sometime before 330. When his bishop was transferred to the great see of Antioch, Aetios went with him. Paulinos, however, lived only a few months as bishop of Antioch; his successor, Eulalios (331–32), disliked the abrasive young Aetios and forced him to leave the city. From 332 until 344, Aetios roamed through Cilicia; he returned once to Antioch and finally journeyed to Alexandria. During his years in Cilicia and Syria he studied the Holy Scriptures under a number of teachers, all of whom had been disciples of Lukian of Antioch. Once in Alexandria Aetios turned his attention to the study of medicine. Apparently, many of the medical students in the iatreia of Alexandrian physicians favored Arian theology. While studying with them, Aetios picked up Arian doctrines and developed them to an extreme position, his Anomoian formula.[58]

When one of his former teachers, Leontios, became bishop of Antioch in 344, Aetios returned to his old home. With the new bishop's support, Aetios won such favor in the church that Leontios decided to ordain him a deacon.[59] During these years in Antioch, Aetios began to put his medical training to a Christian use, offering free medical care to the poor and needy. It seems that Aetios provided his free medical aid in the name of the Antiochene church.[60] No sources describe where or how Aetios practiced his philanthropic medicine. Since his friend and bishop Leontios was renowned for his interest in xenodocheia, it is at least possible that Aetios' medical missions in the service of the Antiochene church took him to the beds of the sick who were staying in Christian hostels.[61]

Additional evidence does indeed support the hypothesis that Aetios was among the first to practice medicine in the poorhouses of the Christian church at Antioch. Aetios' superior, Bishop Leontios, built one of his hostels in Daphne, a suburb of Antioch famous for its healthful climate and salubrious waters, and frequented as a spa by the aristocrats from the Eastern provinces.[62] It is likely that Leontios located a hostel at Daphne for the advantage of the sick among the poor so that they might recuperate in the same healthful environment which the rich had always been able to enjoy. Such a hostel would have offered Aetios an ideal opportunity to practice philanthropic medicine. Moreover, in a bitter attack against Aetios, Gregory of Nyssa ridiculed his opponent's medical practice. "So that he [Aetios] would not be completely bereft of sustenance," Gregory sneered, "he wandered about under the pretext of practicing medicine visiting rather obscure houses and the outcasts [*aperrimmenoi*]."[63] It is tempting to interpret Gregory's account as a veiled reference to Aetios' service in the hostels of Leontios— refuges for Antioch's outcasts. In summary, Aetios and his followers might have taken the practice of philanthropic medicine into the xenodocheia of Antioch. Perhaps during the years of their influence (344–64) they helped to establish particular hostels which specialized in offering medical care to the destitute sick. This would explain the xenon reserved for those stricken with disease which Chrysostom described at Antioch in 381.[64]

During these same years, Aetios enlisted some talented supporters. He made contact with Theophilos Indus, a man renowned for his personal holiness, his miraculous deeds, and his extreme Arian theology. During the early 350s Aetios, Theophilos, and a young student named Eunomios began to build an ecclesiastical party which extended outside Antioch to aid them in counteracting what they considered to be the heretical theology of Nicaea. These Anomoians reached their height of power in 360, when the emperor Constantius made their ecclesiastical ally Eudoxios bishop of Constantinople in place of their bitter enemy Makedonios. Within a few months of their victory, however, Aetios' extreme ideas and refusal to compromise led to his exile and the gradual dissolution of the alliance which supported him.[65] Nevertheless, he remained extremely popular; at his death in 365 his supporters in Constantinople gave him a triumphant funeral.[66] His popularity in the Antiochene church after his return in 344 and his later prominence in Constantinople probably stemmed in great part from his reputation as a physician who treated patients free of charge.

Among the Anomoian leaders, only Aetios is known to have completed medical training and to have practiced philanthropic medicine. Since Aetios personally tutored Eunomios, it is possible that he shared his medical knowledge with his student.[67] Although no sources indicate that Theophilos Indus, the third Anomoian leader, ever practiced medicine, they do reveal him as a miraculous healer.[68] In fact, several of the principal Anomoian figures, including Aetios, were supposed to have worked wondrous cures. Apparently, curing the sick by natural or supernatural means was part of the Anomoian propaganda effort, a campaign which included in its sphere much of Asia Minor.[69]

The first opponents of the Anomoians coalesced about the powerful bishop of Ankyra, Basil, who with the support of Eusebios of Nikomedeia had come to the episcopal throne of that city in 336.[70] One source claims that Basil, like Aetios, was a physician.[71] In Asia Minor Basil had the strong backing of an ascetic movement, led by a pious man named Eustathios. Basil and Eustathios were united by a moderate Arian formula and a common distrust of the Nicaean Council. But they also objected to the extreme Arian doctrine of Aetios. Sometime after 350, Basil and Eustathios publicly debated Aetios and later denounced the Anomoian leaders before the emperor Constantius.[72] In opposition to Aetios, Basil and his followers developed the term *homoiousion* (of similar substance) to describe the relationship of the Father to the Son, a position similar to that of Nicaea.[73]

Although Eustathios played a leading role in Basil's party and in its theological disputes, he was primarily concerned with the monastic movement then emerging in Anatolia. He and other ascetic leaders of Asia Minor helped to steer this monasticism away from the anchoritism of Egypt and Syria by stressing that the second of the two great commandments—the Gospel demand to love one's neighbor—was central to a monk's life. In accordance with their views, Eustathios and other Anatolian leaders founded their monasteries in or near cities where the monks could minister to the poor.[74] When Eustathios became bishop of Sebasteia in lesser Armenia (357), he built near his see a hostel similar to the xenodocheia of Antioch and placed it in the hands of an ascetic community.[75]

Eustathios designed his hostel specifically to serve persons afflicted with disfiguring or disabling diseases.[76] There is, however, no direct evidence that physicians attempted to treat the residents of Eustathios' hostel for their ailments. Both the usual name of this institution—*ptochotropheion* or *ptocheion*—and the casual references to it in the sources imply only that it fed and housed the sick. One should recall, however, that the Greek terminology for charitable institutions was still undeveloped during the fourth century and had not yet devised specific words to describe specialized hostels. Since Eustathios designed his institution in Sebasteia especially for the diseased and the disabled, it is not far-fetched to assume that he encouraged physicians to treat the sick in his ptocheion. Moreover, when Basil, bishop of Caesarea (371–79), built in his city a ptocheion modeled on the hostel of Eustathios, he definitely included physicians as part of the staff.[77] In addition, Eustathios opposed the Anomoians, who were certainly emphasizing some form of free medical care and spiritual healing as part of their evangelization program both in Syria and Asia Minor.[78] Supporting some system of philanthropic health care would have been a natural response on the part of Eustathios to Anomoian proselytism.

Before he attained the episcopal throne of Sebasteia, Eustathios had sojourned in Constantinople. There he had converted to an ascetic way of life and to fervent philanthropic activity a former bureaucrat named Marathonios.[79] An excellent organizer, Marathonios quickly formed in Constantinople a number of urban monastic communities, usually called *synoikiai*, on the Anatolian model. United in these communities, Marathonios and his ascetic brethren served both the poor and the sick.[80] In describing these synoikiai, however, the two historians Sozomenos and Socrates do not mention any medical practice connected with these early Constantinopolitan philanthropies.[81]

During his stay in the capital Eustathios also succeeded in forging an alliance between the Anatolian *homoiousion* party and the controversial bishop of Constantinople, Makedonios. A clever politician, Makedonios realized the importance not only of joining a larger theological party of the church universal, but also of gaining popular support among the people of Constantinople. He therefore became a champion of Anatolian monastic communities and their charities in the capital. Moreover, he ordained Eustathios' disciple, Marathonios, as a deacon of his church and placed him in charge of all the city's urban ascetic communities and their charities.[82] The bishop's alliance with the urban monks succeeded in winning the hearts of the demos in Constantinople. Despite his persecution of rival ecclesiastical factions in the capital, Makedonios and his party achieved fame for their modest and pious behavior, their monklike demeanor, and their great philanthropy toward the poor.[83] When the emperor Constantius exiled Makedonios from Constantinople in 360, a crowd of the lesser people followed him out of the town, hailing him as *philoptochos* (lover of the poor).[84] Even opponents of Makedonios and his party praised their charitable activities.[85]

When the church historians Socrates and Sozemenos mention the philanthropic projects of Makedonios and his deacon Marathonios they describe them in terms too vague to establish whether or not their charitable institutions included a staff of physicians, although their accounts do make clear that these foundations offered some special care to the ill.[86] But while the historical sources fail to reveal any practice of charitable medicine under Makedonios, hagiographical traditions may have preserved the shadows of philanthropic medical activity in the *homoiousion* institutions in Constantinople during the 350s. These traditions center on the good Christian physician named Sampson.

From the several sources which refer to Saint Sampson one cannot determine exactly when this physician lived in Constantinople. All versions of the *Vita Sampsonis* claim that he cured Justinian (526–65);[87] the tradition preserved in the *Synaxarion* of the Great Church of Hagia Sophia, on the other hand, asserts that he came to the new capital when Constantine first dedicated his city (330).[88] The most reliable sources to mention the saint himself, the *De aedificiis* of Prokopios and Novel 59 of Justinian, establish that he had lived sometime before Justinian's accession (526). Indeed, Prokopios implies that Sampson had flourished long before 532, the year when the Nika fire destroyed the hospital which the saint had founded, along with many other buildings at the center of Constantinople.[89]

In the novels of Justinian and in the *Book of Ceremonies,* a tenth-century compilation of court ceremony drawing on traditions from earlier centuries as well, several passages regarding Sampson's hospital, the Sampson Xenon, offer additional evidence that the saint had established his medical facility in the capital years before 526. In Justinian's legislation the Sampson Xenon always received the first rank among the city's hospitals. In referring to the xenones of Constantinople, Novel 59 singles out only the Sampson Xenon and its administrator by name.[90] Such special status could well reflect the greater age of the Sampson among the hospitals of the capital. From among the many charitable foundations in the city, Novel 131 grants the privileges of the Great Church of Hagia Sophia only to the Orphanotropheion and to the Sampson Xenon.[91] Since the Orphanotropheion was a prestigious institution in the capital by the mid-fifth century, it surely had been founded sometime before 450.[92] By recognizing the Sampson Xenon as an institution with the same privileges as the orphanage of Constantinople, Justinian confirmed that this hospital also enjoyed similar prestige, an honor due most probably to its age.

The *Book of Ceremonies,* however, presents the most convincing evidence for placing the foundation of Sampson's hospital in the years before 450. In describing the Palm Sunday celebration in the ninth-century imperial palace, it lists the directors of the principal hospitals in Constantinople as they were to appear before the emperor. Their order of entrance reflected their official rank. With the exception of the xenodochos of the Theophilos hospital, who was classed apart from the other xenon directors, their rank depended upon the age of the hospitals they supervised.[93] It is easiest to demonstrate this order by beginning with the last director to approach the emperor—the xenodochos of the Irene. His xenon was a relatively recent institution in the ninth century, since it owed its foundation to the empress Irene, who had died in 802.[94] Just before the xenodochos of the Irene, the director of the Narses Xenon had come before the emperor. A general of the emperor Maurice had built this hospital toward the end of the sixth century.[95] Ahead of him was the director of the Irene in Perama, whose xenon had been opened by the priest Markianos in the mid-fifth century.[96] Before him, two other directors had entered the hall; the xenodochos of the Euboulos and ahead of him the xenodochos of the Sampson. Since the court ceremonial required that the last three hospital directors approach the emperor according to the age of their institutions, it probably applied the same rule to these two directors as well. Thus, the Sampson Xenon must have opened before the Euboulos, which in turn was older than the hospital which Markianos established just after 450. The Palm Sunday list, therefore, agrees with the evidence presented by Justinian's novels that the physician Sampson had organized his hospital long before 526, indeed sometime before 450.

While the *vitae* of Sampson assert that he cured the emperor Justinian, other details in these same stories support the conclusions derived from Prokopios and the legal sources and, in fact, provide some basis for placing the doctor's life before 400. One version on the *Vita Sampsonis* implies that Sampson had been a pioneer in medical philanthropy. By following Christ's commands to feed and shelter his patients, he added something totally new to the practice of medicine.[97] By the episcopacy of Chrysostom (398–404), however, Constantinople had several nosokomeia where physicians practiced their art in a Christian context, obeying both the rules of proper medical treatment and the Gospel norms regarding feeding and sheltering the needy.[98] Thus, if this version of the *Vita Sampsonis* is accurate in portraying its hero as the first physician to offer lodging and food as well as medical treatment to his patients, Sampson must have done this before the end of the fourth century, by which time a number of nosokomeia were already providing such services.

In addition, all versions of the *Vita Sampsonis* state that Sampson was

buried at the Church of St. Mokios because he was related to Mokios, a man
martyred in Bithynia by Diocletian.[99] A number of other sources confirm that
Sampson's relics were indeed in the Church of St. Mokios, but the story
concerning a family connection between Sampson and the martyr would
seem to be pure invention, since the authors of the *vitae* begin by claiming
that their hero was born and bred in Rome.[100] No doubt, the hagiographers
fabricated Sampson's family relationship with Mokios to explain the curious
fact that the saint was buried so far away from the xenon that bore his name.
Both the old xenon of Sampson and the new structure, which Justinian
erected, were located in the center of old Byzantium, next to the Great
Church of Sancta Sophia. The Church of St. Mokios, on the other hand, lay
several kilometers away, in the southwest section of the city outside of the
Constantinian walls.[101] If one discounts the family connection, then why were
Sampson's relics at St. Mokios' church and not at the institution which he
founded? An examination of the emperor Theodosius' settlement of the Arian
schism at Constantinople in 380–81 should provide the answer to this question.

When the Nicaean emperor Theodosius gained control of the Eastern
capital in November 380, he offered Bishop Demophilos and his clergy,
Arians of the Homoian party, the option of accepting the Nicaean creed or
of surrendering the churches of Constantinople to the orthodox faction in
the city. Demophilos chose to reject Nicaea and accept exile. As he left Sancta
Sophia, he told his supporters that they would reassemble their Arian congregation outside the city.[102] Theodosius allowed them to do this, assigning
them a church beyond the fourth-century walls of Constantinople, St. Mokios.[103] In the process of moving from inside Constantinople to their new
place of worship in exile, perhaps the Arians took with them relics of their
most popular saints, among whom might well have been the physician
Sampson. Since the Patrographs reveal that the Arians buried many of their
dead close to St. Mokios, it is easy to believe that they would have placed
the remains of some of their saints inside the church itself.[104] If this explanation of Sampson's burial place at St. Mokios is correct, then the revered
physician must have lived some time before 380. Possibly he served under
the Homoian episcopacies of Eudoxios or Demophilos.

It is much more likely, however, that his philanthropic medical practice
formed part of the charitable programs fostered by Makedonios during his
second episcopacy (350–60). As we have seen, Socrates and Sozomenos both
indicate that under Makedonios the deacon Marathonios organized his philanthropic institutions around urban monastic communities called synoikiai.
Shunning the solitude of the wilderness, these ascetics lived in Constantinople, where they dedicated themselves to prayer and to the service of the
poor. The oldest version of Sampson's vita clearly pictures its subject pursuing this same path to holiness. Sampson arrived in Constantinople with

only a single cloak, a hallmark of men who heeded the advice of the greatest ascetic, John the Baptist. He took up residence in a simple house, where he lived in the greatest piety and humility. The hagiographer adds that the original dwelling of the saint was still standing in eighth-century Constantinople, where it shone as an example of Sampson's angelic lifestyle.[105] In addressing the emperor, Sampson himself declared that he had renounced the riches of the world.[106] Finally, when he died, he joined the ranks of those who dwelled in the immaculate monasteries of heaven.[107] The whole vita presents Sampson as a monk who had left the world; yet nowhere does it describe him fleeing to the quiet of the desert or the mountains, nor does it associate him with a well-ordered cenobitic monastery. Rather, he lived in a humble residence while laboring in the service of the sick among the demos of Constantinople, a lifestyle which fits perfectly the ideals of the urban monastic movement Marathonios had introduced into the capital in the 350s.

Sampson thus belonged to the urban monks, but later his relics fell into the hands of the Homoian Arian party of Demophilos. The best explanation of these facts is as follows. Sampson was a physician who joined the Marathonian monks of Constantinople. He opted to serve the poor by offering his medical expertise free of charge and by opening extra rooms in his iatreion where he could feed and house his destitute patients.[108] When the Homoian Arians gained control of Constantinople in 360, they either convinced Sampson to join their ranks, if he was still alive at the time, or they used their control of the official church to gain custody of his relics. Thus, in 380 they were able to translate Sampson's remains to their only church, St. Mokios, outside the walls.

There is still another argument for assigning Sampson to the ranks of the Arians or Makedonians (*homoiousion* party) in the Constantinopolitan church of the fourth century. Later Constantinopolitans listed Sampson together with other doctor-saints as anargyroi, a class of Eastern holy men whose cults were discussed in Chapter Four. At least one of these anargyroi, Saint Artemios, clearly belonged to an Arian party. Since his biography, the *Martyrium Artemii,* claims that Eusebios of Nikomedeia had trained and baptized him and that he had been a trusted companion of the Arian emperor Constantius, he surely held a heretical definition of the faith.[109] During his life Artemios had served as a high-ranking military man with no apparent connection with the medical profession. After his death for the faith at the hands of the emperor Julian and the translation of his relics to Constantinople, however, people began to associate him with the practice of medicine.[110] His devotees usually saw him dressed as a physician, often carrying a bag of medical instruments as he made his rounds among the sick at his shrine.[111] It is difficult to see why people would confuse a military man like Artemios with a physician. That Artemios healed the sick at his shrine would not be enough to explain this metamorphosis, since many relics of saints who were clearly not physicians possessed healing powers. The only apparent explanation for such a change would seem to be Artemios' creed. Thus, in Constantinople, at least, the popular imagination tended to associate Arian holy men with the practice of medicine.

After the victory of Nicaean orthodoxy, the church continued to permit the veneration of famous Arian Christians such as Artemios. Moreover, hagiographers of later centuries did not shrink from writing accounts of their deeds. Artemios' biographer made no attempt to hide his subject's obvious Arian associations unabashedly including them in his narrative. In writing Sampson's vitae, however, the hagiographers seem simply to have recast the story in much later days—the reign of the orthodox Justinian—to free their subject from any taint of heresy.[112]

To summarize the arguments regarding Arianism and the first hospitals, no extant source credits any one Arian holy man or any single Arian party with establishing the first medical centers to offer food, housing, and a doctor's care. Although Aetios practiced medical philanthropy in Antioch, it cannot be shown conclusively that he did this in a xenon. Although Eustathios built a great hostel in Sebasteia for the sick and disabled, there is no indisputable evidence of physicians in his establishment. Although Makedonios emphasized philanthropy in Constantinople, not enough detailed information survives to establish that medical services for the poor were part of his program. It seems certain that Sampson opened his iatreion for the poor of Constantinople sometime in the late fourth century, but it is not yet possible to determine precisely to which ecclesiastical party he belonged. In isolation each fragment of evidence has its weaknesses. Taken together, however, all these scattered examples present a definite pattern. Arian leaders were frequently interested in philanthropic institutions, and among their ranks were many who seem to have been physicians or to have studied medicine. As early as the 330s the medical students of Alexandria found Arian ideas appealing. Aetios, the founder of the Anomoian sect, certainly practiced medicine; his opponent, Basil of Ankyra, was perhaps a physician. Moreover, the personal physicians of Constantius played active roles in the Homoian party of Eudoxios, bishop of Constantinople.[113] When one considers all these indications and recalls too that hospitals were well established in Constantinople and Antioch by the end of the fourth century—that is, at the close of the Arian controversy—it seems likely that one or other of these contending ecclesiastical parties encouraged physicians in their ranks to offer free medical care to the poor. Some of these men turned to the sick who were staying at the xenodocheia or ptochotropheia maintained by the local church and thus took the first step in setting up hospitals. That the sources do not speak clearly of such an achievement and only indicate it in shadowy legends or in vague references is the natural result of the final defeat of Arian beliefs and the subsequent hostility shown by the Nicaean victors toward heterodox leaders.

THE *PTOCHEION* OF BASIL OF CAESAREA

The Orthodox sources through which one must view Arian activities necessarily omitted or distorted details regarding beneficial programs which heretical bishops had promoted. These sources, however, did not obscure the achievements of Basil, the bishop of Caesarea (370–79). They reckoned him a champion of Nicaean doctrine in the East, a great theologian, a monastic leader—in short, one of the Fathers of the Greek Church.[114] They also credited him with founding during his episcopacy a large philanthropic institution to serve his city of Caesarea, an institution which he placed in the care of a monastic community. This large charitable facility—Gregory of Nazianz called it a veritable city of piety—forms a link between the charitable operations of Arian sects in Asia Minor and Nicaean orthodoxy.[115]

Almost all scholars of Eastern monasticism agree that the moderate Arian Eustathios and his ascetic ideas helped to shape Basil's views of the ideal Christian life.[116] First, Basil himself admitted that he had been attracted to Eustathian monasticism.[117] Second, his ascetical works reveal a number of similarities with tenets held by Eustathian monks.[118] Finally, in the fifth century Sozomenos mentions that a book containing ascetical works of Basil circulated under Eustathios' name.[119] Since legitimate works of Eustathios or of his disciple Marathonios have not survived, it is impossible to tell how exactly Basil's monastic ideals paralleled those of the moderate Arian monks. Certainly Basil's views differed from those of the more radical Eustathians, principally by emphasizing the bishop's authority over all monastic communities of his city.[120]

Since Basil established the New Testament as the essential rule of his monasteries, he required that his monks carry out the corporal works of mercy, the practical application of Christ's command to love one's neighbor.[121] So that the monks could serve the needy, especially the suffering demos of the cities, Basil located his ascetic communities in or near towns or large villages. Thus, he built a monastery just outside the gates of Caesarea so that the monks could easily minister to the poor of the Cappadocian metropolis. Basil also joined specialized facilities, his ptocheion, to the monastery, so that his monastic brothers could offer shelter and care to the needy.[122]

Basil surely adopted his practice of locating his monasteries near population centers from the Eustathians, who always founded their monasteries, or synoikiai, close to large settlements. Moreover, it is likely that Basil patterned the structure of the charitable foundations attached to his monasteries on those built by Eustathios. Sozomenos certainly viewed Basil's city of phi-

lanthropy at Caesarea as part of the wider Cappadocian-Pontic ascetic movement.[123] In addition, Basil chose to call his facility a *ptochotropheion* or a
ptocheion—terms preferred by the Eustathians over *xenodocheion,* a name
used by the Antiochenes for their centers of charity.[124] Finally, in his eulogy
of Basil, Gregory of Nazianz heaped every sort of praise on his old friend,
especially regarding his ptocheion, but nowhere did he imply that Basil's
charitable foundation was something new among ecclesiastical organizations.[125]

Since several surviving sources describe Basil's ptocheion at Caesarea,
it would be well to consider their accounts carefully, for they not only reveal
what sort of an institution Basil provided for Caesarea during the 370s, but
they might also help to supplement our lack of information regarding earlier
Arian charitable institutions. The details which these sources provide concerning Caesarea most likely apply as well to the hostels that Eustathios and
Marathonios built to serve Constantinople, Sebasteia, and other towns of Asia
Minor during the 350s and 360s and perhaps reflect, too, conditions in the
Antiochene xenodocheia where Aetios had labored.

Although Gregory of Nazianz wrote in a highly rhetorical style, es-
chewing concrete descriptions, his eulogy of Basil includes some useful
information regarding the ptocheion near Caesarea. First, he referred to it
as a city, indicating that it housed a large number of people in a collection
of buildings.[126] Since Basil's monastic communities were not to be very
large—thirty men would seem to have been the maximum—most of the
citizens of this philanthropic city must have been those in need.[127] Among
these men and women, Gregory listed the poor and the sick; he added that
disease received special attention.[128] A second source, a letter written by
Basil himself, states that the institution employed both physicians and nursing
attendants—no doubt the men who, according to Gregory, showed special
concern for the sick.[129] Gregory described too how the lepers and crippled
whom society had rejected found shelter, food, and treatment at the ptocheion. Amid his episcopal duties Basil found time not only to visit the sick
at his institution, but also to minister to their suffering. He greeted them with
a kiss, treated their physical ailments, and dressed their wounds.[130] Clearly,
Basil was putting into action the study of medicine which he had pursued
while a student at Athens during the 350s.[131] His service to the sick of the
ptocheion reminds one of Aetios, who during the 340s had offered his medical training to the destitute of Antioch.

Basil's letter describing his ptocheion specifies that it included lodgings,
pack animals, and guides for strangers, as well as a separate hostel for those
who needed care because of some illness. In the building for the sick Basil
provided both doctors and nurses.[132] Since both Basil and Gregory refer to
physicians at the ptocheion and emphasize care for the sick over any other
form of charity performed at the facility, it would seem that Caesarea had a

hospital in the 370s. Basil thus opened his hospital several years before Chrysostom would visit a xenon reserved for the sick in Antioch and twenty years before he would build his nosokomeia, staffed with physicians, in Constantinople.[133]

Although a number of scholars have indeed counted Basil's ptocheion at Caesarea as the first hospital, more recent studies have classified it as a mixed institution serving a great variety of needy people and thus not focusing its resources on treating the ill.[134] That the poor, the aged, and the crippled received help at Basil's foundation along with those who suffered from disease, however, would not in itself exclude the possibility that a well-organized hospital was functioning as a part of the facility at Caesarea. If no typikon had survived to reveal the several distinct institutions that composed the Pantokrator complex, it would be difficult from the allusions to that foundation in the twelfth-century narrative histories or from the letters of John Tzetzes to establish the presence of a hospital there. Indeed, it is possible that Basil's ptocheion closely resembled the Pantokrator complex. First, it was centered on a monastery and a monastic church, as was the Pantokrator. Second, it included at least two structures serving the needy: one equipped for travelers and one for those who were sick. Similarly, the Pantokrator had its xenon for the sick and its gerokomeion for the old and infirm. Third, it also provided other structures to house ancillary services, as did the twelfth-century institution of Constantinople. It would seem, then, that Basil's foundation at Caesarea formed a cluster of monastic buildings and separate philanthropic houses under the supervision of a single superior (*proestos*). Such a physical plant fits perfectly Gregory's curious description of the institution as a new city.[135]

Although there are good reasons to believe that Basil patterned this monastery and ptocheion as a whole on Eustathian communities and their hostels, it is possible that the hospital facility at Caesarea was Basil's own innovation. That Basil had been especially interested in medicine during his student days and had studied the subject with zeal, that his sermons and theological writings reflected a strong attraction to the Greek medical system, and that he himself applied his medical expertise in treating the patients of his hospital, all support such a conclusion.[136] It is conceivable, then, that Basil alone decided to set aside a hostel or xenon solely for those who were suffering from disease and that he first equipped such an institution with beds, medicines, and a staff of physicians. Against such an argument, however, one should recall how much Basil had admired Eustathian monasteries and how his ascetical writing incorporated much of the moderate Arian ascetic lifestyle into its system. Moreover, the eulogy composed by Gregory of Nazianz nowhere indicates that Basil had established anything new at Caesarea when he opened his city of philanthropy. Finally, in defending his ptocheion before the provincial governor, Basil himself did not claim that his hostels at Caesarea represented an innovation of any kind.[137] It thus seems more likely that Basil adopted his city of philanthropy, including its medical hostel, from Eustathian models both because he believed that such charitable operations truly followed Christ's commands and because he wanted to put the orthodox faction in Asia Minor squarely behind popular charities such as the ptocheia. A holy man with a clear head for practical politics, Basil no doubt saw the political implications of the Arians' elaborate charitable facilities.[138] Founding a great ptocheion at Caesarea which included a hospital and establishing similar institutions throughout Cappadocia formed part of Basil's campaign in Asia Minor on behalf of Nicaean orthodoxy. His efforts gained for the Nicaeans a strong base of support in Anatolia, paving the way for the complete triumph of the *homoousion* party under Theodosios I.

With the support of the imperial government after 380, the Nicaean party reestablished control of episcopal offices throughout much of the East. Although Arian factions were still strong enough to harass Bishop Nektarios in Constantinople, they had lost their leadership in the official church forever, both in the capital and in the other major sees of the East.[139] In many respects the Arian dispute revealed the debilitating weaknesses of Eastern Christianity: its failure to establish a reliable source of authority and its inability to enforce a measure of discipline among its bishops. On the other hand, the conflict stirred the church to action and roused her to meet the needs of the growing mass of urban poor, especially the many sick and infirm. Once peace was restored, most Arians eventually rejoined the established church so that the movement and its theology evaporated. Its medical hostels, however, remained. Basil enshrined them in his monastic movement and John Chrysostom placed the episcopal church of Constantinople firmly behind the new nosokomeia.

CHAPTER SIX

City, Church, and State

By the first decade of the fifth century hospitals were admitting the sick in Constantinople, in Caesarea, and possibly in other cities of Asia Minor and the East. The Pantokrator *Typikon* of the twelfth century proves that medical centers for the public were still operating in the Byzantine capital seven hundred years later. Born in the tumultuous years of the Arian crisis, these institutions not only survived the dramatic changes of later centuries; they experienced a remarkably vital development from 400 to 1204, the year in which Constantinople fell to the knights of the Fourth Crusade. Indeed, they came to occupy a significant place in the Byzantine conception of the polis. Since the East Roman Empire did not remain static during the centuries from the death of Chrysostom in 405 to the Latin conquest of Constantinople, it is necessary to look more closely at the individual xenones and nosokomeia during this long period in order to understand both the hospitals themselves and the shifting society which supported them.

Establishing a continuous tradition of Byzantine hospitals from Chrysostom's nosokomeia to those of twelfth-century Constantinople requires that one identify some concrete examples of hospitals both in the capital and in provincial cities of the East Roman Empire. To open the xenon door onto Byzantine society as a whole, however, one must venture beyond identifying hospitals to examine why these institutions flourished not only during the prosperous days of late antiquity, but even after the catastrophic events of the seventh century.

We have already discussed a fundamental reason for their survival—the attitude of Eastern Christianity toward medicine and physicians. Since the practice of medicine came to epitomize philanthropia in the sermons and treatises of Greek theologians and pastors, Christians naturally promoted medicine and institutions which dispensed it as fitting ways to express charity.[1] Thus, the Eastern churches, spurred on by the Arian conflict, had developed hospitals as one of the institutions which translated the commands of Christ into action.[2] After the victory of Nicaean orthodoxy, the church's teaching regarding philanthropia continued to sustain a concern for hospitals for the poor and anyone else in need until the Fourth Crusade and even afterward under the Palaeologan emperors.

Within this general framework of Christian social doctrine, which elements of Byzantine society actually provided the material support xenones
needed to carry out their philanthropic mission? Since Christian pastors had
taken the lead in establishing hospitals during the fourth century, one would
expect them to continue supporting such institutions in the centuries that
followed. As a survey of the sources will show, bishops did indeed keep
alive the hospital traditions of Basil and John Chrysostom at least until the
thirteenth century. Christian xenones, however, struck such deep roots in
the polis of the late ancient world that they were able to draw sustenance
from secular institutions as well. Ancient notions of civic pride as well as
concepts of imperial philanthropia motivated both private persons of wealth
and the emperors themselves to foster hospital care for the cities of the
empire. Indeed, the xenones became such vital fibers in the fabric of East
Roman society that they continued to flourish even after the drastic upheavals
of the seventh century. Nevertheless, the ways in which the church, the state,
and private citizens patronized hospitals changed significantly during these
many years, a process which did not always encourage the survival of well-
equipped xenones.

Although Byzantine sources illustrate that hospitals expanded their services and multiplied in number from the year 400 until 1204, xenon development occasionally experienced periods of difficulty. Just as the East Roman
Empire as a whole suffered many changes of fortune during these eight
centuries, so too the xenones would wax and wane in response to shifts in
the empire's political stability and economic prosperity. The greatest turning
point in the long life of the Byzantine state came in the first four decades
of the seventh century, when Persians, Avars, and the Moslem armies of the
Arabs ravaged the provinces. Since the society that survived these onslaughts
was markedly different from the prosperous world of late antiquity, we will
consider first the references to hospitals in the Eastern cities during the fifth
and sixth centuries and then direct our gaze at those xenones which operated
after the upheavals of the seventh century. We shall begin the inquiry with
the early hospitals of Constantinople.

EASTERN HOSPITALS IN THE FIFTH AND SIXTH CENTURIES

The capital of the East Roman Empire—the city of Constantine, the New
Rome—was famous for its philanthropy by the fifth century. The historian
Sozomenos claimed that the first Constantine had instituted philanthropic
services in his new capital so that it would surpass ancient Rome in glory.[3]
Fifth-century sources, however, offer very little evidence that many hospitals
were among the charitable institutions of the capital. Chrysostom's biographer, Palladios, provides the sole contemporary reference to fifth-century
nosokomeia which maintained physicians for their patients.[4] Additional evi-

dence must come from a much later source—the tenth-century *Book of Ceremonies* with its chronological list of ancient Constantinopolitan xenones.[5]

The first three xenones mentioned by the *Book of Ceremonies*—the Sampson, the Euboulos, and the Irene in Perama—were all built before about 450. These institutions certainly offered hospital services in the ninth century, when this chapter of the *Book of Ceremonies* was composed. But were these places hospitals in the fifth century?[6] It is possible to make the strongest affirmative case on behalf of the Sampson. All the extant sources describing this philanthropy—the versions of the *Vita Sampsonis,* the *De aedificiis* of Prokopios, and the novels of Justinian—agree that a physician first founded the Sampson as a hospital for the poor of Constantinople.[7] Moreover, when the Nika fire destroyed the institution in 532, it was housing only the sick.[8] Since Saint Sampson surely lived long before Justinian's reign and probably before 380, the hospital he founded must have served the poor sick of Constantinople throughout the fifth century. The older *Vita Sampsonis* and the *Miracula Artemii* demonstrate beyond doubt that the Sampson Xenon which Justinian restored after the Nika fire maintained an elaborate staff of physicians and surgeons and even accepted patients of the middle class.[9]

Regarding the Euboulos and the St. Irene in Perama, much less information has survived. Like the Sampson, the Euboulos sheltered the sick at the time of the Nika fire.[10] Moreover, Justinian built a church dedicated to the anargyros Tryphon next to it, a good sign that this institution served as a hospital as did so many other Byzantine philanthropic institutions linked with the shrines of the doctor-saints.[11] In the second half of the sixth century, the Monophysite missionary John of Ephesus described a staff of *hyperetai* (servants) at the Euboulos to assist the sick.[12] Although none of the extant sources mention staff physicians, there is no reason to believe that the Euboulos Xenon differed in this regard from the Sampson, a philanthropic institution with which it was often associated.[13]

Later tradition also assumed that the third xenon—St. Irene in Perama— had always been a hospital. The Patrographs recount how the saintly priest Markianos built a nosokomeion by this name in the mid-fifth century.[14] Moreover, the oldest version of the *Vita Marciani* contains indirect evidence that this priest had indeed founded a hospital and not a simple shelter for the poor. In recounting his efforts to restore the Church of St. Irene in Perama, where both the *Book of Ceremonies* and the Patrographs locate his xenon, the vita omits any reference to a hospital. It does, however, mention that many people afflicted with diseases and other physical sufferings sought relief at Markianos' holy house (*oikos*).[15] This Greek term could refer to the church itself, in which case the people would have been seeking miraculous cures. *Oikos,* however, could also mean a hospital where the sick would be seeking the treatments of secular medicine.[16] Since churches with famous shrines of healing were usually associated with xenones in Constantinople (recall the Church of Cosmas and Damian in Kosmidion), the vita offers some supporting evidence for the existence of a xenon at the Perama church, whichever meaning *oikos* has in this passage.

As additional evidence for the existence of a widespread network of hospitals in Constantinople before the reign of the emperor Justinian, it is useful to consider his reform of the public physicians—the archiatroi.[17] By removing the archiatroi from the jurisdiction of municipal officials and placing them in the wards of the Christian xenones, Justinian demonstrated that he and his contemporaries already considered these philanthropic institutions medical centers, not simple houses of charity. By his act, he also guaranteed that these hospitals would in the future provide their patients with access to the top echelon of the medical profession. As a result of Justinian's legislation, the simple doctors of Chrysostom's nosokomeia were replaced by a phalanx of specialized physicians and assistants.

In addition to the Sampson and the Euboulos, sixth-century Constantinople could claim several other hospitals. The famous monastery of Cosmas and Damian—the Kosmidion—maintained a xenon just outside the city walls that included a separate room for surgical operations and a bathing facility.[18] It is probable that this hospital had opened in the fifth century when the courtier Paulinos founded the Kosmidion complex.[19] Sometime in the sixth century if not before, the Christodotes Xenon must have opened. With its staff of archiatroi working in monthly shifts, its professional hypourgoi, and its hyperetai, this institution reveals most clearly the elaborate development of medical centers after Justinian's reorganization.[20] The *Book of Ceremonies*—supported this time by the reliable chronicle of Zonaras—reveals that a general named Narses founded a new hospital in Constantinople toward the close of the sixth century.[21] He dedicated it and an adjoining church to the anargyros Panteleemon. Again, no contemporary reference to physicians at the Narses Xenon survives, but the institution's later association with other Constantinopolitan hospitals as well as its dedication to the doctor-saint Panteleemon indicate that it served as a hospital.

Besides the xenones named in the sources, many others must have cared for the sick of Constantinople. According to Palladios, Chrysostom had opened several hospitals at the beginning of the fifth century. None of these have left any further traces in later sources.[22] The historian Sozomenos emphasizes the important role which the empress Pulcheria played in constructing shelters for the poor and for strangers.[23] The *Epitome of Theodore Anagnostes* refers to some of Pulcheria's philanthropic houses as *xenones.*[24] Given the ambiguity of this term before the sixth century, it is impossible to determine whether or not any of Pulcheria's foundations included medical services, but it is conceivable that some of them resembled Chrysostom's nosokomeia, which had hired professional physicians.

Constantinople was not the only city of the East to have hospitals in the fifth century. Jerusalem also opened philanthropic institutions with hospital services before the year 500. As early as 450 the empress Eudocia had built a number of pious houses in and around the Holy City. Although the sources describe some of these institutions as *nosokomeia* or *xenones,* there is no evidence that they offered professional medical care.[25] During the second half of the century, however, the monastic leader Theodosius constructed three separate houses (*oikoi*) for the ill, five kilometers south of Jerusalem: one for sick monks, one for the sick poor, and one for sick laymen above the poverty level. Theodosius' biographer, Theodore, states that the saint had designed these houses to provide medical care.[26] He either hired lay physicians or trained some of his monks in medicine to treat the patients with professional care. Since Theodosius immigrated to Jerusalem from a town in Cappadocia not far from Caesarea, it is likely that he had seen Basil's hospital there and patterned his charities near Jerusalem on that famous model. At the beginning of the sixth century, another monastic leader, Saint Sabas, persuaded the emperor Anastasios to build a huge nosokomeion of one hundred beds to treat strangers who fell ill in the Holy City. These patients would have come both from among the many tourists who flocked to Jerusalem to visit the holy places and from the poor immigrants of the countryside.[27]

At Alexandria, the metropolis of Egypt and still the center of Greek medical wisdom in the late ancient period, indisputable evidence of hospitals surfaces only in the early seventh century. Although the Arian bishop of Alexandria, George of Cappadocia, introduced xenodocheia for the poor and strangers into the Egyptian capital as early as the mid-fourth century, one can find no statement that these institutions offered any special care to the sick.[28] It is worth noting, however, that George had been an associate of the Anomoian leader Aetios, who had set about providing free medical care for the poor in Antioch.[29] In the fifth century the *acta* of the Council of Chalcedon mention that the patriarch Dioskoros (444–51) imprisoned an opponent in a xenon for the maimed. This account, however, offers too little information to establish that physicians practiced at this institution.[30] A hundred years later, when the orthodox patriarch Apollinarios constructed a church dedicated to the Three Children of the Fiery Furnace, he added to it both a gerokomeion and a nosokomeion. Once again, the sources contain no references to physicians.[31] Not before the seventh century is there a clear statement that doctors worked in Alexandrian hospitals. *The Life of John the Almoner* by Leontios of Neapolis refers to some of the patriarch's hospitals where physicians treated the sick in 612.[32] On the other hand, a fascinating papyrus from Antinoopolis, dated 570, illustrates that an archiatros governed a xenon for the sick in that city and that his father before him, also an archiatros, had managed the same hospital.[33] If a physician supervised medical treatment for xenon patients of provincial Antinoopolis a generation before 570 (i.e., ca. 550), patients at hospitals in the Egyptian capital surely enjoyed the same services at least as early as the mid-sixth century. Moreover, in listing professional guilds in Alexandria another papyrus document from the early seventh century mentions a fully developed association of medical assistants (*hypourgoi*) who worked in the city's hospitals.[34] Such a guild proves that organized medical staffs similar to those we saw in sixth-century Constantinople had been working in Alexandrian xenones for some time before the beginning of the seventh century, probably since Justinian's reforms regarding city archiatroi. Other papyri from the late sixth and seventh centuries provide ample evidence that nosokomeia and xenones had become common not only in Alexandria, but also in the smaller towns of Egypt.[35]

With regard to Antioch, where the first efforts were made to organize Christian philanthropic medical care, there exist only very brief references to hospitals of the sixth century and none to any of the fifth century. When Justinian rebuilt the city after the Persian sack of 540, he constructed a hospital for the citizens together with other public buildings. In his account of the rebuilding project Prokopios implies that nosokomeia had contributed to the quality of life in the Syrian capital in the years before the Persian attack.[36] According to the ecclesiastical historian Evagrios, Daphne, Antioch's fashionable suburb, also possessed a facility for the sick in the mid-sixth century, for the monk Thomas was taken to it for the treatment of severe injuries about 550.[37] (Thomas had received these wounds at the hands of the orthodox *oikonomos* Anastasios, who had struck him in an angry fit.) Perhaps this nosokomeion at Daphne was the same institution which Bishop Leontios had opened there in the fourth century.[38] Although neither Prokopios nor Evagrios mention doctors or hypourgoi at these Syrian institutions, they probably differed little from the hospitals of Constantinople and Alexandria, with their physicians and complex support personnel. Indeed, Justinian's reorganization of the public physicians applied to all the poleis of the empire, not just to Constantinople. Thus, cities such as Antioch as well as provincial Antinoopolis in Egypt must have had full-scale hospitals with physicians of the highest quality after Justinian's changes, if not before.

Very few surviving sources offer evidence of hospitals functioning in the smaller, provincial cities of the East Roman Empire. The fifth-century version of the *Vita S. Danielis Stylitis,* however, does include a vignette briefly referring to a nosokomeion at Ankyra. After falling among thieves, an unfortunate traveller was left for dead by the side of the road. Some men later rescued him, took him to nearby Ankyra, and entrusted him to the bishop. He, in turn, handed the injured man over to the city's nosokomeion for medical treatment.[39] Nothing in the story suggests that this hospital at Ankyra was something extraordinary. In addition, a simple gravestone found near Dervisos in Asia Minor commemorates a doctor named Theodore who worked for a provincial nosokomeion sometime in the fifth or sixth century.[40] Both the story about Ankyra and the gravestone indicate that hospitals had become common during the period before 600, not only in the great metropolises such as Constantinople and Jerusalem, but even in regional centers.

HOSPITALS AFTER 610

The first three decades of the seventh century visited a series of disasters upon the East Roman Empire that not only deprived the Byzantine state of its wealthiest provinces—Syria, Palestine, and Egypt—but also sapped many of its ancient cities of their vitality.[41] Despite the catastrophic invasions and the radical changes in economic and social life which began in the seventh century, Byzantine society still continued to support its hospitals. As with every other aspect of East Roman history after 600, we know most about the xenones in Constantinople.

Again, the *Book of Ceremonies* demonstrates that at least four Constantipolitan xenones survived the upheavals of the seventh and eighth centuries—the Sampson, the Euboulos, the Markianos (St. Irene), and the Narses (St. Panteleemon).[42] As one might expect, some hospitals, such as the Christodotes Xenon described in the *Miracula S. Artemii,* were apparently no longer functioning by the ninth century. Sources from the tenth through the twelfth centuries prove that the Sampson and the Narses continued to serve the sick until the sack of the city in 1204.[43] The last reference to the Euboulos, however, comes from the tenth century,[44] while no documents other than the *Book of Ceremonies* refer to the Markianos.

While some old hospitals of Constantinople vanished after 600, new ones were always opening up. The empress Irene founded a hospital together with other charities at the end of the eighth century.[45] Thirty years later, the emperor Theophilos opened a spacious xenon which afforded patients fresh air and a beautiful view of Constantinople along with healing medicines.[46] At the dawn of the Macedonian Renaissance, Basil I (867–86) constructed new nosokomeia and restored old ones.[47] In the early tenth century Romanos I Lekapenos founded the Myrelaion Xenon;[48] during the prosperous decades of the mid-eleventh century Constantine IX (1042–55) included a hospital in his extravagant Mangana complex.[49] We have already seen how John II Komnenos established the Pantokrator Xenon in the twelfth century. Even in the troubled years preceding the Fourth Crusade the emperor Isaak II Angelos found the resources to open the Nosokomeion of the Forty Martyrs.[50]

References to hospitals outside Constantinople are harder to find, but even in the provinces, Byzantine society continued to support xenones in the changed conditions which followed the Avar, Persian, and Moslem invasions. On the island of Crete in the eighth century, Archbishop Andrew founded a hospital which offered patients both comfort and medical care.[51] At the beginning of the ninth century, Metropolitan Theophylakt built a two-story hospital at Nikomedeia, providing it with a staff of physicians.[52] During the twelfth century, Thessalonica had a hospital which sheltered bed-ridden patients and distributed medicine to walk-in patients.[53] In 1156 Isaak Komnenos, the nephew of John II, opened a hospital offering limited medical services to the men in the Thracian town of Ainos.[54] Finally, in praising his native city of Nicaea, the thirteenth-century intellectual Theodore Metochites boasted that the Bithynian capital also had a hospital.[55]

THE HOSPITAL IN CIVIC LIFE

In his paean to Nicaea, Metochites reveals that he considered a xenon one of the hallmarks of urban life, just as ancient writers like Pausanias had counted aqueducts, theaters, and gymnasia as essential elements of a true polis. Conceiving of hospitals and other philanthropic institutions as integral parts of the polis did not begin with Metochites, or even with men who lived in the Middle Byzantine era (610–1204); rather, the notion first took shape as early as the late fourth century and assumed a definitive form by the sixth century.

The spiritual revolution of the fourth century not only affected men's religious beliefs; it profoundly changed the political organization of Greco-Roman society and its physical setting, the ancient city. We have already considered the process by which the local Christian church, represented by the bishop, came to hold a crucial position in the Greek polis of late antiquity.[56] As Christianity increased its influence over city governments during this century, it began to reshape the urban environment of the Eastern provinces. Studying the ruins of the great Christian basilicas reveals most strikingly the effect of the fourth-century synthesis of Christianity and classical culture on the physical city. In the East archaeologists have found these churches usually at the very center of the ancient polis, often replacing the old pagan temples. In 370 the church of Alexandria built its cathedral on the ancient agora.[57] During the reign of Theodosius I, the Christians at Damascus converted the old temple of Jupiter into a church.[58] This process gained momentum during the fifth and sixth centuries. Of the 245 churches from the late antique epoch which Professor Zakythinos examined on the Greek peninsula and the islands, 124 were erected on or very near the ruins of pagan temples in the very heart of the classical city sites.[59]

This same spiritual revolution introduced the hospitals onto the urban scene. As we saw in Chapter Five, during the second half of the fourth century, the Eastern churches developed xenones and other charitable institutions in response to demographic changes, to new political and social patterns, and to the internal ecclesiastical pressures generated by the Arian conflict. Once established, these institutions assumed an important place in the Eastern church's conception of a Christian community—the polis of God.

As the Christian churches shouldered ever greater responsibilities inside the polis, their leaders had to develop new concepts along with new institutions to express the Gospel message. In response to the tremendous changes both in society as a whole and within the church itself during the fourth century, Eastern bishops came to see the practice of philanthropia no longer confined to serving the brethren of a limited Christian community; rather, they conceived of it as a force which aimed at transforming the pagan world, represented by the ancient polis, into a truly Christian society, a heavenly city. In a sermon he delivered to his flock while still bishop of Constantinople, Gregory of Nazianz urged the citizens of the capital to make their polis a city of God (*Theou polis*) by turning away from the idle pleasures of pagan urban life—the races, the theater, the animal fights, corrupting luxury of all kinds—in order to aid the poor and care for the sick. Such philanthropia should guide a truly virtuous city. At the close of his sermon Gregory stirred his Constantinopolitan flock to greater acts of charity by appealing to their civic pride. They had already surpassed Rome itself in expressing philanthropia; he now urged them on to even more heroic acts of Christian love.[60] As bishop of Constantinople, John Chrysostom also encouraged the Christians of the Eastern capital to build a new society. They should follow the example of the early Christian community at Jerusalem, contributing their wealth to the common good so that all the poor of the city could eat.[61]

Neither of these sermons specifically mentioned the new charitable foundations as agents of civic philanthropia. In his funeral oration in honor of Basil, however, Gregory of Nazianz referred to his friend's ptochotropheion at Caesarea as a new city; he hailed it as a wonder of the world surpassing such marvels of civic achievement as the seven gates of Thebes, the Colossus of Rhodes, or the great temples of the pagan world. Here Gregory clearly expressed the new spirit of Christian civic pride and its relationship to charitable institutions. By supporting such philanthropies as Basil's ptochotropheion, the wealthy citizens of the Greek cities could win for themselves a reward far more enduring than the worldly renown which the grandees of the pagan past had gained when they had beautified their native towns.[62]

As a result of their fervent preaching and their own example, Eastern bishops were able to motivate wealthy Christians of the late fourth and fifth centuries to establish charitable institutions in their native cities. At Constantinople, a close friend and courtier of Theodosius II named Paulinos dedicated a shrine to the doctor-saints Cosmas and Damian which included a monastery, a hospital, and a public bath.[63] Sometime during the first half of the same century, a man named Euboulos founded his famous hospital.[64] Under the emperor Markianos the priest Markianos used his own resources to set up the nosokomeion that bore his name.[65] During these same years, a wealthy citizen and clergyman at Ephesus, Bassianos, provided the resources to build a ptocheion with seventy beds for his fellow citizens—most likely a hospital modeled on Basil's house outside Caesarea. Bassianos' ptocheion along with his other benefactions gained him great popularity among the people of Ephesus, just as the munificence of pagan aristocrats had won for them influence and renown in the Greek cities of the Antonine Age.[66] By the sixth century so many men and women of wealth were founding hospitals and other kinds of charities that the emperor Justinian had to draw up a number of guidelines in 544 and 545 for establishing such institutions.[67]

By the reign of Justinian charitable institutions had assumed a permanent place alongside theaters, baths, stoas, and other public buildings as essential features of a true polis. In describing Justinian's repairs at Antioch in 540, Prokopios mentions that the emperor not only provided the Syrian capital with a strong defensive wall, agoras, and graceful stoas, but also with beautiful churches and a large hospital for the sick.[68] In praising Justinian's building project in Cappadocia, Prokopios adds that the emperor expanded the simple fort of Mokesos into a true city by building churches, public baths, and xenones.[69] Again the emperor provided the Thracian settlement of Kiberis with baths, xenones, and other buildings such as befitted a city.[70] Justinian himself expressed the important position of hospitals in the polis when he issued a constitution in 530.[71] Citizens of any city had a right to interfere whenever a philanthropic institution failed to carry out its duty, since by its nature such an institution belonged to the community. Although Justinian drafted his legislation for all charitable foundations, he clearly had hospitals foremost in mind, since, in all the clauses of this constitution, he refers in detail only to one kind of philanthropic house—a xenon with beds for the sick. The sixth-century notion that the hospital helped to form a fitting polis survived the catastrophes of the seventh century, and was still alive in the mind of Theodore Metochites.

Philanthropic institutions in general took root in the Greek cities of late antiquity because they met the critical social needs of the local community. Hospitals, in particular, provided a valuable service by extending medical and nursing care to those who otherwise would have had no professional treatment. Christian xenones alone provided the members of the new demos of the fourth, fifth, and sixth centuries with access to trained physicians of the secular Greek tradition; they alone offered a patient of any class a chance to recuperate under professional medical supervision. As a result they rapidly eclipsed the older civic institutions of the medical profession—the public physicians or archiatroi—finally replacing them in the sixth century. Thus, a hospital of Justinian's reign with its highly skilled archiatroi and professional nurses had inherited not only the mantle of the early Christian deacons on their visits to the sick, but also that of the pagan doctors from Kos or Knidos who labored as public physicians for the poleis of classical Greece.

Although medical care for the sick first brought the hospitals to the attention of urban society in the East and remained the principal service which they offered the citizens of their poleis, they also fulfilled other civic functions. Justinian's Novel 59 reveals that the Sampson Xenon along with other hospitals had come to play a significant role in the free burial program of the sixth century, a system which apparently Constantine had instituted for all citizens of his new capital. Constantine had ordained that rents from 950 shops in his city be used for maintaining a corps of public pallbearers. By the time of the emperor Anastasios, the Great Church of Hagia Sophia collected the rents from these shops and supervised the city's funeral workers, men drafted primarily from the *collegii*—the guilds of the capital.[72] As Justinian reorganized the system, the *oikonomoi* of Hagia Sophia (the managers of the Great Church's resources) were to distribute money from the funeral fund to the administrator of the Sampson Xenon and to the heads of other hospitals so that they, in turn, could organize and pay the *asketriai,* communities of ascetic women who sang at the burial services and funeral processions.[73] Probably the xenones had begun their role in burying the city's dead by providing funerals for the poor who had expired in their wards. In carrying out this corporal work of mercy the xenones must have developed some system for conducting dignified services which the government later incorporated into its plan for publicly financed funerals for any citizen.[74] By the time of Leo VI (886–912), however, Justinian's complex system of free funerals had broken down.[75] The hospitals must have reverted to their former custom of burying only those who died while patients. To meet these more limited needs, the twelfth-century Pantokrator Xenon maintained only a special cemetery and chapel together with a cadre of pallbearers for some of its patients.[76] So, too, during the thirteenth century, the provincial town of Philadelphia had a cemetery for the poor attached to its hospital.[77]

As often happened in Byzantine society, political and social realities of late antiquity shaped the development of court ceremonies for centuries afterward. Thus, several celebrations at the imperial palace during the ninth and tenth centuries reflect the close relationship between hospitals and the great polis of Constantinople and its demos as that relationship had developed by the sixth century. On Palm Sunday, for example, the emperors of the ninth century greeted a number of officials who seem to have represented the people of Constantinople—citizens of the New Jerusalem. The list included the *demarchoi* of the city and the *demokratai* of the coastal districts (both regional officers of the people), but also the xenodochoi of six major hospitals, the head of the city's orphanage, and two financial officials of the church.[78] A similar ceremony took place on the Feast of the Prophet Elijah (July 20).[79] Moreover, on the tenth day of the Christmas celebration, the emperor received the administrators and archiatroi of the city's hospitals at a state banquet together with the Domestic of the Noumeron and the

Count of the Walls with all their subordinates—officers who policed Constantinople and defended its walls.[80] In all these ceremonies the xenodochoi of the hospitals appear along with dignitaries who either represented the people of Constantinople or ensured their security.

CONTROL OF HOSPITALS IN THE SIXTH CENTURY

THE BISHOPS, PRIVATE CHARITIES, AND JUSTINIAN'S NOVELS

From the fifth century hospitals occupied an increasingly prominent place at the heart of East Roman civilization, the Christian polis. Whether Constantinople or a provincial town like the Egyptian Ansinoë, the city had a strong interest in opening, maintaining, and regulating xenones.[81] But who spoke for the local community with regard to xenones? Who in the final analysis was responsible for securing continuous hospital services for the citizens of the polis? Historically, the bishops had played the leading role in organizing Christian charity. We have seen how they opened and supervised the early xenodocheia, ptochotropheia, and nosokomeia of the fourth century. The great promoters of permanent philanthropic houses—Leontios of Antioch, Makedonios of Constantinople, Eustathios of Sebasteia, Basil of Caesarea—all held episcopal seats.[82] Their successors in the fifth and sixth centuries continued the philanthropic building tradition. Bishop Rabbula constructed a xenodocheion for both the sick and the healthy in his Syrian city of Edessa.[83] A Palestinian inscription commemorates a bishop named Peter who founded a xenon for the town of Soada.[84] In the sixth century the orthodox patriarch of Alexandria, Apollinarios, constructed both a nosokomeion and a gerokomeion for his metropolis.[85]

As a result of their prominent role in opening philanthropic agencies, both the church universal and the state soon expected local bishops to secure hospitals and xenodocheia for their poleis. A fifth-century collection of ecclesiastical regulations from Syria included a paragraph which required the local bishop to maintain facilities for strangers, the sick, and the poor and to appoint a man to administer them.[86] The Fourth Ecumenical Council at Chalcedon (451) placed all ptocheia and xenodocheia inside a bishop's see under his jurisdiction, a rule which applied to hospitals as well.[87] A century later, in 544 and 545, the emperor Justinian issued two novels (nos. 120 and 131) which were supposed to give the canons of the church regarding episcopal jurisdiction over all charitable institutions the force of Roman law and also aimed at defining more precisely what the jurisdiction entailed.[88] In these two novels and others he issued Justinian treats all philanthropic agencies as a single class. From the lists of the various kinds of charitable foundations which he frequently incorporates into the text of his legislation and from the priority he assigns to xenones in his constitution on unspecified gifts to the poor, we know that he was often thinking of hospitals first.[89]

Although Justinian's legislation confirmed the Canons of Chalcedon by recognizing the bishop's ultimate responsibility for hospitals and other charitable institutions, it set some limits to his jurisdiction. Novel 120 recognized two classes of philanthropic institutions. Following Chalcedon, the first class stood directly under episcopal administration. Presumably, these were the nosokomeia, gerokomeia, and ptocheia which the bishop or one of his predecessors had founded with the resources of the episcopal church or with his own personal property. Institutions of the second class had independent status—their own administration (*dioikesis*) in the words of the novel. The director of such an independent house (the xenodochos or nosokomos in the case of a hospital) could lease or exchange the institution's property with the advice of his administrative assistants, called *chartoularioi*. Justinian did not require that the local bishop consent to the transactions of such independent houses, only that he be present when the director made such contracts.[90]

Novel 120 does not specify what sort of institutions had independent administrations. Novel 131, however, indicates that these self-governing institutions owed their existence to the wills of wealthy benefactors, private citizens who wished to establish specific philanthropic institutions in their own names.[91] Stirred by the example of bishops, by the vigorous sermons of men like Gregory of Nazianz and John Chrysostom, and by a Christian civic pride, sixth-century aristocrats were setting aside a portion of their estates in their wills to construct and maintain such institutions. In his will a benefactor could determine what sort of charity he wished to open, whom he wished to act as its director, and finally who would be responsible for its functioning after his death—usually the heirs of his estate. The heirs could even appoint directors after the death of the founder.[92] Following the Council of Chalcedon, however, Novel 131 gave the bishop some significant rights in the life of such an independent foundation. First, he played the leading ceremonial role in dedicating the new institution; second, he could compel the heirs of the testator to carry out the terms of the will within a year of the founder's death; third, he had the right to intervene whenever a private foundation ceased to carry out its stated purpose—in the case of a hospital, providing good medical and nursing care for the sick. Under such circumstances, the bishop could appoint a new administrator.

In the final analysis, Justinian's legislation upheld for the most part the role of the bishop in supervising all the charitable agencies of his diocese as the Council of Chalcedon had required. Although the bishop did not have rights of ownership over private foundations, the law still recognized his authority to intervene in these independent houses if he deemed that they were falling short of their philanthropic purpose. Thus, the local bishop continued to bear the ultimate responsibility for ensuring that his polis had adequate charitable institutions, a list which by the sixth century placed hospitals at the very top.

Justinian's novels, however, demonstrate that wealthy individuals were claiming a substantial role in supervising charities through the terms of their wills. When as a priest Chrysostom had urged the wealthy Christians of Antioch to contribute at least a tenth of their income to support those in need, he had in mind that they would donate gifts to the episcopal church for the bishop to administer as he and his clergy saw fit.[93] So, too, the fifth-century collection of ecclesiastical canons from Syria required that the xenodochos, an episcopal appointee, make collections from the faithful to supplement the income of the hospice. It did not consider the possibility that the donors would place conditions upon their gifts.[94] In the case of such general collections, clearly the donors had no mechanism to oversee the bishop's use of their gifts. In the spirit of these general collections, some individuals continued to leave legacies to the local church or named it as the heir, renouncing any right to control the use of their gifts. Justinian assumed that these testators who simply willed their property to Christ intended the local bishop to exercise control over their gifts.[95] But some testators wished to retain some control over the use of the gift. Like their classical forefathers, who had employed their wealth to build baths, stoas, and theaters for their fellow citizens, they wished to endow specific institutions to dispense philanthropia in their native poleis. We have already seen how Paulinos, Euboulos, and Markianos founded hospitals for the poor demos of Constantinople. Some of these Christian benefactors even tried to exclude the local bishop from any influence whatsoever over their foundations.[96] Justinian's Novels 120 and 131 helped to curb such tendencies by setting limits to the independence of private philanthropic foundations and by reaffirming the claim of the Universal Church, speaking at Chalcedon, that the bishop had to bear the ultimate responsibility for maintaining adequate charitable foundations.[97]

By allowing private persons to establish independent hospitals, old-age homes, hospices, and orphanages for their cities, Justinian and his imperial predecessors had given ample room to the ancient Hellenic ethos of civic pride, helping to direct the old habits of the pagan Greek polis into Christian channels. Such independent charities also released the bishop and his clergy from the burdensome task of overseeing every Christian institution within their see and probably provided more efficient and expert management for individual institutions, an especially important consideration with regard to hospitals, which required special managerial skills. Moreover, such independent institutions did not necessarily weaken the position of the episcopal office within the local church so long as the bishop could exercise a right of supervision. Constantinople offers an example where the bishop—here the patriarch—avoided any direct ownership of the city's many charities while maintaining a close relationship with the executives of the most prominent charities. As we have seen, several bishops of that city had supported charities; Chrysostom had clearly used episcopal revenues to finance new nosokomeia for the city.[98] Nevertheless, Novels 120 and 131 indicate that by the sixth century patriarchs of the capital no longer claimed any ownership over the city's extensive system of philanthropic institutions. Even two of the oldest and most prestigious among Constantinople's charities, the Orphanotropheion and the Sampson Xenon, had a status independent from the Great Church of the patriarch.[99] On the other hand, the patriarch exercised considerable authority over the Sampson Xenon as well as over the other hospitals of the capital. Through his officials, the oikonomoi and ekdikoi (lay business managers) of the Great Church, he coordinated the efforts of all xenones to ensure proper funerals both for patients who died in the hospitals and for any citizen of Constantinople whose relatives opted for a publicly financed burial service.[100] Moreover, in the reign of Justin II, we find the Euboulos Xenon at the disposal of both the emperor and the patriarch when they wished to imprison the Monophysite John of Ephesus there.[101] Finally, in the seventh century, the xenodochos of the Christodotes Xenon served in the patriarch's retinue, where he no doubt both advised his superior and also received direction in administering his hospital.[102]

IMPERIAL PHILANTHROPIA

Beside such local figures as the bishop and prominent individuals of the Christian community, the emperor himself assumed an ever-growing role in promoting and shaping the hospitals of the Greek cities. The predecessors of the Roman emperors in the East, the Hellenistic kings, had often financed building projects for cities which acknowledged their sovereignty or which simply allied with them. For example, Attalos II, king of Pergamon, constructed a graceful stoa for his allies, the second-century (B.C.) Athenians.[103] The Roman emperors continued this tradition of royal munificence. Also in Athens, Hadrian completed an immense temple to Zeus northeast of the Acropolis.[104] Such projects not only displayed the ruler's power; they also demonstrated his care for his subjects. Once the emperors became Christians, it was only natural for them to express their traditional munificence in Christian forms. Thus, Constantine not only built great churches for his new capital of Constantinople, but also constructed the famous basilica of St. Peter's in Rome and the Church of the Anastasis in Jerusalem.[105]

In addition to the tradition of public building, the Christian Roman emperors inherited the concept of royal virtue from their pagan predecessors. As Herbert Hunger has demonstrated, Greek and Hellenistic society had developed the notion that the good ruler ought to possess philanthropia. With its doctrine of agápe, Christianity only served to strengthen this old Greek concept.[106] The great rhetorician of the fourth century, Themistios, could tell the Christian emperor Constantius II that of all the virtues philanthropia most befitted the imperial office.[107] Thus, the first Christian emperor,

Constantine, was conforming not only to the dictates of his new religion but also to the traditional classical concept of the good ruler when he allotted a share of the *annona* collected in Syria to the clergy and xenodocheia of Antioch for the victims of famine.[108]

Although pagan tradition associated philanthropia particularly with the royal or imperial office, it also linked it directly to the practice of medicine. Thus, it venerated the god of medicine, Asklepios, as a deity who most expressed divine philanthropia. As Aristides declared, Asklepios was "the most philanthropic of the gods."[109] So, too, orthodox Christian tradition in the Greek East emphasized medicine as the very embodiment of philanthropia in action. When one considers that both pagan and Christian traditions exalted philanthropia as the emperor's especial virtue and that both considered the practice of medicine an ideal expression of such love for men, there should be no surprise that the emperors soon assumed a prominent role in supporting hospital care. As early as the 370s the emperor Valens patronized a Christian hospital by giving a substantial grant of land to Basil's ptochotropheion in Caesarea even though Basil was among Valens' theological opponents.[110] Subsequent emperors continued this tradition.

Unlike other benefactors, emperors could express their philanthropia toward hospitals in several ways. First, they could donate money or lands from their personal resources to establish or assist xenones just as private founders did. In such a manner, the emperor Valens had donated several villages from the *res privata* to support Basil's famous ptochotropheion. So, too, the powerful fifth-century empresses Pulcheria and Eudocia employed their share of the imperial estates to finance ptocheia, gerokomeia, xenones, and monasteries in Constantinople and Jerusalem.[111] In the sixth century the emperor Justin II apparently established a hospital from his private resources over which he continued to exercise rights of ownership along the lines of the private foundations described in Justinian's Novel 120.[112]

As the sole independent executive of the state and the undisputed master of the state's financial resources, the emperor could also apply public revenues to support hospitals. Constantine had done just this with the annona of Syria when he authorized a share of it for the xenodocheia.[113] So, too, at the request of Saint Sabas, Anastasios allotted a portion of the public revenues to construct and maintain a hospital at Jerusalem.[114] The greatest of the imperial benefactors, Justinian, used government funds to found, repair, or enlarge xenones in many cities. After he restored the Sampson Xenon in Constantinople with the wealth Belisarius had won from the Persians and the Vandals of Africa, he assigned tax revenues to the hospital and granted it landed estates to cover the daily expenses of maintaining medical services.[115]

Finally, as the source of law, the emperor could legislate to benefit both Christian philanthropic institutions in general and hospitals in particular.

Through the imperial constitutions of the two centuries from Constantine to Justinian, the Roman law came to the aid of all charitable houses by allowing them to accept legacies and to receive inheritances.[116] Imperial legislation also extended certain exemptions from extraordinary taxes and *munera* to the estates of the churches, philanthropic institutions, and monasteries.[117] Finally, beginning with Leo I, the emperors tried to protect churches and charitable foundations from unscrupulous magnates and corrupt administrators desirous of their extensive lands. They did this by forbidding alienation of any church property and by strictly defining the percentage of the estates which bishops or administrators of charities could lease and the terms of such leases.[118] By the time of Justinian's novels, Roman law both favored the estates of Christian philanthropic institutions with certain immunities and protected them from rapacious laymen.

Moreover, Justinian's legislation had profound effects on the development of hospitals in particular. First, when he reassigned the civic archiatroi to the hospitals, he not only provided the Christian xenones with society's leading physicians; he also assigned them civic and imperial funds which the curial councils had received to pay the public physicians.[119] Second, in Constantinople at least, Justinian provided the xenones with a stipend administered by the patriarch to pay for public funerals and with special authority over the *asketriai* of the city to conduct proper liturgies for the dead.[120] As a result of Justinian's reforms the hospitals became the largest of the Christian charities. To pay their elaborate staffs of archiatroi, assistant physicians, hypourgoi, servants, chaplains, and administrators (chartoularioi), they needed greater financial resources than did simple ptocheia or gerokomeia. As an example, the Pantokrator *Typikon* assigned far greater resources to maintain its xenon than it did to run its gerokomeion.[121] Though this typikon is dealing with twelfth-century philanthropic agencies, it probably reflects the relative expenses of sixth-century houses as well. In any case, as a result of Justinian's reorganization, hospitals came to outrank all other kinds of philanthropic institutions in Constantinople with the exception of the Orphanotropheion, an institution whose antiquity and significance in Late Roman law gave it special honor.[122] Justinian indicates that hospitals ranked first among charitable institutions in other Eastern poleis as well.[123]

THE DISMANTLING OF THE JUSTINIANIC SYSTEM

Justinian's legislation succeeded in achieving a delicate balance of forces with regard to founding and supervising charitable institutions. It allowed private donors a sufficiently large role in such endeavors as to keep alive the ancient tradition of civic munificence; at the same time it enabled the local bishops to exercise their canonical supervision over all Christian institutions of their sees. Finally, by its very concern for the empire's philanthropic agencies, Justinian's legislation emphasized the responsibility of the emperor himself in assuring that the cities had adequate charities. After Justinian's death, however, the East Roman state underwent a series of devastating shocks which totally altered Byzantine society and especially afflicted urban life. The provincial cities of Asia Minor almost disappeared, and even Constantinople never recovered the glory of Justinian's age.[124] These shocks never crushed the xenones; they survived in the capital and in provincial centers as well. The Justinianic system for administering hospitals and other philanthropies, on the other hand, vanished completely. When the emperor John II established the Pantokrator monastery, xenon, and gerokomeion in the twelfth century, he specifically excluded the patriarch—the bishop under whose jurisdiction the Pantokrator would have fallen according to Novel 120—from any role in administering the monastery or its dependent charities.[125] Moreover, the emperor's nephew, Isaak Komnenos, founded a monastery and hospital at Ainos which he too freed from any ties with the local bishop, the metropolitan, or the patriarch himself.[126]

Some contemporaries of John and Isaak Komnenos were aware that private foundations such as the Pantokrator complex or the monastery and hospital at Ainos violated both the church canons and the constitutions of Justinian. According to Theodore Balsamon, a learned canon lawyer of the twelfth century, Canon 8 of the Council of Chalcedon had granted authority to bishops both over the clergy and monks of pious houses and also over the institutions themselves. Indeed, Justinian had so interpreted this canon in his novels. Balsamon boldly asserted that monks and clerics of private monasteries and philanthropic houses of his own day were violating the canons when they denied the authority of the local bishop and claimed that the founders of their institutions and their heirs alone had jurisdiction over them.[127] A more conventional scholar, Zonaras, on the other hand, supported twelfth-century mores in his interpretation of Canon 8. He saw it as applying only to the clergy of philanthropic foundations who had responsibility for the spiritual care of the patients or guests of the houses. The bishop had to license the priest who performed the liturgy or heard the confessions of the patients.[128] This would seem to have been the standard interpretation of Canon 8 by that time, for the emperor John II did in fact allow the patriarch one function in his Pantokrator Xenon, the licensing of a chaplain to hear confessions.[129]

Why did Justinian's system of private foundations under episcopal supervision collapse so completely? Several reasons emerge from a careful consideration of sixth-century attitudes expressed in both private documents and in Justinian's laws themselves. First, the private founders did not firmly separate their institutions and the estates which supported them from the rest of their private property. Consider a papyrus from Oxyrhynchos dated 587. The heirs of the great Apion had donated 371 *artabae* of wheat to the

Nosokomeion of Abbot Elias. Menas, the administrator of the hospital accepting the gift, also worked for the donors as a *notarios*. Although the
editors of the Oxyrhynchos papyri admit that Menas could have held both
the hospital job and the notary post by chance, they do not rule out the
possibility that he filled these two positions because of some relationship
between the hospital and the Apion estates. Most probably the great Apion
had founded the Nosokomeion of Abbot Elias and left the appointment of
its supervisor to his heirs; they in turn chose a trusted employee of theirs,
Menas, to administer the hospital.[130] Menas' appointment did not violate the
regulations of Justinian, but it surely tended to confound the line between
the hospital and its property and the strictly private property of the Apion
family. Let us consider a second document, the will of the archiatros Flavianos
from Antinoopolis, dated 14 November 570, a document we have already
studied regarding the institution of the archiatroi. This testament not only
indicates something about public physicians, but also reveals how closely a
founder and his heirs linked private hospitals to their own property. Flavianos
names his children as the heirs of his estate and then designates his brother
John as the administrator of the xenon which their father willed to them.
Although Flavianos' will clearly dealt with the xenon separately from the rest
of his property, still he considered it family property—part of the patrimonial
land (*kata patroas paradoseis*)—and appointed a family member to oversee
its revenues and supervise the care of the sick; his brother John was probably
a physician, as he and his father were.[131] Here as with the Apion nosokomeion, the line distinguishing the hospital from the rest of the family's private
property was exceedingly thin.

   Second, Justinian's legislation failed to establish private philanthropic
foundations like the two Egyptian hospitals as self-governing institutions. The
thrust of the regulations in *Codex* 1.3.45 and Novels 120 and 131 was to
protect the founder's will, not to incorporate the privately founded charitable
agencies as independent legal entities. Even when Justinian authorized the
local bishop to intervene in private charities and to appoint new directors,
he was concerned with preserving the founder's will against negligent heirs,
not in protecting the hospital or old-age home from private control.[132] But
what was the bishop to do if the founder had expressly forbidden him to
intervene in any way? Indeed, Justinian dealt with such founders in his legislation. Novel 131 mentions testators and donors who had established special funds for redeeming prisoners of war and who had added clauses to
their bequests which specifically excluded the local bishop from any role in
administering the fund. Justinian declared that such exclusions were invalid
and that the bishop should intervene whenever he saw that the private
administrator of the fund was not carrying out the philanthropic purpose.[133]
Codex 1.3.45 refers to wills which excluded the bishop from any supervision
of a philanthropic institution such as a xenon. Here, too, Justinian ordered
the local bishop to ignore these clauses. Yet this particular constitution, issued

in 530, clearly demonstrates that the bishop intervened primarily to defend the wishes of the testator and only secondarily to represent the interests of the local community, the polis, in preserving charitable institutions.

In the final analysis Justinian's constitutions regarding private philanthropic houses suffered an internal contradiction. The emperor and his legal advisors had designed their legislation to defend the wishes of pious testators from negligent or dishonest heirs; yet in pursuit of this goal, they authorized the local bishop to ignore clauses in a founder's will or benefaction which specifically excluded episcopal intervention. Though no evidence has survived from the four tumultuous centuries between Justinian's death and the eleventh century, one can imagine that this contradiction together with the military and political crises which swept the empire after 565 gave rise to frequent disputes and litigation.[134] Moreover, some bishops no doubt abused the power of supervision, deposing private administrators on the slightest complaint. In such cases the heirs would have sought the intervention of the magistrate. In addition, some testators probably continued to include clauses in their wills which excluded the local bishop from any interference in their foundations. Such exclusions still provided heirs with a weapon against episcopal supervision which magistrates were willing to consider despite the rules which Justinian laid down against such provisions. The *Synopsis major* of the *Basilika,* a practical digest of the Justinianic corpus in its Greek redaction, indicates that the courts had robbed the bishops and their administrators of any real jurisdiction over private foundations well before the mid-tenth century. In summarizing Justinian's rules regarding private foundations, the *Synopsis* mentions only the bishop's right to demand that a founder or his heirs fulfill their promises; it omits any reference to the bishop's authority to intervene directly in the institution's administration by removing incompetent supervisors.[135] We have concrete evidence that the courts had completed the process of dismantling episcopal supervision of private philanthropic institutions by the reign of Basil II. In his decision regarding a private monastery, the most famous judge and jurist of the eleventh century, Eustathios Romaios, clearly stated that the patriarch of Constantinople had absolutely no jurisdiction over religious houses in his see over which his patriarchal church did not exercise property rights. Eustathios classified philanthropic institutions together with monasteries as religious houses.[136]

Further evidence from the eleventh century indicates that the principal weapon in fending off the bishop's claims remained an exclusion clause in wills or typika. In founding his ptochotropheion centered at Raidestos, the bureaucrat and lawyer Michael Attaleiates carefully banned the local bishop, the metropolitan, and the patriarch from any role in his foundation.[137] The oldest male heir of each generation was to assume the task of supervising the ptochotropheion. If he was suspected of mismanaging the foundation, his brother was to replace him.[138] Here the decision regarding the manager's capabilities or honesty had become a family affair in which the bishop had no place. Attaleiates' exclusions blatantly violated Justinian's rules, which were technically still in force as part of the *Basilika,* but the decision of Eustathios Romaios demonstrates that in practice the rights of the private founder had triumphed completely in civil law.[139] The twelfth-century commentaries to the Canons of Chalcedon indicate that most canon lawyers also recognized the exclusive rights of founders over all pious houses—monasteries and philanthropic agencies alike.

The eleventh-century typikon of Attaleiates excludes not only the bishop from any role whatsoever in his ptochotropheion, but also the emperor himself and his officials. Attaleiates wanted his agency to be free and totally self-governing save for the ordinary jurisdiction of the courts over any private property.[140] The twelfth-century *Typikon of the Kosmosoteira* contains similar clauses directed against imperial interference in the monastery and hospital at Ainos.[141] If a trained lawyer and experienced bureaucrat like Attaleiates added such clauses against any supervisory power which the state might claim over philanthropic agencies, it is probable that the courts often supported the wishes of such private founders even against official supervision.[142] Indeed, the twelfth-century emperor John II exempted his own Pantokrator complex from the jurisdiction of the ordinary state offices and from those which managed his palace estates.[143] Such exemptions again contravened Justinian's constitution of 530, which empowered the civil magistrate—usually the local civil governor—to assist the bishop in ensuring that all privately founded philanthropic institutions faithfully carried out their pious works.[144] Reinterpretation by generations of magistrates had freed private charities from any control other than that of their founders and their heirs, certainly by the eleventh century if not before.

That such private charities fell outside any public supervision no doubt weakened the network of Byzantine hospitals. First, since the heir of the founder had gained unlimited control over his foundation, he could mismanage the pious house in any way he wished. He could pocket revenues, cut services, and even close the institution completely without fear of civil or ecclesiastical authorities. Northern Italy provides a good example of how such unlimited private control over philanthropic agencies could destroy them. Since Italy formed part of Justinian's empire, it received the same laws regarding ecclesiastical organizations which the emperor had established to regulate the independent philanthropic institutions of the Eastern provinces. With the eclipse of East Roman authority on the Italian peninsula after 568, the Justinianic system of administering charities rapidly disintegrated. No ecclesiastical or civil power made any sustained effort to oppose the rights of private individuals over their charitable or monastic foundations.[145] In 850 the Synod of Pavia complained bitterly about the fate of philanthropic institutions in particular. It described how rapacious heirs systematically pillaged the xenodocheia and other pious houses over which they exercised own-ership.[146] There is no evidence of similar rapacity on the part of Byzantine owners. Perhaps public opinion restrained such excesses; perhaps too East Roman society considered such dealings totally within both civil and canon law in the centuries after Justinian's death and simply did not register any complaints.

As the system of totally independent, private foundations evolved under Justinian's successors, it threatened the quality and even the survival of public hospitals in the Byzantine Empire. Because the founders of such independent charities often had family interests foremost in their minds in establishing and governing their agencies, they relegated philanthropic goals to second place. As Paul Lemerle had observed, Attaleiates founded his ptochotro-pheion at Raidestos not just for his spiritual benefit, but for temporal gain as well. By supporting such a private charity, he organized his family's prop-erty as a more stable unit which now enjoyed certain legal advantages. More-over, it might attract unconditional gifts from others in future years.[147] Once the expenses of the ptochotropheion and its monastery had been met, At-taleiates and his heirs could claim any surplus revenues. If a founder placed a high priority on such motives, he would certainly not choose a xenon as a pious front for his schemes. Maintaining a hospital and its expensive staff of physicians, medical assistants (hypourgoi), and servants would no doubt have convinced self-seeking founders to opt for simple hostels or poorhouses as their family's investment in the future, institutions with much less over-head. The records of Eustathios Romaios indicate that some privately founded hospitals did in fact exist in the eleventh century, but they have left almost no traces in the sources before the Palaeologan period.[148] I have found only two private hospitals founded after 600 and before 1261. One of these hospitals—the institution which Isaak Komnenos financed at Ainos in the mid-twelfth century—employed only one physician and ten medical assis-tants, a small staff when compared to the nineteen physicians and thirty-four medical assistants who worked at the imperial Pantokrator Xenon.[149] It seems safe to assume that private xenones were either less numerous than ptocho-tropheia such as Attaleiates' foundation or of such a limited nature that they differed only slightly from simple ptochotropheia or gerokomeia. Indeed, Isaak called his small hospital at Ainos a gerokomeion although it admitted sick men of any age.[150]

HOSPITAL ADMINISTRATION AFTER 600

The collapse of ancient society at the end of the sixth century radically altered the nature of the Greek polis and of local aristocracies. The changes this collapse wrought, including the shifts in Byzantine law which we have just discussed, greatly limited the role of private support for hospitals after 600.

The local bishops and individual emperors, however, retained their interest in maintaining public hospitals during the centuries of changing fortunes which the reign of Herakleios ushered in and thereby guaranteed their survival.

Despite the loss of public authority which the bishop suffered at the hands of magistrates in the years after 565, he still represented the local Christian church, he still controlled the institutions and property belonging to the episcopal office proper, and he still had ownership of his personal property. As the visible representatives of the church, Eastern bishops after 600 did not abandon their traditional role in supporting public hospitals, even if they had to use their personal property. In the eighth century, Saint Andrew, archbishop of Crete, employed his own resources to build a hospital for the sick of his flock.[151] Surely control of this institution remained in the hands of Andrew's episcopal successors. In the ninth century Theophylakt, metropolitan of Nikomedeia, displayed his philanthropia by building a well-equipped hospital for his city, perhaps with his own resources.[152] Indeed, such philanthropia on the part of Eastern bishops struck contemporary Christians of the Latin West as distinctively oriental. When Bishop Praeiectus of Gaul financed a hospital for twenty patients in his city of Clermont with his own property, his biographer emphasized that he was following the regular practice of Eastern bishops.[153] Visiting Antioch in 1049, the renowned Arab physician Ibn Butlan noted that the city's hospital was directly under the patriarch's care.[154] When Thessalonica fell to the Norman Sicilians in 1185, the only hospital in the second city of the empire belonged to the episcopal church.[155] In the new world which followed the Persian and Arab invasions of the seventh century, Eastern bishops continued to view medicine and the Christian institutions which dispensed it as ideal vehicles to express the central Christian virtue of charity. According to his biographer, Bishop Theophylakt's hospital at Nikomedeia perfectly reflected his love and care for those in need.[156]

Episcopal support seems to have played the leading role in ensuring hospital facilities in provincial towns like ninth-century Nikomedeia. Even in the troubled thirteenth century Bishop Phokas of Philadelphia labored to build a xenon for his town. But the emperors shouldered the heaviest share of the burden in financing public medical institutions in Constantinople and probably assisted a number of provincial towns as well. Their unflagging patronage of hospitals guaranteed the survival of these expensive institutions in the face of military, political, and economic crises. Moreover, their strong support guaranteed an adequate system of hospitals even after the legal system ceased to protect the public interest from the whims of those powerful men and their heirs who controlled private philanthropic institutions.

The emperors after Justinian continued to use their absolute authority over all public revenues to provide adequate resources for the empire's xenones. The eleventh-century Ashburner Treatise states that emperors up to Leo VI had often given hospitals tax exemptions to help them maintain their charitable activities. To ensure that these xenones were no longer bothered by the tax collectors, the emperors had the exempt estates of privileged hospitals struck from the local tax register.[157] They also authorized regular distributions from the public treasury to pay hospital officials and other staff.[158] As part of this system, rulers after Justinian began to absorb xenon administrators into the imperial bureaucracy, so that by the time Philotheos prepared his *Kletorologion* in the ninth century, xenodochoi held regular positions in the government. In his list of offices, Philotheos ranks them as subordinates of the administrative assistant (*chartoularios*) of the central treasury (the *sakellion*) along with imperial *notarioi*, the *protonotarioi* of the themes, gerokomoi, and a number of other officials.[159]

Although the term *xenodochos* could refer to directors of xenodocheia just as well as to the chiefs of medical xenones, a careful comparison of passages within the *Kletorologion of Philotheos* and an appeal to the tenth-century *Book of Ceremonies* will establish not only that the xenodochoi under the chartoularios of the sakellion (the administrative assistant of the central treasury) governed hospitals but also which hospitals these men supervised. First, the *Kletorologion* refers to the administrative assistant of the treasury toegether with the subordinate xenodochoi in two pasages besides the roster of officials just cited. Where it describes the court ceremonial on Palm Sunday and on the Feast of Elijah (20 July), the *Kletorologion* stipulates that on both days the administrative assistant of the treasury and the xenodochoi—presumably those who reported to him—should present crosses to the emperor.[160] The *Book of Ceremonies* describes the Palm Sunday commemoration in greater detail. In listing the xenodochoi who participated, it indicates the institutions they directed—the Theophilos, the Sampson, the Euboulos, the Markianos, the Narses, and the Xenon of St. Irene.[161] All of these, as we have seen, were prominent medical xenones, not simple xenodocheia. Moreover, in its rules for the banquet on the tenth day of the Christmas celebration, the *Kletorologion* itself links to hospitals the *xenodochoi* having sufficient rank to participate in imperial ceremonies. There it describes the xenodochoi not only in the company of their superior, the treasury's administrative assistant, but with their subordinates—the archiatroi and legal officers of their medical xenones.[162]

The hospital xenodochoi under the chartoularios of the sakellion no doubt reported to him because they received substantial, regular disbursements from the central treasury. Probably they collected the annona grants which the government paid to the archiatroi on the hospital staffs.[163] In the prosperous days of the Late Roman Empire the archiatroi of Constantinople and Rome had received their annona allotments directly from the treasury of the praetorian prefect, as had professors and other municipal officers.[164]

When Justinian placed the archiatroi under the jurisdiction of the Christian hospitals, it was logical that their new supervisors, the hospital xenodochoi, thereafter reported to an official of the central state treasury. Thus, in the ninth century we find xenodochoi under the jurisdiction of the chartoularios of the sakellion, the second officer of the central treasury at that time.[165]

The *Kletorologion of Philotheos* reveals that xenodochoi usually held the honorary imperial rank of *spatharios*.[166] As holders of this rank, they themselves received regular government stipends as well as irregular donatives.[167] A lead seal from the ninth century proves that at least one xenodochos at the provincial town of Loupadion had received the higher title of *protospatharios*, the lowest grade of senatorial rank.[168]

The *Kletorologion* also presents evidence of a significant change in the method the emperors used to organize and finance philanthropic institutions, a change which parallels the evolution in the legal status of private philanthropic houses. According to the *Kletorologion* three xenodochoi— most probably the supervisors of medical xenones—reported, not to the administrative assistant of the central treasury, but to the *megas kourator*.[169] Since this last official supervised most of the imperial estates and palaces throughout the empire, it seems reasonable to assume that the three pious institutions which these particular xenodochoi governed were considered to be divisions of imperial property and were financed by revenues from the emperor's private estates, organized in the ninth century as the *kouratori-kion*.[170]

During the tenth century, this novel method of imperial patronage was used to finance all of the new hospitals in Constantinople. The emperor Romanos I established his famous monastery and xenon at the Myrelaion by remodeling one of the imperial palaces.[171] Rather than setting up the new hospital as an independent legal entity represented by its director, he conceived of the Myrelaion Xenon and the other institutions of his complex as simple divisions of his private property. As a result, all references to the Myrelaion complex in the narrative sources refer to it as a palace belonging to the emperor Romanos.[172] One never finds such expressions of ownership in documents describing the Sampson Xenon restored by Justinian or the hospital built by Theophilos in the early ninth century. Since the Myrelaion was a division of the imperial estates, the megas kourator no doubt continued to manage its resources, just as he did the property of all other imperial palaces with the exception of the Mangana.[173] Thus, in establishing the Myrelaion Xenon, Romanos employed the same system which recent emperors had used to support the three xenones or xenodocheia which the *Kletero-logion* listed under the megas kourator.[174]

The evidence indicates that the Myrelaion Xenon had a different status from the older hospitals: it was the emperor's private foundation, not a public institution of Constantinople. By the eleventh century Eustathios Romaios classified the Myrelaion and other private imperial foundations as privileged pious houses which alone enjoyed the rights of the *demosion*—in this context, no doubt the rights of the imperial estates. It is significant that he did not list as an example of an imperial foundation any of the older xenones, such as the Sampson or even the Theophilos; these did not owe their foundation to an endowment from the *kouratorikion*, even though emperors or empresses had established several of them.[175]

The Myrelaion Xenon of Romanos and the three earlier hospitals or hospices listed under the office of the megas kourator thus represent philanthropic agencies with a new legal status: those ranked as divisions of the emperor's private estates. By founding xenones in this manner, Leo VI, Romanos, and subsequent emperors were acting as other individuals of the empire were doing when they assigned a section of their estates to support charitable institutions. Theophilos seems to have been the last emperor to open a large xenon in Constantinople supported with public revenues (either by tax exemptions or direct disbursements) or with outright gifts of land, endowing ownership. When Romanos opened the Myrelaion Xenon a hundred years later, the new system of imperial foundations was firmly established. It is thus likely that the ninth century also saw the final steps in the process by which the magistrates redefined hospitals and other pious houses of nonimperial founders as private property instead of the independent, quasi-public institutions that Justinian had considered them to be.

During the tenth and eleventh centuries the emperors frequently rearranged the offices which managed their private estates including the property assigned to the imperial xenones. By 1019 they had reorganized the estates of hospitals and other philanthropies under a new official, the *oikonomos* (manager) of the pious houses (*oikonomos tōn euagōn oikōn*).[176] Although this official managed the estates of all imperial xenones to ensure the necessary revenue, he probably had little role in supervising the daily routines of the hospitals.[177] These were still subject to xenodochoi or nosokomoi, now relieved of legal and financial responsibilities. At some point in the eleventh century, the imperial government once again reshuffled the imperial estates so that now the Myrelaion complex had its own office. Two hagiographical texts refer to provincial officials in the Thrakesion theme who oversaw the estates of the Myrelaion only.[178] So, too, the Petrion complex— a monastery, xenon, and gerokomeion founded by Constantine VII as a replica of Romanos' Myrelaion—also had obtained a separate office to manage its lands by the time Emperor Nikephoros III issued a chrysobull to the lawyer Attaleiates in 1079. The same document mentions a separate official in charge of the estates supporting a prominent imperial gerokomeion in Constantinople.[179] Despite this great flexibility in estate management, the imperial lands, both those supporting palaces and those financing philanthropic houses, never lost their status as the emperor's private property. Thus, individual emperors or their advisors could combine the estates of imperial xenones with those of the *megas kourator* or separate them under independent bureaus without affecting their legal status.

In the twelfth century, the whole system of managing the resources of imperial philanthropic agencies changed. When John II Komnenos founded the Pantokrator complex, he exempted the institution and its estates not only from all public officials, including the collectors of the regular state tax, but also from the officials of all the offices which supervised imperial lands, the welter of bureaus which the tenth and eleventh centuries had spawned.[180] The emperor placed the management of the Pantokrator's estates directly under the superior of the monastery and his four oikonomoi. They in turn made sure that the xenon received the necessary resources to fulfill its mission as outlined in the emperor's typikon.[181] The Comnenian system must have halted the proliferation of central bureaus to manage the resources of imperial charitable agencies, and also have saved the emperor money, since the superior and his assistants did not receive regular government salaries.

To determine why emperors after Theophilos abandoned the older method of establishing autonomous hospitals, subject only to the public power of the local bishop, in favor of private imperial foundations, one must examine the problem of private ecclesiastical foundations in general, a vast subject outside the scope of the present work. The shift, however, had one important effect on hospitals and the medical profession in general which is visible in the twelfth-century Pantokrator Xenon. The director of this hospital—the nosokomos—had no financial or legal responsibilities in managing the hospital's properties; these the superior and his oikonomoi shouldered, leaving the nosokomos free to supervise the staff and the provision of essential supplies.[182] This contrasts sharply with the xenodochoi in Justinian's legislation, who were constantly absorbed in legal activities—land sales, land transfers, and other problems involving the properties of the hospitals.[183] As a result, the xenodochoi of the earlier period were not physicians. The sources usually indicate that they were both ecclesiastics and men with some legal training.[184] By the twelfth century the nosokomoi were regularly selected from the medical profession.[185] Moreover, the chartoularioi, the legal advisors so prominent in the independent xenones of Justinian's time, have disappeared at the Pantokrator and other twelfth-century hospitals.[186] Although I have no textual evidence for placing the change in the professional expertise of hospital directors any earlier than the Comnenian age, it seems likely that the shift from legal to medical leadership must have taken place when the emperors ceased creating independent xenones on the model of Justinianic philanthropies and began to establish hospitals as subsidiaries of the imperial estates.

Despite the many changes in the form of imperial support for xenones between the sixth to the twelfth centuries, emperors never failed to use their vast powers and material resources to provide medical care for the public. Whether they authorized disbursements from the public treasury for hospital salaries, granted property together with rights of ownership, or simply set aside particular lands from the imperial estates, they recognized the obligation which rested on the office to insure that the citizens of their empire had access to hospital care. Indeed, patronizing hospitals seems to have become a particularly conspicuous and appropriate means of displaying imperial philanthropia. Emperors were especially anxious to link their names and their families to prominent xenones. Theophanes Continuatus mentions that the new emperor Theophilos manifested his care for the city of Constantinople first by repairing its walls and second by establishing a xenon.[187] So that the citizens would have a clear sign of his philanthropia, Theophilos named his richly adorned hospital after himself. In founding the Myrelaion Xenon, Romanos also wanted to link his own name and that of the Lekapenos family to a hospital. Not only did he finance the xenon and the other institutions of the Myrelaion complex from imperial lands, but he also ordained that he and his children should be buried at its church. The Myrelaion complex thus served as a living monument to Romanos' philanthropia.[188] Thereafter, pious foundations which included xenones often housed the tombs of the emperors. When Constantine IX Monomachos died in 1055, he was buried at the Mangana Palace, which he had reorganized to support both a xenon and a gerokomeion.[189] In the next century John II designed the Pantokrator on the model of the Myrelaion. It too consisted of a public church, a monastery, a hospital, and an old-age home, as well as the mausoleum of the Komnenoi family. The Palaeologan house followed the same tradition in the thirteenth century. The wife of Michael VIII, the empress Theodora, founded a monastery for women together with a xenon, a complex which she, too, designed as the imperial mausoleum.[190]

In summary, the imperial office remained a firm supporter of xenones in the Eastern Empire. Although private persons continued to found philanthropic institutions after the collapse of the Late Antique world, it is doubtful that they were ever willing to commit enough resources for such purposes to maintain the kind of elaborate institutions of medical care which the sources depict during the centuries from the reign of Justinian to 1204. The large hospitals of Constantinople—those institutions which one medical treatise calls the great xenones—were surely imperial foundations, xenones like the Myrelaion or the Pantokrator.[191] Some of the public xenones of the ancient days, such as the Sampson and the Panteleemon, no doubt achieved the same grandeur as the private imperial foundations, but it is unlikely that these venerable houses of charity could have survived the five centuries from Justinian's death to the Latin conquest if the emperors had not showered them with tax exemptions, land gifts, and regular disbursements from the public treasury. So long as the emperors continued to express philanthropia by supporting old xenones and founding new ones, the Byzantine Empire was assured the luxury of hospital care of the quality we have seen described in the Pantokrator Typikon.

During the prosperous days of the late ancient world hospitals assumed a central place in the Christian notion of a city. By the reign of Justinian, a true polis had to have first its church, but next its hospital, followed by other philanthropic institutions. When the urban culture of the late ancient world of the East collapsed in the seventh century, Christian doctrine regarding the practice of philanthropia combined with notions concerning the duties of bishops and emperors so that both the civil government and the official church channeled sufficient resources to assure the survival of well-staffed hospitals.

Eastern Christianity also provided another rich source of enthusiasm for xenones—the monastic movement, a movement which tapped both the material and spiritual strengths of Byzantine society for the benefit of hospitals. Almost from the very first, the ascetics of the Eastern church involved themselves not only in organizing and administering xenones but also in serving their patients personally. In order to understand better the xenones of the Byzantine Empire as well as the ascetic impulses which helped to sustain them, we must now consider the complex relationship between public hospitals and Orthodox monasticism.

CHAPTER SEVEN

Monasticism

When Basil opened his hospital at Caesarea, he designed it as an integral part of his monastery.[1] An ascetic community also governed Eustathios' ptochotropheion at Sebasteia; its administrator, Areios, was a fervent monastic leader.[2] Regarding Constantinople, the historians Socrates and Sozomenos always associated Marathonios with charitable houses, including those for the sick, and with ascetic communities.[3] Among the fourth-century promoters of philanthropic medical care, only the Anomoians functioned outside of the monastic milieu.[4] Once the bishops of the homoiousion party and their ascetic supporters began to eclipse the radical Arians during the 360s, the monks of Asia Minor came to dominate hospitals and other charitable institutions, a domination which continued until the Council of Chalcedon in 451. Thereafter, the monks still played an important part in maintaining xenones until the very last days of the East Roman Empire.

The role of monks in Byzantine hospitals is closely associated with one of the major questions in Orthodox Christian monastacism, the relationship between *praxis* and *theoria*. Some monastic leaders thought that praxis, the practice of Christian charity in the world, threatened the ascetic life of prayer and contemplation, or theoria; others believed that praxis was essential to any true Christian asceticism. Whenever monks stressed praxis, the way was open to their work in hospitals; whenever they emphasized pure theoria, they withdrew from hospital service. Even when monks turned away from praxis, however, they did not necessarily sever all ties with public hospitals. Monks were involved in Byzantine xenones in two ways: they worked in them as doctors or nursing attendants, as they did at John Chrysostom's nosokomeia in Constantinople, or they simply supported a xenon with some of their endowment and supervised its financial side, as the superior and oikonomoi of the Pantokrator managed their hospital in twelfth-century Constantinople. In order to follow the shifting relationship between Eastern monks and xenones, let us begin by studying some of the early Greek Fathers of monasticism and their views regarding Christian praxis.

PRAXIS AND THEORIA

The first monk of the Byzantine tradition, Anthony of Egypt, took no interest in carrying out any of the corporal works of mercy—Christian praxis. His response to the Gospel message was to flee the world. Upon hearing Christ's command, "Go and sell all that you have and give to the poor; . . . and come follow Me" (Matt. 19:21), Anthony rid himself of all property with no thought of how it would be used. He abandoned even the care of his sister to some pious women so that he could flee into the desert.[5] He desired pure theoria—prayer and contemplation in solitude—not Christian praxis. As one might expect, Anthony played no part in the formation of philanthropic institutions, although his life spanned much of the fourth century.

About 320, one of the Egyptian solitaries, Pachomios, decided that the life of the lone hermit lacked the opportunities of Christian fellowship. At Tabennesi, he established the first cenobitic monastery, a community of monks living and praying together.[6] Although they were located away from the cities, the fourth-century Pachomian monasteries maintained simple xenodocheia to house guests of the community, just as the episcopal churches of the towns did.[7] These xenodocheia, however, never became active agents of charity. Their purpose was to house people from outside the monastery in a place apart from the monks, that is to preserve the ascetics from contamination with the world.[8] There was thus little chance that these Egyptian xenodocheia would evolve into specialized charitable agencies. Pachomios saw his cenobitic communities as great fortresses whose walls and communal fellowship offered a defence against the assaults of the devil, not as communities to carry out the Christian duties toward the unfortunate.[9]

To such solitaries and cenobitic communities the young Basil of Cappadocia came about 358 in search of the perfect Christian life.[10] A man trained in the best analytic tradition of Greek philosophy and science, Basil had studied the Holy Scriptures with great care. When he saw the monks of Egypt, Palestine, and Syria, he was amazed by their ascetic heroics, but he was struck too by their failure to carry out the corporal works of mercy. Basil understood that Christ expected his followers to clothe the naked, to feed the hungry, to visit the sick—in short, to carry out Christian philanthropia.[11]

Basil found the monastic movement of his native Anatolia much more appealing. Here the ascetics had not fled to the mountains or the desert wilderness; rather, they had chosen to live in or near towns.[12] They considered serving the poor and the needy among their primary duties. As we saw in Chapter Five, one of their leaders, Eustathios, established a large ptochotropheion in Sebasteia that probably included medical facilities for the sick. His colleague, Marathonios, carried out a similar program in Constantinople. This urban monasticism of Anatolia and the regions around Byzantium Basil adopted and enshrined in his ascetical works.[13]

Basil and his friend Gregory of Nazianz considered it necessary that the truly Christian life incorporate both theoria and praxis, both prayer and the works of mercy. Gregory believed that action in the world should be the serving brother of the spiritual life.[14] Basil expressed this idea more force-fully: "This life of ours [the monastic life] is not only valuable for mortifying the flesh, but also for loving our neighbor in order that God might offer sufficiency through us to the sick among the brethren.[15] Thus, Basil designed the monastic communities he founded so that his followers would have the opportunity both for quiet prayer and for active philanthropy. Under his ascetic system the contemplative life would complement the life of service just as the sea enhanced the dry land.[16]

Two of the giants in the Orthodox tradition, Basil of Caesarea and Gre-gory of Nazianz wrote sermons, tracts, and letters recommending an ascetic life nourished by contemplation yet active in the world. Moreover, Basil established his vast ptochotropheion with its hospital as one of the organs through which his monks could express their active philanthropia.[17] The writings and actions of these leading Fathers helped give momentum to the active monastic movement. Twenty years after Basil's death in 379, monks worked as nurses in the hospitals of Constantinople under John Chrysostom's episcopacy.[18] During the fifth century monks supervised or worked in many of the charitable agencies in the Christian churches of the Eastern provinces. Bishop Rabbula of Edessa found pious ascetics to care for patients in the hospital he had opened.[19] The customs of the Syriac church, collected some-time during the same century, stipulated that the local bishop should appoint a monk to supervise his church's xenodocheion.[20]

The active ascetic life which Gregory and Basil championed had devel-oped out of a movement Gilbert Dagron has called Anatolian monasticism or the urban monastic movement. In their early days in Anatolia, however, the urban monks had displayed a number of traits which irritated the epis-copal leadership of the church. The Council of Gangra (ca. 340) had con-demned some of them for their extreme views on asceticism and their failure to recognize the established church.[21] Under the leadership of Eustathios and Marathonios, men closely tied to the episcopal structure, the monks had worked in relative harmony with the established local churches, though even Eustathios had had trouble with the ascetic director of his ptochotro-pheion.[22] Basil, too, was able to harness the enthusiasm of the Anatolian monks for the work of the episcopal church in Caesarea. Before his election as bishop, however, while still the spokesman of the local monastic move-ment, Basil himself had quarreled with his bishop Eusebios.[23] After Basil's death, his successor on the episcopal throne, Helladios, fought with the monk he himself had appointed to supervise the city's ptochotropheion and mon-astic community.[24]

The struggle between the episcopal office and the urban monks reached serious proportions in Constantinople when John Chrysostom was appointed bishop of the capital. Chrysostom began a major campaign to impose disci-pline on ascetic groups in his city. As Dagron has emphasized, the urban monks of Anatolia and Constantinople did not usually live in stable cenobitic monasteries. Rather, they lived celibate lives in smaller communities (*syn-oikiai*), while they worked in charitable foundations, served in *martyria*, or simply walked the streets of the town. Such communities had fluid populations and often included women.[25] As bishop, Chrysostom set down stricter guidelines for this restless group of active men and women. He wanted them either to live in cloistered, cenobitic houses or to withdraw into the wilderness as the earliest monks had done.[26] He also wanted to halt the practice of both men and women living in the same ascetic community.[27] Since Chrysostom perceived the active monks as a source of trouble regarding both matters of discipline and doctrine, he began a program which encouraged them to return to theoria and leave praxis to the bishop and his clergy.[28]

As one might expect, Chrysostom's program encountered stiff opposition from the urban monks of Constantinople, who were now organized under a leader, Isaak the Syrian, a man described as "always plotting against the bishops."[29] Although Isaak succeeded in deposing Chrysostom with the aid of the patriarch of Alexandria, the good bishop's concept of the proper monastic life—withdrawal from the world, including church affairs, and total devotion to prayer and contemplation—was gaining ground not only among his fellow bishops but also among some of the monks themselves. Even before the beginning of the fifth century, Evagrios of Pontos, a man trained in the best circles of Anatolian Christianity, a pupil of both Basil and Gregory of Nazianz, found a spiritual life untenable in the world, even when he was laboring in the service of the church. Evagrios fled the temptations of Constantinople and retreated to the Egyptian desert, where he studied the ways of the early monks. His writings represent a return to the ideals of the early Egyptian ascetics and a major step away from the Anatolian monasticism of Eustathios and of Basil.[30] According to Evagrios, the monk should strive after *apatheia* and the *gnosis* of God, a process which precluded any involvement in the cares of the world or even any personal part in the chores of philanthropia. Evagrios' mysticism fit well with Chrysostom's concept of monastic peace (*hesychia*). Although the Orthodox church condemned Evagrios' writings in the sixth century for their Origenist tenets, they had already circulated widely throughout the world of Eastern Christendom; they were able to survive their condemnation and to reach far beyond the fifth century to influence orthodox writers such as Maximos the Confessor and representatives of the later Byzantine mystical tradition.[31]

Neilos of Ankyra, an associate of John Chrysostom, not only recommended the life of pure theoria as the proper ascetic road; he openly attacked the urban monks.[32] In one of his tracts, Neilos accused the Anatolian ascetics of having no experience of spiritual things. Since they were always exposed to the temptations of the world, the seductions of fame and renown, of wealth, and of the flame of sexual desire, they were constantly distorting their souls. In the furor of their philanthropic duties, they could not even recognize their own sins or hear the soft promptings of the Spirit. Finally, in practicing charity, they resembled men who tried to rescue people hanging from dangerous precipices: in attempting such rescues, they were risking their own salvation.[33] Neilos carried his attack against the urban monks so far that he seems to deny the practice of philanthropia as a requirement of a Christian life. Save oneself, Neilos advises, and avoid the mire of the world.[34] In sum, he recommended that those men and women who truly wanted to be perfect flee all contact with the world and seek out the desert in the footsteps of Anthony.

While these movements away from urban monasticism and its ideals of Christian praxis were gaining momentum in monastic circles, the bishops were growing increasingly concerned with the power the urban monks could exert on the church. During the Christological disputes of the fifth century, these groups represented a constant source of disturbance, especially in the church of Constantinople.[35] Finally at the Council of Chalcedon, the bishops of the East took a united stand against monastic independence. Canon 4 of the council required that monks stop troubling the harmony of both the church and state by wandering uncontrolled through the cities and by forming monastic communities when and where they wished without episcopal approval. From now on, the monks were to be strictly subjugated to the local bishop. They were to obtain his permission to form any new communities and were to obey his commands. Moreover, they were not even to leave their cloister except on business approved by the bishop.[36] The Council of Chalcedon thus put into action a program similar to the one Chrysostom had advocated to control the urban monastic movement in Constantinople.

THE HIGH POINT OF MONASTIC CHARITIES: 350–451

The hundred years from Eustathios' episcopacy in Sebasteia (ca. 350) to the Council of Chalcedon marked the most dynamic era of monastic praxis in the world. From their inception in the cities of Asia Minor to their period of greatest influence in the mid-fifth century, the Anatolian monks dedicated themselves to the practice of philanthropia on behalf of the urban demos. These same years saw them closely involved with almost every hospital in the Eastern Empire concerning which we have any substantial information.

To demonstrate the close relationship between the urban monks and the new nosokomeia, we shall examine the references to hospitals at Constantinople and Jerusalem, emphasizing the evidence for monastic participation in these philanthropies. The earliest leader of urban monks in Constantinople, Marathonios, organized ascetic communities which he called *synoikiai*, a term which the Anatolian monks under Eustathios had favored to describe their loose communities.[37] Sozomenos also associated Marathonios with organizing ptocheia for the poor of the capital. As we have seen, some of these ptocheia surely offered care for the sick, as Eustathios' ptochotropheion had done at Sebasteia, and some might have offered medical services, as Basil's philanthropic complex did at Caesarea.[38] Following Marathonios' example—perhaps as one of his disciples—the physician Sampson instituted a ptocheion in Constantinople during the late fourth century which clearly served as a hospital. The oldest Sampson vita leaves no doubt that this doctor belonged to the urban monastic movement. Living not in an organized cenobitic community or in a place of retreat in the countryside, but in a humble house amidst the poor of Constantinople, Sampson dedicated his life to both theoria and praxis.[39]

Coming to the episcopal throne of the capital at the close of the century, Chrysostom took an active interest in promoting hospitals. According to his biographer Palladios, he reallocated funds from his personal account to refurbish an existing nosokomeion and to open additional ones to meet the city's growing demand for hospital care. As part of his program to subject all ecclesiastical activities to the bishop's supervision and control, Chrysostom not only financed these nosokomeia but also appointed two priests to supervise them and hired both the physicians and the cooks to staff them. Palladios' account, however, indicates that even Chrysostom did not totally divorce the capital's hospitals from the urban ascetic movement, for he allowed the monks—those workers Palladios calls the unmarried ones—to serve as assistants in his nosokomeia.[40] Nevertheless, his reorganization of the capital's hospitals was probably part of his plan to strengthen episcopal power over the local church and particularly over the urban monks.[41]

After Chrysostom's fall one would expect renewed leadership on the part of the urban monks in the hospitals. Although we have almost no information concerning nosokomeia in Constantinople during the fifth century, what evidence does survive supports such a hypothesis. Sozomenos and Theodore Anagnostes both emphasize how the empress Pulcheria fostered the monastic movement in and around Constantinople. Although the *Vita Hypatii* illustrates the empress also could support anchorites, Sozomenos' account stresses her patronage of urban monks. As part of her efforts on their behalf Pulcheria financed xenones and other philanthropic institutions.[42]

The urban monastic movement of the fifth century also played a leading part in the founding of one of Constantinople's long-lived hospitals, the Markianos, or the Xenon of Irene Perama, as the tenth-century *Book of Ceremonies* lists it. As we have seen, the priest Markianos opened this nosokomeion in conjunction with the Church of St. Irene in the Perama district.[43] Although the several accounts of Markianos' life do not refer to any monks or *synoikiai* in connection with either the hospital or the church, details from his vitae together with information in the ecclesiastical histories and other hagiographical records definitely link him with the Anatolian ascetics of Constantinople. The historian Sozomenos relates that, before Markianos joined the patriarch's administration as oikonomos of the Great Church, he had associated with urban ascetics. His friend Auxentios had an uncle who had served as a priest in the Macedonian church—the old party of Marathonios—and maintained ties to an ascetic community of Macedonian women in nearby Bithynia.[44] Moreover, Auxentios himself sang at Markianos' church with people called the *spoudaioi* (the zealous ones), a term often used to describe the ascetics of the Anatolian movement.[45] Another friend of Markianos, Anthimos, also belonged to the spoudaioi and won renown in Constantinople for organizing joint choirs of men and women, a practice popular with the urban ascetics of the Anatolian movement since Basil's day.[46] With these two men Markianos had frequented the Church of St. Irene before his ordination as presbyter and continued to associate with them after he joined the patriarch's administration.[47] Versions of Markianos' vita include vignettes which clearly picture him practicing the lifestyle of the Anatolian ascetics. In the company of others—presumably his companion spoudaioi— he would roam the streets of Constantinople at night to distribute copper coins to the poor and also to wash and bury the indigent who had died in the alleys and byways of the city.[48] He also frequented brothels to preach to the prostitutes.[49] Finally, all versions of his vita hail him as a man who nourished the poor while leading a life of great moderation. Even as oikonomos, he owned but one cloak.[50] Markianos' life, given to serving the demos of Constantinople, fits the pattern established by Marathonios almost a century earlier.

The patriarch appointed Markianos oikonomos of the Great Church in 458. It is possible that Markianos received this influential appointment not only as a reward for his benefactions to the church and people of Constantinople, but also in an attempt to integrate one of the leaders of the urban ascetics into the established church government. After his appointment, Markianos continued to associate with the spoudaioi. They sang in his church, and one can reasonably assume that they also worked in his nosokomeion, especially since such hospital service had been part of the urban monastic tradition from the time of Marathonios and Sampson.

About 439 a prominent member of Theodosios' court, the emperor's friend and companion Paulinos, seems to have established a hospital under the direction of a monastic community. The Patrographs record only that Paulinos constructed a church later called the Kosmidion, which he dedicated to the doctor-saints, Cosmas and Damian.[51] Evidence from the sixth century, however, indicates that a monastic community serviced his church and that a xenon for the sick formed part of this foundation.[52] The miracle tales which mention the xenon describe it as composed of several rooms, including a surgery and bathing facilities.[53] Thus, by the sixth century Paulinos' foundation was a complex of buildings—a central church, a monastery, a hospital, and a public bath, a small campus strikingly similar to the Pantokrator complex of the twelfth century.

Although evidence from the fifth century is lacking, there are reasons to suppose that the Kosmidion complex visible in the sixth century represents the original institution. First, such a complex in the fifth century would not have been without a precedent, since Basil had constructed a similar city of philanthropy at the gates of Caesarea under monastic leadership in the 370s.[54] Paulinos was perhaps following Basil's example in placing his foundation outside the Theodosian wall of Constantinople.[55] Second, since Paulinos had dedicated his church to the most illustrious of the doctor-saints, Cosmas and Damian, he might have attached a nosokomeion to it.[56] Third, in the sixth century, tradition regularly referred to the monastic community at the Kosmidion as Paulinos' monastery, a good indication that it at least owed its origins to the man who had financed the church.[57] Finally, since Paulinos founded the Kosmidion during the decades when the urban monastic movement exercised its greatest influence in ascetic circles and in the practice of philanthropia, it seems likely that a loosely knit group of urban monks first staffed his church and xenon as they did the institutions which the empress Pulcheria founded in Constantinople and those which the empress Eudocia supported a little later in and around Jerusalem.[58]

After Constantinople, Jerusalem offers the best opportunity to observe the relationship between hospitals and the urban monastic movement. Jerusalem had become a focal point of the Christian world after the conversion of Constantine. The Holy Land and its shrines eventually drew every form of Christian piety to its shores. Early in the fourth century, anchorite monks from Egypt had established their austere life of withdrawal in the hills and rocks east of Jerusalem.[59] By the mid-fifth century, Cappadocians had brought the urban monasticism of their Anatolian homeland with them to Palestine. Early in the century, a monk from Cappadocia named Longinos had come to Jerusalem. By the time of the Council of Chalcedon, Longinos had joined a large group of Anatolian monks who served the famous Church of the Anastasis. In Palestine, the urban ascetics, like the ascetic group around Markianos in Constantinople, also called themselves *spoudaioi.*[60] One of the men who was to become a leading figure in orthodox monasticism, Theodosios the Cenobiarch, began his career in Jerusalem as a spoudaios. Like Longinos he hailed from a small village in Cappadocia within the see of Caesarea. During his early years in Cappadocia, Theodosios had come to know the urban monastic movement. When he reached Jerusalem about 451, it was only natural that he first associated with his countryman Longinos and later joined a community of spoudaioi organized by a pious woman named Ikelia.[61]

With the urban monastic movement, one would suppose that charitable foundations like those of Caesarea and Constantinople also came to Jerusalem. Indeed, the first references to specialized philanthropic institutions appear among the recorded deeds of a woman close to the urban monastic life, the empress Eudocia. When Eudocia arrived in the Holy Land on her second visit about 443, she found a bewildering variety of ascetic groups in and around the Holy City: strict cenobitic communities, bizarre forms of anchorite life, and the urban monks.[62] Although she financed all sorts of monastic communities, she associated herself especially with the urban monks and built or restored for them residences and various specialized charitable institutions: ptocheia, xenones, nosokomeia, and gerokomeia.[63] Because the urban monks of Jersualem were especially zealous in aiding the sick, nosokomeia and xenones with special facilities for patients must have been prominent among their organized charities.[64] Although no sources mention that physicians worked with these monks or that any of the monks themselves practiced medicine, we have seen that physicians were employed in some of the hospitals of Constantinople and Asia Minor, the homeland of urban monasticism. It is reasonable to suppose that physicians also served in these early Jerusalem hospitals, especially since the nosokomeia which the former spoudaios Theodosios set up very near the Holy City during the second half of the fifth century did in fact include professional medical treatment in their programs.[65]

THE DECLINE OF THE URBAN MONASTIC MOVEMENT

The relationship between hospitals and urban monks changed completely when the Council of Chalcedon issued its canons. As part of its campaign to regulate all forms of asceticism by subjecting monks and their communities to episcopal authority, the Fathers of the Council required that local bishops gain control over the philanthropic institutions of their cities.[66] During the decades after Chalcedon, the emperors expanded Roman civil law to include the decrees of Chalcedon. In giving final form to this process, Justinian confirmed the local bishop's authority over all hospitals in his city, even those which were legally independent from the episcopal church.[67] Parallel to these developments in ecclesiastical and legal administration, we have observed that the weight of monastic opinion shifted into new directions which opposed the active life of the urban ascetics. A close look at hospitals and the monastic movement in Constantinople after 451 will prove that the bond between xenones and the urban monks did not long survive in the new climate following the Council of Chalcedon.

Opening in Constantinople just about mid-century, Markianos' Xenon of Irene reflects the changing conditions at the time of Chalcedon. We have seen that its founder, Markianos, along with a group of spoudaioi, actively followed the urban monastic life. On the other hand, Markianos also came to represent the episcopal power. He served the patriarch both as a priest and as an oikonomos of Hagia Sophia.[68] Although the patriarch never controlled Markianos' church and xenon as the property of the episcopal office, through the oikonomos he could exercise the kind of influence over the institution which the Council Fathers wished.[69]

From the second half of the fifth century, we have no information regarding either xenones or urban monks in Constantinople. When the sixth- and seventh-century sources again shed light on the capital's hospitals, the Anatolian monks have vanished from the wards of the xenones. Thus when the Syrian holy man Isaak gained too much fame as a member of a Monophysite ascetic group, he left for humility's sake and found a job as a salaried *hyperetes* (servant) in a hospital just outside Constantinople. The short account of Isaak's life emphasizes that he viewed his hospital service as a religious calling but that his co-workers found him exceptional. Most of them had chosen to wait on the sick simply to make a living.[70] So, too, at the Christodotes Xenon, the medical assistant (hypourgos) who accompanied the archiatros on his morning rounds conceived of his job as a lay profession, as did the physicians.[71] Finally, the miracle tales of Saint Sampson dating from the sixth through the tenth centuries mention staff doctors, legal experts called chartoularioi, salaried clerks, and a married *hyperetes* at the saint's xenon, but not a word about monks or ascetics such as those Chrysostom had installed in his nosokomeia.[72]

So too, at the Euboulos xenon only laymen were employed by the second half of the sixth century. The fascinating account of John of Ephesus provides a glimpse inside this famous hospital during the reign of Justin II (565–78). Arrested for his staunch support of Monophysite beliefs, John was imprisoned in a small jail attached to the Euboulos Xenon. John describes in lurid detail his sufferings while confined in his cell. Immobilized by gout, he lay helpless, while flies, gnats, and fleas, attracted by the hospital odors, tortured him. Although employees of the hospital guarded him constantly, neither they nor the nurses who cared for the sick made any attempt to aid him. Finally, John asserts that an angel in spotless white clothes came to his rescue, a man John at first believed to be a hospital servant until he later had an opportunity to meet all the employees in a futile effort to locate his benefactor. Throughout his account, the author gives no indication that these servants working at the Euboulos were ascetics of any kind.[73]

Although xenones such as the Sampson and the Euboulos had no relationship to monks by the reign of Justinian, some hospitals, such as the Kosmidion Xenon next to the Church of Cosmas and Damian, were probably under the jurisdiction of a community of monks and their superior. By the sixth century, if not before, the Kosmidion complex included a monastery, a church, and a xenon.[74] Despite the administrative link between the Kosmidion monastery and its xenon, the single piece of evidence surviving from the sixth century suggests that by that time even in this hospital lay employees had replaced monks. Here salaried workers were serving as bath attendants—jobs which urban monks had especially relished in their vigorous days on the eve of Chalcedon.[75]

Although monasteries such as the Kosmidion still owned and probably supervised xenones, the urban monastic movement had retreated from laboring in the public hospitals of Constantinople by the sixth century. Surely, these monks withdrew as a result of external pressure exerted by the bishops and the legislation of the state. But developments within the monastic movement itself may have had an even greater impact on altering the active ascetic life which had flourished in the early fifth century. By about 450 the anchorite impulse, which had gained such eloquent spokesmen in Evagrios of Pontos and Neilos of Ankyra, was capturing the minds and hearts of the most fervent ascetics again. At Constantinople, the prominent spoudaios and close associate of Markianos, Auxentios, fled the active praxis of an urban monk in the capital to seek out a lonely place in the mountains of Bithynia. Other spoudaioi followed him, so that he eventually founded a cenobitic community for his many followers.[76] The same years saw the flowering of the cenobitic monasticism at the Monastery of the Sleepless Ones (*akoimetoi*) at Irenaion. The monks of this community dedicated themselves to constant liturgical prayer, rather than to the active life of philanthropia.[77] Under Abbot Markellos, the monastery grew so rapidly that it needed totally new quarters to house its many members. Moreover, it founded daughter monasteries or reorganized older communities in Constantinople and its environs along the lines of its liturgical routine.[78] Men like Auxentios and Markellos surely helped to redirect ascetic enthusiasm away from the active life into more disciplined forms which were also much more removed from contact with the world.

Under pressure for the church, the state, and its own prominent men, the urban monastic movement rapidly withered in Constantinople. In the course of its retreat, it surrendered its serving role in xenones to laymen. One novel of Justinian, however, indicates that remnants of the urban monastic movement in the Eastern capital still retained a foothold in the city's hospitals. Novel 59 describes communities of pious women called *asketriai* who were under the authority of Constantinopolitan xenones. Whenever the hospital directors had to organize free burial services according to the system Justinian had devised, the asketriai were to sing at the services.[79] It is likely that these women descended from the old Marathonian synoikiai, since Anatolian ascetics such as the Marathonians had been famous for their choirs of men and women from their earliest days in Cappadocia.[80] Moreover, the fourth-century synoikiai which Marathonios had founded had been closely associated with philanthropic organizations, just as these asketriai of Justinian's reign were bound to the city's xenones.[81] After the Council of Chalcedon had imposed new discipline on the monastic movement, female ascetics were no longer permitted to live in loose communities like the synoikiai, but were reorganized in cloistered monasteries of one sex. Some of these communities, however, were apparently able to preserve their old practices of Christian philanthropia.

Novel 59 also mentions *dekanoi,* men who were recruited from the city's guilds to serve as pallbearers.[82] These dekanoi also seem to have originated in the urban ascetic milieu. The fifth-century *Vita S. Hypatii* describes as dekanoi men who served the *martyria* of Constantinople and associated with the poor, activities typical of Marathonian monks.[83] Moreover, one of the oldest vitae of Saint Auxentios refers to the urban ascetic Anthimos as a dekanos.[84] Finally, urban ascetics like the famous Markianos had always considered the proper burial of the poor and homeless as one of their special works of mercy.[85] Their sixth-century descendants—the asketriai and dekanoi of Novel 59—simply carried on the tradition, now in the service of the official church and the imperial government.

The surviving sources indicate that the Anatolian monastic movement at Jerusalem also declined rapidly after the Council of Chalcedon. Before 451 these monks had dominated the ascetic world of Palestine. Evagrios Scholastikos provides a fascinating picture of monasticism in and around the Holy City in the mid-fifth century. He describes cenobitic communities and strange anchorites who grazed on grass like cattle or wore ponderous chains. In his view, however, the holiest of Jerusalem's monks were the spoudaioi. They led lives of the strictest asceticism while living in the midst of urban commotion. They considered all human beings their fellow travellers. Thus, they conversed with everyone, frequenting taverns, brothels, and baths. So completely did they control their passions that they dared to bathe with women. At the same time they constantly toiled in the service of the sick—bending, stretching, and stooping in their ministrations.[86]

The colorful lifestyle of these urban monks did not escape the censure of some monastic leaders, however. The very practices which Evagrios Scholastikos painted in such glowing colors had led Neilos of Ankyra to condemn the movement.[87] By the mid-fifth century more prominent monks were seeing the dangers of uncontrolled exposure to the world, even in carrying out the duties of Christian praxis. Although the renowned ascetic Theodosios had first joined a small community of Jerusalem spoudaioi, composed of both men and women in the Anatolian tradition, he yearned for pure theoria, the opportunity to contemplate and pray in total silence free from the distractions of the world. For fifteen years the conflicts surrounding the Monophysite question prevented him from pursuing his goal. Finally, about 465, he was able to leave Jerusalem to seek out a place of solitude. He found a cave five kilometers south of Jerusalem on the road to Bethlehem where he could practice a life of quiet prayer. As with so many other prominent ascetics, Theodosios began to attract followers. Gradually his small retinue grew into a large and prosperous cenobitic community, a community which became a model for subsequent generations of Byzantine monks.[88]

Following the guidelines established by the Council of Chalcedon, the episcopal church at Jerusalem also took steps to control the uninhibited ways of the urban monks. At the close of the fifth century, the patriarch Elias forced the large group of spoudaioi attached to the Great Church of the Anastasis to abandon their scattered synoikiai and to take up residence in a more tightly organized cenobitic monastery close to the episcopal palace.[89] Thereafter, we no longer hear of urban monks in Jerusalem who lived in synoikiai while giving themselves to the life of praxis in the streets of the city.

The urban ascetic movement did not vanish totally from the East Roman Empire, however. During the late fifth century, two cities still had active groups of spoudaioi who preserved the traditions of the Anatolian monks in ministering to the sick and aged among the urban poor. In his life of the monophysite leader Severos of Antioch (465–538), the Syrian writer Zachariah mentions spoudaioi at Alexandria, where they were customarily called *philoponoi*. Zachariah portrays these philoponoi of the early sixth century spending many hours in prayer at local churches in Alexandria. They lived in great simplicity, remained celibate, and gave themselves over to works of philanthropia on behalf of the poor.[90] In other words, they observed the same lifestyle which the Anatolian ascetics had championed since they first achieved prominence at the Council of Gangra about 340.[91] These philoponoi especially devoted themselves to helping those who suffered from disease. Sophronios of Jerusalem called them the strength of the sick. In Alexandria and its suburb Menuthis, they stood ready to carry the ill to and from the church of the Egyptian anargyroi, John and Cyrus.[92]

The philoponoi of fifth- and sixth-century Alexandria, however, seem to have had no direct relationship to the nosokomeia of the city. As at Constantinople, hospitals now employed lay professionals, both physicians and medical assistants. The medical assistants who worked in the nosokomeia of the Egyptian capital were numerous enough by the end of the sixth century to have organized their own guild alongside other lay professions.[93] Probably, the philoponoi limited their role in the city's hospitals to carrying the sick to the infirmary doors, just as they transported them to and from the Church of John and Cyrus at Menuthis.

Zachariah also describes an active group of spoudaioi working in contemporary Antioch. After an accident at the games, Zachariah's friend Evagrios had experienced a deep conversion and joined the spoudaioi, who chanted in the Church of Stephen Protomartyr while devoting themselves totally to Christian praxis. In the words of Zachariah, "they ceded nothing to the monks."[94] Zachariah's account demonstrates that by the late fifth century, the spoudaioi no longer considered themselves monks; they now formed a separate group of pious laymen who labored in the streets of Antioch. The monks, on the other hand, led lives of greater isolation from the turmoils of the world.

These late-fifth-century spoudaioi and philoponoi usually supported the Monophysite party. Indeed, Zachariah and his spoudaioi companions all belonged to the Monophysites who followed Severos of Antioch.[95] In the sixth century, Paul, later the Monophysite bishop of Antioch, came to prominence in his city as one of the spoudaioi leaders. He gained renown by carrying the old and sick to the baths, washing and anointing them, and giving them some food and clothing. He would also distribute copper coins to the destitute, a custom which had also made Markianos famous in fifth-century Constantinople.[96] Paul required the spoudaioi under his direction to wear distinctive dress, including a hood which hid their faces.[97] Paul not only promoted the spoudaioi of Antioch, but he sponsored the movement in Constantinople and other cities as well.[98] Paul's spoudaioi, however, did not perform any services to benefit the old xenones. Both at Antioch and later in Constantinople, Paul founded new institutions called *diakoniai,* where spoudaioi carried out their acts of philanthropia.[99] These new charitable institutions formed part of Paul's program to strengthen the Monophysite cause in Constantinople itself and in other urban centers, just as the various Arian sects had opened philanthropic agencies to advance the popularity of their factions in the fourth century. Indeed, the official Chalcedonian church considered Paul's diakoniai to be nests of heresy.[100]

It is perhaps significant that Paul's diakoniai did not include medical services. The Monophysite historian John of Ephesus emphasized that the diakoniai observed the word of God, offering his rest. Perhaps John is contrasting here the Christian philanthropia of the diakoniai—the washing and feeding administered by Christian volunteers—with the medical treatment of the xenones, a treatment based not strictly on the Word of God, but on the doctrines of the pagan luminaries Hippocrates and Galen.[101] When the Monophysite organization was crushed in Constantinople, the diakoniai and their spoudaioi remained.[102] The seventh-century author of the *Miracula S. Artemii* describes such an organization of Constantinopolitan philoponoi; indeed, he himself might well have belonged to a circle of these men.[103] If he did, it would be an ironic ending to the urban monastic movement which had fostered hospital development in the fourth century, for the *Miracula S. Artemii* contains some of the harshest attacks on the secular medical profession found in any Byzantine literature.[104]

Although it is impossible to prove that the spoudaioi fostered the sort of hostility toward medicine in general and toward xenones in particular which surfaces in the *Miracula S. Artemii,* they surely abandoned any direct connection with public hospitals. As the result of Justinian's reorganization of public physicians in the cities, xenones became the preserve of professional medical men, from the leading archiatroi to the humble hyperetai, while the spoudaioi, the direct heirs of the Anatolian monastic tradition, now worked in separate institutions which did not offer treatment based on secular medicine.

HOSPITALS AND CENOBITIC MONASTERIES

It is one of the fascinating paradoxes of Eastern Christian asceticism that the spoudaioi and philoponoi, dedicated to Christian praxis, shunned the hospitals by the seventh century, while the cenobitic monasteries, developed initially as refuges from the confusion and temptations of the urban ascetic lifestyle, came to support them. Although the austere cenobitic communities aimed primarily at the primitive monastic ideal of pure theoria, they did not abandon the xenones; in fact, their most influential leaders incorporated public hospitals into the fiber of cloistered monastic life. As an example, let us consider the famous Monastery of the Sleepless Ones at Irenaion. Here the monks had developed a life which stressed communal prayer as the central aspect of the ascetic life. Their highly structured days of perpetual liturgy about the altar made impossible the heroic praxis of the urban monks.[105] Nevertheless, as early as the mid-fifth century their monastery included a hospital for the sick from outside the monastic community. Moreover, when Abbot Markellos expanded the community's physical plant, he enlarged both the quarters for the monks as well as the facilities which housed healthy guests and the building which sheltered the sick.[106] Markellos played a leading role not only in the monastery at Irenaion but also in many daughter communities throughout the Constantinopolitan region.[107] His support of xenones as part of the cenobitic movement helped to win hospitals a place even in monasteries, where the monks themselves practiced the rituals of ceaseless prayer rather than the duties of active philanthropia.

Although fifth-century Constantinople and its *akoimetoi* (sleepless ones) were influential in steering Eastern asceticism along new paths, the monks of Jerusalem stood at the cutting edge of monastic development. Among these, the Cappadocian Theodosios shone the brightest, so brightly that later generations gave him the honorary title of cenobiarch (leader of the cenobites). Like Evagrios of Pontos and Neilos of Ankyra, Theodosios rejected the life of the urban monks because of its constant exposure to the spiritual dangers of the city, but he did not abandon their concept of ministering to the sick. Thus, in expanding his cenobitic community outside Jerusalem, Theodosios decided to include three separate hospital buildings: one for sick monks, one for laymen of some wealth, and one for the poor. From the brief description of these hospitals in the *Vita Theodosii* of Theodore, it is clear that the separate infirmary for monks stemmed from Theodosios' desire to erect a barrier between monks and laymen in opposition to the open lifestyle of the Jerusalem spoudaioi. On the other hand, he welcomed laymen of all ranks to the two remaining facilities which his monastery supported.[108] In this he did not deviate from the monastic ideal of Basil the Great. Indeed, Theodosios' cenobitic community with its three hospitals, removed but five kilometers from Jerusalem, does not differ much from Basil's monastery and its ptochotropheion just outside of Caesarea. Although Theodosios championed an asceticism which sought to steer monks away from the entanglements of the world—his flight from Jerusalem into the wilderness reminds one of Anthony's escape into the desert—he preserved the notion that monks should support hospitals which served people from beyond the monastery's walls. As Eastern monks were forming much more disciplined communities during the late fifth century, Theodosios provided a model of a cloistered monastery which nevertheless continued the hospital tradition of Saint Basil.

As monks continued to raise greater barriers between their life and lay society in the years after Theodosios, tensions concerning their relationship to the public hospitals and the work connected with them naturally arose. How could a monk withdraw from the world and practice perfect theoria if he had to trouble himself with the duties of a hospital and even mix with laymen? During the sixth century, the pious monk Dorotheos from a monastery near Gaza addressed just this question to his spiritual father, Barsanouphios.[109] The leaders of Dorotheos' monastery had ordered him to take charge of the nosokomeion, an institution which served primarily the monks of the community, but also offered some services to the men of the world.[110] This institution included laymen on its staff, some of whom were physicians.[111] Dorotheos complained constantly about his hospital duties. Contact with the laymen who came to the nosokomeion for treatment troubled him deeply; the hospital staff—both brother monks and laymen—pestered him with questions even during his prayer time; the frustrations of dealing with staff members and fussy patients occasionally drove him to the sin of anger.[112] He longed for quiet contemplation, for the peace to find the Lord. His advisor Barsanouphios, however, reminded him that the Lord requires mercy; that mercy is greater than any sacrifice. Contemplation, he added, could lead to the arch-sin of pride.[113] In sum, Barsanouphios recommended that Dorotheos continue to direct the hospital and to serve the sick, both monks and laymen, although, of course, he should restrict his conversation with the worldly to what was strictly necessary.[114]

Dorotheos also worried about his study of scientific medicine. As part of his duties in the nosokomeion, he had to consult the medical books; he feared that time so spent might distract him from spiritual matters. He asked Barsanouphios whether he ought to abandon medicine and use only the remedies of faith. Barsanouphios told him to continue studying the medical texts and even to consult with the physicians, remembering that all cures came ultimately from God.[115]

Theodosios and Dorotheos helped to forge a tight bond between the cenobitic communities stressing withdrawal from the world and the public hospitals, a bond which was to survive until the very last days of the East Roman Empire. The cenobitic traditions of Palestine, embodied in the customs of Theodosios' community and in the writings and questions of Dorotheos, acquired great respect throughout the East and came to dominate the Orthodox monastic movement during the later centuries of the Byzantine era. When the early-ninth-century reformer Theodore the Stoudite revived cenobitic life in Bithynia and Constantinople, he turned, of course, to Basil, the traditional father of Greek monks, but he also relied on the works of the fifth- and sixth-century superiors of Palestine. For the typikon of the Stoudion he borrowed from the customs of Theodosios, while many of his catechetical themes he adapted from the writings of Dorotheos.[116] Following these Palestinian fathers, Theodore emphasized the practice of charity as an integral part of the monastic vocation. His monks were to direct their efforts to gain enough both for themselves and also for the sick and the strangers.[117] Theodore even composed didactic poems to motivate the supervisors of the nosokomeia and the xenodocheia attached to his monasteries.[118] Besides these short poems, we have no evidence regarding hospitals or hospices attached to those monasteries Theodore reformed or founded. Nevertheless, the sources provide enough references to establish that Theodore did not reject the principles of Basil or the Palestinian ascetics which sanctioned hospitals as part of the monastic life.

In the tradition of the Palestinian monastic leaders, another giant figure in the history of Byzantine monasticism, Athanasios the Athonite, promoted hospitals at the great cenobitic institution which he formed in the late tenth century on Mount Athos. In his younger days Athanasios had striven after the primitive monastic ideal of perfect theoria. He had originally sought out Mount Athos in Macedonia because it offered such splendid wilderness for the hermit's life of prayer. At some point after 961, however, Athanasios changed his mind. Perhaps under the influence of the general and future emperor Nikephoros II, he decided to build a great cenobitic community on Athos which was to become known as the Great Lavra—a name borrowed from the Palestinian communities of the fifth century.[119] Athanasios included as part of the Lavra complex a xenodocheion for guests, a nosokomeion for both sick monks and laymen, and a bath.[120] He appointed a monk to serve as nosokomos and other brothers to tend the sick. He himself often treated the wounds of patients and relieved the monks, permanently assigned to hospital duty, when they were overcome by the noxious odors.[121] Although there is no evidence of professional physicians at the Lavra nosokomeion, it is possible that Athanasios hired a physician from the outside to treat his patients, as did the twelfth-century monastery of Isaak Komnenos at Ainos for its small hospital.[122] Or perhaps some of the monks studied secular medicine themselves, as Dorotheos had done in the sixth-century Gaza monastery to prepare for his duties as nosokomos. In any event, the Athonite nosokomeion represented an institution solely for the sick, not a hospice or a rest home.

After the founding of the Great Lavra, Mount Athos became the home par excellence of Byzantine monasticism, setting an example of the monastic ideal throughout the Orthodox world. Despite the isolation offered by a remote location like Athos, the mountain's greatest leader, Athanasios, insisted upon continuing the hospital tradition of Basil the Great and even bent his back in personally serving the sick as Basil himself had done so many centuries earlier.

The hospital at the Great Lavra demonstrates that Athonite monks in the tenth century continued both to finance hospitals for the public and to work personally in the service of the patients. Athanasios himself provided an example of the ideal monk's commitment to helping the hospital's sick. When one considers that all the major figures of Byzantine monasticism from Basil through Theodosios to Athanasios incorporated public nosokomeia into their cenobitic programs, it should occasion no surprise that so many hospitals in Constantinople and elsewhere inside the empire were attached to monastic communities.

The relationship between cenobitic monasteries and xenones on the administrative level seems to have been especially close with regard to private foundations. The older hospitals of Constantinople such as the Sampson or the Markianos had developed out of the urban monastic movement, but by the sixth century they had severed their ties with monastic communities of any kind. They appear in the sources as independent legal entities under their directors, deacons or priests, who in turn often held influential positions in the patriarchal church.[123] When the private imperial xenones opened in the tenth century, however, they were always closely associated with monasteries. For example, in the 920s Romanos I founded the Myrelaion Xenon together with a monastic community. Indeed, most of the sources refer to the whole complex only as Romanos' monastery. The superior of this community surely had important responsibilities in administering the xenon, though at this time the financial bureau of the *megas kourator* probably managed the foundation's estates.[124] Several decades later, Constantine VII followed the same system in opening the Petrion complex; so did Constantine IX at the Mangana in the eleventh century.[125] At the Pantokrator, John II Komnenos took the final step in the development of monastic supervision of hospitals by removing the whole complex from the authority of any government office, including those which managed the imperial estates.[126] The superior and the household managers (oikonomoi) of the Pantokrator community assumed full responsibility for governing the resources of the entire institution, including the xenon.[127] Private citizens too subjected their independent charitable foundations to monastic communities. We have the examples of Attaleiates' ptochotropheion in the eleventh century and of the hospital which Isaak Komnenos opened at Ainos in the twelfth century.[128] Private citizens instituted monastic communities to manage their pious foundations because such religious communities formed more stable units than did the directors, physicians, and support staff of a xenon or the supervisor and assistants of a ptochotropheion.

WITHDRAWAL

Following the example of Basil and Theodosius the Cenobiarch, monastic leaders were willing to cooperate with both emperors and private founders in establishing and managing hospitals as well as other philanthropic agencies. Some communities assumed ultimate responsibility for the financial side of their subject hospitals. These same monastic leaders, however, were less willing to follow Barsanouphios' advice to Dorotheos or the vivid example of Athanasios the Athonite regarding personal service in the xenones. The twelfth-century Pantokrator Typikon clearly shows that the monks performed no services in their xenon. From the nosokomos (hospital director) to the hyperetai (servants) the staff of the Pantokrator Xenon was composed of professional laymen, not members of the monastic community.[129] Moreover, the monks had their own infirmary so that they did not need to use the xenon whenever any one of them fell ill. In this the Pantokrator monastery was following the precedent set by Theodosios when he had established separate hospital facilities for monks at his cenobitic community outside Jerusalem.[130] On the other hand, John II Komnenos was ignoring ancient cenobitic tradition when he assigned his monks no duties in the service of the hospital sick, save the liturgical footwashing which the superior carried out for patients on Holy Thursday.[131] In excluding the monks from Christian praxis in the xenon, John II might simply have thought that professional lay employees at all levels of his hospital guaranteed the best possible medical care. Then, too, John and his monks might have considered service in the xenon unsuitable for the former aristocrats who doubtless made up a substantial proportion of the monastic population in a rich, imperial foundation such as the Pantokrator.[132] In isolating the monks from the xenon, however, the emperor and his monastic advisors were probably influenced most by the old conception of the true monastic vocation, the view which saw it as a call to pure theoria free from disturbances and contact with worldly duties.

The contemporary hospital in provincial Ainos displays the same pattern as the Pantokrator, even though it provided medical care of a much lower quality than that of the great Constantinopolitan xenones. The founder-restorer of the Ainos hospital, Isaak Komnenos, established it as part of a monastic community. According to the typikon, the superior and his monks were to see that the hospital always had enough resources—food, medicine, and fuel—to meet the needs of its patients. Besides ensuring the supplies of the hospital, however, they performed no work of mercy—no work of Christian praxis—for the sick laymen. The monastery hired a single physician to treat the hospital's thirty-six patients and paid the salaries of ten hypourgoi, but not one of the twenty-four serving brothers among the monks held a post which had any relation to the duties of the public hospital.[133] In the same fashion, when the empress Theodora established the Lips Monastery with its dependent xenon in the thirteenth century, she carefully stipulated that salaried laymen were to staff her hospital, from the professional iatroi to the washerwoman.[134] The empress expressly designed her monastery to offer its nuns an opportunity to separate themselves completely from the world, a place where they could take up the cross and follow the Lord. Theodora believed that her nuns would best follow the Lord by liturgical prayer and contemplation, not by praxis in the public hospital.[135] On the other hand, she warned the superior of the Lips Monastery never to neglect her financial duties toward the patients of the xenon.[136]

The typika of these three monastic complexes indicate that in practice monastic patrons and the monks themselves often felt uncomfortable with personal service in the xenones. In his questions to Barsanouphios Dorotheos had confirmed the propriety of hospital service for monks, while Athanasios had taught the same lesson when he himself succored the patients in his hospital on Athos. Nevertheless, the old notion that the ascetic should be free of such duties to pursue union with God in liturgy and private contemplation remained strong. The dichotomy between theoria and praxis ever plagued the ascetic world of the East Roman Empire. Even Athanasios had not been able to establish his monastery with its hospital and hospice without criticism. The anchorites who had followed the life of pure theoria on Athos long before Athanasios set foot on the peninsula were steadfastly opposed to the kind of cenobitic monastery with its public philanthropies which Athanasios sponsored. Upon the death of Nikephoros II in 969, these anchorites appealed to the new emperor, John Tzimiskes, in a bid to halt Athanasios' progress. The emperor summoned both Athanasios and his opponents to Constantinople and conducted a hearing. Athanasios eventually gained the confidence of the new emperor and, according to his two biographers, even won over the anchorites to his views.[137] Although the incident did not halt the spread of cenobitic communities on Athos as Athanasios conceived of them, still it revealed again the ancient split in the monastic world.

Despite their defeat at the hands of the great leaders of cenobitic monasticism such as Athanasios, the proponents of pure theoria never abandoned their position that the life of silence (*hesychia*) alone led up the narrow path to God. In the eleventh century they found their most aggressive spokesman in the revolutionary Symeon, called the New Theologian. Symeon not only exalted the life of theoria, but he also attacked the compromise between praxis and contemplation which Theodosios and Dorotheos had forged in Palestine more than 500 years earlier. He dared to challenge the very basis of Christian praxis by reinterpreting Matthew's Last Judgment scene (Matt. 25:31–46), a text of prime importance to a theology of active charity.

Symeon had at first joined the Stoudite monastery in Constantinople; when he later quarreled with the monks of that prominent community, he withdrew to the Mamas Monastery. There he began his career as a spiritual director and writer.[138] Dualistic ideas dominated Symeon's world view. He firmly believed that the enemies of God controlled the visible world.[139] Man must seek to free himself from this *kosmos* by a series of ascetic exercises in an effort to behold the divine light.[140] In Symeon's ascetic program, the practice of charity played a very small part. In a sermon on mercy, he introduced his novel interpretation of Matthew's Last Judgment scene. When Christ mentions those who hunger and thirst, he cannot mean those who desire physical sustenance, but rather those who desire spiritual food. According to Symeon, when Christ says that he hungers, he could not possibly mean that he, the Lord of Heaven, could suffer a human desire for food; rather he wants to show how he hungers and thirsts for our salvation.[141] In the same sermon, Symeon reminds his hearers of Saint Maria of Alexandria. When she had served her fellow men, she had received them in a shelter of sin—a house of prostitution. Her salvation came only when she fled into the desert.[142] In discussing the Lord's command to sell all and give the proceeds to the poor, Symeon shifts the emphasis from giving or helping the poor to divesting oneself of the burden of wealth. Yet even this unburdening is only a preparation for the real business of salvation—shouldering one's cross, a task which Symeon understands as beginning the severe exercises of penance and mystical prayer.[143] Finally, as a precondition for his hesychastic discipline (the way to silence), Symeon demands complete separation for his monks from the world, including any contact with the sick and needy.[144]

Symeon saw positive danger for the monks if they personally participated in any form of active charity such as serving the sick in hospital wards. Moreover, he recognized no real value in monastic support for hospitals. In short, his theology of asceticism revived the old spirit of flight from the world and its responsibilities which Anthony had enkindled in the fourth century.

Symeon's writings gained great popularity in Byzantine monastic circles. His doctrines helped to shape the hesychast movement which came to dominate not only Byzantine monasteries, but the Orthodox church as a whole during the fourteenth century.[145] His ringing appeals for a return to the ancient theoria of the desert Fathers surely influenced lay founders and monastic superiors in the years after his death (1022). Thus some typika of the twelfth and later centuries discouraged or even barred monks from personally nursing the sick or performing any other function in public hospitals. As we have seen, this was the case with the Pantokrator *Typikon* and with the Lips *Typikon* of Empress Theodora. So, too, at the monastery of the Kosmosoteira, the hospital stood outside the cloistered precinct of the monks.[146]

Symeon the New Theologian thus convinced many monks to ignore the words of Basil the Great and the example of Athanasios the Athonite regarding personal labors on behalf of the sick. Symeon exhorted them to embrace pure contemplation free from the distractions of Christian praxis. On the other hand, Symeon and even more extreme hesychasts never gained such a hold on the Byzantine monastic movement that the monks refused to share their resources with xenones or to assume the financial supervision of dependent hospitals. Thus, the superior of the Pantokrator and his financial assistants willingly accepted the responsibility for ensuring adequate revenues for the imperial xenon under their care, a job formerly shouldered by the bureaucrats who managed the emperor's estates.[147] Moreover, despite the strident appeals of men like Symeon and the subsequent strength of the hesychastic movement in the Byzantine church, the sources provide a few glimpses of monks who still labored in public hospitals even in the last centuries of the East Roman Empire.

A medical manuscript executed in 1323 presents the best evidence that some monks were intimately involved in the operation of xenones as late as the fourteenth century. In a colophon to this manuscript, the copyist George declares that he is both a monk and a physician in the imperial xenon (he does not include the actual name of the institution).[148] Here the fourth-century tradition of the urban monks of Anatolia is still flourishing. Just as Basil the Great and the physician Sampson employed their medical training in the service of their hospital patients, so too this fourteenth-century George worked as a physician on the staff of a Constantinopolitan xenon and copied medical texts, probably for the xenon library, while wearing the cowl. Another manuscript note, this time from the early fifteenth century, reveals that a monk named Nathaniel headed the staff of the Krales Xenon as nosokomos, a position that salaried laymen had filled at both the Pantokrator Xenon of the twelfth century and at the Lips hospital of the thirteenth century.[149] These two notices should warn against generalizing too widely from the three surviving typika that describe hospitals in detail. Since in the tradition of Eastern monasticism each community could design its own rules within certain limits, it is entirely possible that while some monasteries such as the Pantokrator forbad their members to serve in public hospitals, others encouraged their monks to undertake such work. The two notices we have just considered indicate that some communities still permitted monks to assist xenon patients in the last two centuries of the Eastern Empire. Even though Symeon and his heirs within the monastic world attempted to steer asceticism away from Christian praxis toward the life of pure theoria, some monks of the late Byzantine centuries continued to reject Anthony's path into the desert and to follow instead Basil's road of Christian praxis nourished by contemplation.

The fourteenth-century romance *Emperios and Margarona* proves that the popular notion of the monastic life still included hospital service among the duties of monks and nuns. According to the romance, when the abbess Margarona received a mysterious treasure of gold ducats, she ordered that a xenon of a hundred beds be built for the sick. There, she and her nuns not only nursed the sick, but they stood ready to meet their every wish.[150] Margarona's monastery existed only in fiction—indeed, the romance places it in far-off Provence—but the picture the poem presents reflects the reality of Athanasios' great Lavra of the tenth century, Dorotheos' monastery in sixth-century Gaza, or even the nosokomeia of John Chrysostom in fourth-century Constantinople.[151] The monastic ideal never completely lost its commitment to serving hospital patients. Despite continual pressure from proponents of total theoria, some monks of the Byzantine Empire refused to renounce a life of active philanthropia in the xenones.

CHAPTER EIGHT
The Hospital in Action

The imperial government, the episcopal organization, wealthy citizens, and the monastic movement supported not only hospitals in the Byzantine Empire but also a multitude of other charitable organizations. These shared the same legal status, the same ecclesiastical standing, and similar internal administrative structures with nosokomeia. Thus, the legislation of Justinian classified all philanthropic foundations as pious houses (*euageis oikoi*) with no legal distinctions within that category. Throughout the Byzantine centuries, the emperors and private founders felt free to select institutions to express their love of neighbor from a whole range of these pious houses; monasteries too could opt to practice philanthropia by supporting one or several charitable institutions. Some, such as the Kosmidion, chose to establish hospitals, others gerokomeia or xenodocheia, while a rich community like the Pantokrator in Constantinople could afford to support both a nosokomeion and a gerokomeion. What set the Byzantine hospitals apart from other philanthropic houses were the medical services these institutions offered to the people of the empire. The hospital in action thus won a unique status among pious houses as well as the admiration of contemporaries and later historians.

This chapter will attempt to reconstruct how the hospitals of the Byzantine Empire actually functioned in fulfilling their mission to heal the sick. By drawing on monastic typika, hagiographical texts, imperial legislation, literary sources, and some archaeological and iconographic evidence, it is possible to obtain a picture of these hospitals: what they looked like, whom they received as patients, how they organized their staffs of physicians and nurses, and finally what sort of treatment their medical personnel offered the patients entrusted to them. In discussing this last question, it will be necessary to consider whether or not the hospital affected the traditional practice of Greek medicine as it had been enshrined in the works of Galen and Hippocrates.

We have already examined in detail one prominent Byzantine hospital, the twelfth-century Pantokrator Xenon as it appears in the typikon issued by the emperor John II Komnenos. Although this document provides the best illustration of the hospital in action, it ignores some areas of hospital administration, staff organization, and patient care and mentions others only briefly.

Although none of the other sources present as full a picture of a hospital as the Pantokrator *Typikon* does, some do provide details which supplement its information. A careful examination and collation of these sources will help to complete our knowledge of Byzantine hospitals. Moreover, the striking picture which the Pantokrator *Typikon* paints of the xenon of John II has led some historians to focus solely on this document and to view the Comnenian hospital as an institution peculiar to the twelfth century, an institution with features Constantinople must have adopted from the flourishing hospitals among the Moslems.[1] A cursory review of the sources has already illustrated that the Pantokrator Xenon did not suddenly appear on Byzantine soil in 1136, but had developed from earlier philanthropic institutions. It remains, however, to analyze the historical process by which East Roman hospitals expanded the quality and variety of services they offered the sick, a process which does seem to have reached its peak in the Constantinople of the Comnenian emperors.

THE BUILDINGS

From the information in the Pantokrator *Typikon* it is impossible to determine what a Byzantine xenon actually looked like; no extant copy of the *Typikon* includes an illustration of the hospital's exterior or a diagram of its interior floor plan. And indeed, no other document from any period of the empire's long history describes hospital buildings in sufficient detail so that one can visualize the physical plant. To compound the problem, archaeologists have not been able to distinguish the remains of hospitals from the foundations of other sorts of Byzantine buildings nor do manuscript illuminations offer much help. An illustrated codex containing a collection of sermons delivered by Gregory of Nazianz includes a picture of Basil's ptochotropheion outside fourth-century Caesarea. The artist executed this illustration sometime in the late ninth century. From this picture, however, it is possible to say only that the artist conceived of Basil's hospital as a large, oblong building, surrounded by an arched stoa. Through the arches of the porch one can see clearly Basil and Gregory of Nazianz ministering to the sick but no further details regarding the hospital's facilities.[2]

Nevertheless, in his study of monastic architecture, Anastasios Orlandos has managed to shed some light on the hospital building. Among the monasteries of the Meteora in Greece he has identified two ruins which served as hospitals—one at the Barlaam Monastery and the second at the Metamorphosis. While neither of these facilities served as public hospitals, being infirmaries reserved for the monks themselves, and while they date from a period after the collapse of the East Roman state in 1453 and thus were not, strictly speaking, Byzantine institutions, nevertheless, they provide enough information to establish a central feature of earlier Byzantine hospitals: the presence of a large, open hearth. From the ruins still standing, Orlandos has determined that these infirmaries were simple square buildings. At the core of each stood a great fireplace, surrounded by four pillars, also in a square, which supported a cupola with vents to release the smoke. About this central hearth were four aisles where the sickbeds were placed. Orlandos maintains that the fireplace with its cupola chimney represented the distinguishing feature of Byzantine hospitals, whether they were monastic infirmaries or xenones.[3]

The written sources support Orlandos' conclusions. In establishing an infirmary for its monks, the eleventh-century typikon of the Evergetes Monastery in Constantinople stipulates that this nosokomeion must have a large hearth for cooking the patients' food, for proper heating, and for preparing other things the sick might need—presumably medicines. With its eight beds the Evergites nosokomeion easily conforms to the patterns of the later Meteora infirmaries: a central hearth with beds arranged along the four side aisles, in the case of the Evergites infirmary, two beds to a side.[4]

Like the monastic infirmaries, the public xenones also included prominent fireplaces. Although no descriptions of early Byzantine hospitals mention them, Theodore Stoudites included a hearth in his detailed allusion to a well-organized hospital at the beginning of the ninth century.[5] The twelfth-century hospital at Ainos made special provisions to ensure the fuel supply for the patients' hearth.[6] As we have seen, the Pantokrator Xenon in Constantinople had three such fireplaces: one large hearth and two smaller ones for the surgery and for the women's ward.[7] If the Pantokrator Xenon was constructed on the pattern found in the Meteora monasteries, then it is probable that the surgery and the women's ward formed separate wings of the hospital, each built about a hearth, while the other wards were housed in a much more spacious central hall with a correspondingly larger fireplace.

Most modern accounts of the Pantokrator Xenon assume that the hospital had five separate rooms in which it housed its patients. Orlandos, Constantelos, and other researchers have reached this conclusion by focusing their attention on the five *ordinoi* (sections) of the hospital and ignoring the number of hearths.[8] If one follows Orlandos' own arguments, however, a hospital of five nearly equal rooms for patients would require five hearths of similar size. Instead, the *Typikon* provides for only three hearths—one substantially larger than the other two. To reconcile the problems regarding the physical layout of the Pantokrator Xenon, it is useful to consider evidence regarding earlier Byzantine hospitals in conjunction with the *Typikon*.

First, we can be certain that the women's ordinos at the Pantokrator certainly had its own room. The *Typikon* itself demonstrates this in requiring a separate hearth for this particular ward. Moreover, earlier evidence confirms that such an arrangement reflected hospital tradition in the East Roman provinces. When Bishop Rabbula of Edessa constructed his charitable complex in his city at the beginning of the fifth century, he added a separate institution for women; and when the emperor Justinian rebuilt Antioch in 541, he fitted out his hospital there with distinct facilities for men and for women.[9] Since Byzantine society normally maintained strict separation between the sexes, church leaders had from the beginning divided hospitals into two sections, one for men and one for women.

Second, the Pantokrator Xenon certainly had a separate room for its surgery (*trauma*), since here too the *Typikon* requires a hearth. Again, earlier evidence indicates that other major hospitals had traditionally maintained special rooms for surgical procedures. One story from a sixth-century collection of miracle tales describes how Cosmas and Damian carried a sick man through a Constantinopolitan xenon to an operating room (*iatreion* in the words of the text) equipped with a couch for the patient and a special medical chest; in this surgery the two doctor-saints performed their miraculous operation.[10] Most modern treatises on the Pantokrator Xenon do not distinguish between the operating room proper and the ordinos, where patients who needed surgery and those recuperating from surgery could rest and receive medical attention. In fact, the surgery must have been a separate room from the surgical ward in all Byzantine hospitals. The sixth-century miracle tale of Cosmas and Damian described above does not mention any patients housed in the operating room. A seventh-century source relates how a patient awaiting surgery had his bed near the ophthalmic section, not in the operating room itself.[11] Finally, a detailed description of a twelfth-century operating room mentions the blazing hearth, the assistants, the operating table, and the cautery irons, but says nothing about other patients.[12] Indeed, it would have been most disturbing for surgical patients to await their ordeal or recuperate in a room where others were undergoing the pains of the knife or the cautery iron.

When one considers the three hearths and the true nature of the *trauma* as a surgery only, one must conclude that among the five patient ordinoi of the Pantokrator Xenon, only the women's section was assigned to a separate room. Moreover, no descriptions of any other hospitals from the sixth through the fourteenth centuries mention any distinct rooms for patients other than the women's dormitories. In accordance with Orlandos' research regarding monastic infirmaries, it seems likely that a single central hall housed the four remaining ordinoi with each section occupying one aisle about the great hearth. Three additional considerations make this hypothesis even more attractive. First, the Pantokrator *Typikon* divides the thirty-eight beds in these four wards in such a way that they easily could fit into the sides of a large square hall. Three sections have ten beds each; the fourth section for acute cases has only eight to allow the staff more room in which to work.[13] Second, since the *Typikon* required that the main hearth of the xenon be much larger than the other two, it surely kept many more patients warm than the women's hearth did: i.e., thirty-six compared to twelve in the women's ward.[14] Finally, the *Typikon* uses the term *ordinos* to describe its sections. *Ordinos* is rendered most accurately into English as "row" or "rank"—a word which would apply well to four lines of beds on each side of a central hall.[15]

It is doubtful that hospitals adopted the specialized building I have described here from the very first. Since Byzantine nosokomeia had developed from more general Christian charitable institutions of the fourth century, they probably shared a common building plan with these early pious houses. If the ninth-century manuscript illustration of Basil's ptochotropheion represents an accurate iconographic tradition, then these early hospitals occupied simple basilican buildings of some sort. Only gradually did the exigencies of patient care require altering the building plan. Clearly, the need to keep patients warm played a major role in the change from a simple oblong hall to a smaller, square building centered on a great hearth. It is impossible to determine when these changes occurred. Perhaps Justianian introduced the novel hospital building when he rebuilt the Sampson Xenon after the Nika fire at a time when he introduced new elements into the hospital personnel structure. The hospital description of Theodore Stoudites, however, offers good evidence that hearth-centered nosokomeia had become common by the ninth century.[16]

A Byzantine xenon consisted of more than the central structure housing the patients. From the sixth century at least, bathing facilities normally adjoined Byzantine nosokomeia. At the time of Justinian, the Kosmidion complex included a church, a xenon, and a bath with a staff of lay attendants.[17] The seventh-century *Miracula Artemii* mentions a bathhouse belonging to a xenon in Constantinople.[18] Even a rural hospital like the one which Athanasios established on Mount Athos in the tenth century offered its patients bathing facilities.[19] The Pantokrator *Typikon* required the monks to maintain a bath both for the patients of the hospital and for the residents of the gerokomeion.[20] Ordinarily these baths were housed in buildings separate from the nosokomeion proper. Although the baths played an important role in the therapy which hospitals promoted, apparently the general public could also use the xenon facilities. The *Miracula Artemii* describes a woman not a patient who was able to enjoy a xenon's bathhouse.[21] Similarly, the twelfth-century hospital at Ainos kept its bathing facilities open to all Christians.[22]

By the twelfth century Byzantine xenones also set aside a room or perhaps a separate building to treat outpatients. The Pantokrator *Typikon* detailed four physicians and a staff of medical assistants (*hypourgoi*) to examine and treat people who walked in from the streets.[23] Before the twelfth century one can find no references to walk-in clinics at Byzantine hospitals. It seems likely that hospitals introduced them sometime after the mid-tenth century after they ceased maintaining a corps of physicians to roam the streets of

Constantinople and offer medical assistance to the poor and homeless. In a fourteenth-century manuscript containing the famous *materia medica* of Myrepsos (*Paris. gr.* no. 2243), there is a miniature which depicts one of these hospital dispensaries. It represents a typical scene in the clinic: the physician and two assistants admitting two patients. Above them in what appears to be a dome hovers a fresco or mosaic of Christ enthroned with the Gospel Book. Edouard Jeanselme and Lysimachos Oeconomos, who have commented on this miniature, suppose that the fresco in the dome represents Christ as he presides over the physician below and animates his work.[24] In addition, the picture was no doubt meant to emphasize the parallel roles of the doctor, who treats the body with his medicines, and Christ, who cures the soul with the salve of the Gospels, an analogy which, as we have seen, Orthodox Christians had been developing since the third century.[25] This illustration provides a strong argument that the Byzantines decorated the dispensaries of their hospitals, and possibly the central dormitories as well, with wall paintings. A poem from the reign of Andronikos II (1282–1328) adds additional support to such a supposition when it describes a picture of the *Theotokos* with Cosmas and Damian in the hospital of the Glabas family.[26]

In addition to the main dormitories, the surgery, the baths, and the outpatient clinic, a large xenon of the capital also had separate rooms or adjoining buildings for a library, for a lecture hall, for administrative functions and record keeping, for storage, and for other services such as laundry work.[27] Hospitals also included chapels where the ambulatory patients and the staff members could pray and attend the Divine Liturgy. The Pantokrator had two chapels, one for male patients and one for the women.[28] Xenones naturally set aside rooms to serve as latrines, again one for men and one for women.[29] Finally, some also included under their administration rooms or buildings which could serve as jails. Bishop Dioskoros of Alexandria imprisoned his opponent Ischyrion in a xenon during the fifth century; the Orthodox patriarch of Constantinople had the Monophysite leader John of Ephesus incarcerated at the Euboulos Xenon during the reign of Justin II. Since Ischyrion had contact with other patients, he presumably stayed in the dormitory. John, on the other hand, was kept in total isolation in a cell of some sort.[30] No sources from later centuries mention prisoners at xenones. In refurbishing the Lips Monastery sometime after 1282, the empress Theodora describes small cells (*oikiskoi*) in the xenon where the community's spiritual father could stay on his monthly visits to the monastery.[31]

In addition to buildings, the physical plant of Byzantine hospitals included furniture, special equipment, medicines, and supplies of all kinds. The Pantokrator *Typikon* specifies exactly the number and kind of beds which the hospital should provide, the mattresses, sheets, and covers each bed should have, and a routine for replacing worn-out sleeping gear.[32] The concern for proper bedding goes back to the earliest days of Byzantine hospitals and probably to the simple Christian hospices from which nosokomeia evolved. In the early fifth century, Bishop Rabbula of Edessa made every effort to ensure clean beds, sheets, and covers for the guests of his hospice and hospital.[33] Since Basil the Great had deeply influenced Syriac Christianity, it is likely that Rabbula's regulations regarding sleeping accommodations reflect the practices at the ptochotropheion which Basil had built in Caesarea.[34] In the surgeries one could find operating tables, medicine cabinets, and an array of surgical instruments.[35] Similarly, the dispensaries had large medicine cabinets, special vials for urine analysis, and a great *cathedra* for the presiding physician.[36]

THE PATIENTS

The same sources that devote scant space to describing the physical makeup of Byzantine hospitals contain somewhat more information about the patients who occupied the sickbeds, especially regarding the classes from which they came. The earliest Byzantine hospitals were designed exclusively for the poor. After all, nosokomeia had developed out of the hostels for the indigent migrants who began to stream into the cities of the East Roman Empire at the beginning of the fourth century. As we have seen, the first permanent institutions to serve these poor appeared in Antioch and its Syrian hinterland, those xenodocheia which Constantine favored with annona allotments. The first steps from hostel to hospital apparently took place in Antioch under Bishop Leontios, when Aetios began to treat the sick among hospice guests.[37] Some time later at Constantinople, Sampson expanded his iatreion into an institution offering both bed and board to the sick; Sampson clearly designed his new hospital for the poor and homeless.[38] Moreover, Eustathios, Basil, and other Anatolian bishops called the philanthropic institutions which they opened ptochotropheia—shelters for the poor. They surely intended the medical sections of their foundations for the indigent.

The first evidence that the new charitable facilities for the sick accepted any but the poorest patients comes from Edessa in the early fifth century. When Bishop Rabbula of that city established his xenodocheion for both the sick and the healthy, he made sure that its guests and patients would receive excellent food. According to his biographer he provided such good food for the sick that even those who were spoiled enjoyed it.[39] These finicky eaters must have come from classes above the poverty level. Some years later, in the middle of the fifth century, the monk Theodosios founded a hospital complete with physicians not far from Jerusalem with three separate buildings to house the patients: one for monks, one for the poor, and one for men of the world who needed medical attention. The patients in this third group clearly did not come from the destitute demoi collecting in the urban centers of the East, but were men of some substance.[40]

Jerusalem, of course, was a special case. After the conversion of Constantine it became a tourist center for Christians from all over the world and from every rank of society. So many of the poor swarmed there that by the sixth century Justinian had to authorize a special fund to support them.[41] Wealthy tourists such as Jerome's friend Paula also came to visit the famous sites of Christ's passion and death.[42] If these wealthier visitors fell ill in the Holy City, far from home, family, slaves, and friends, they too might need medical and nursing care. Very wealthy tourists could travel with a numerous retinue and bring along a household physician, but the improvident rich and people of moderate means would have been in a difficult position if they fell seriously ill away from home.

From the sixth century comes evidence that, even when staying in their native cities, people of the propertied classes occasionally used the xenones themselves or sent family members there. In a law reissued in 531 Justinian required that slave owners either care for their sick slaves at their homes or entrust them to hospitals.[43] At the beginning of the next century a deacon of the Great Church of Hagia Sophia, named Stephen, fell ill with an infection of the groin. His family recommended that he go to the Sampson Xenon rather than remain at home for treatment. The staff of the hospital admitted him, assigned him a bed, brought him to the surgery, operated on the infection, and allowed him to recuperate for several days. Stephen had a caring family in Constantinople; as a deacon of Hagia Sophia he had enough money to hire a private physician. Still, he chose to enter a nosokomeion.[44] The Sampson Xenon must have been a far different kind of place from the hospitals of the medieval West or even from the *hôtels-Dieu* of Old Regime France.

People from the wealthier classes would have turned to the xenones of the church for medical treatment once Justinian transferred archiatroi from the payroll of the old polis governments to that of the nosokomeia. As a result of Justinian's reform, the best practitioners of Greek medicine now worked in the hospitals, physicians of the quality people of substance sought. Stephen and his family must have believed that the physicians, the nursing care, and the medical equipment of a xenon surpassed any treatment he could obtain at home by hiring a private physician.

The twelfth century still saw Constantinopolitans of moderate means committing themselves to hospitals. The Pantokrator *Typikon* indicates that some patients had enough money to offer physicians extra tips for special treatment.[45] In the same century, a monk of a monastery in the capital mentioned that his superior would allow the brothers to leave the cloister whenever they were sick enough to need the doctors of the xenon. Apparently, some monasteries did not maintain infirmaries for their monks, but simply sent them off to one of the city's public hospitals for treatment.[46] Finally, in comic verse from the Comnenian period, a poet recounted among his many miseries how he had injured his hand and, as a result, had had to spend a month in a xenon. Although the poet constantly complains of his poverty, he was not one of the homeless poor. He had a house or apartment in Constantinople and a family.[47]

But what of the extremely wealthy? One would suspect that they had the means to hire private physicians of a quality equal to those of the hospital archiatroi and to have had at their palaces all the equipment which the public nosokomeia normally maintained for their patients. Such seems to have been the case. During an outbreak of disease in seventh-century Germion, the sick children and relatives of the leading citizens were confined to their homes, but the others—presumably those stricken from the lower and middle classes—were assigned beds in the city's xenones.[48] So, too, toward the close of the ninth century, a high-ranking aristocrat and friend of the empress Theophano called a number of physicians to his house in Constantinople when his son fell ill.[49] In the eleventh century, the peers of the military aristocrat Kekaumenos summoned private physicians to their estates.[50] It is possible that these great men hired the hospital doctors themselves when these were free of xenon duties. The Pantokrator *Typikon* allowed staff doctors to treat private patients provided only that they did not leave the city to visit aristocrats, even if these might be the emperor's relatives.[51]

One hospital, however, surely served the very pinnacle of Byzantine society—the emperor and his family. In the mid-eleventh century, the emperor Constantine IX opened an imperial xenon as part of his vast Mangana complex—an institution which included a monastery, several philanthropic agencies, and a palace. When Constantine fell gravely ill before his death in 1055, he withdrew to this foundation.[52] In their narrative histories, neither Zonaras nor Skylitzes mentions that the emperor sought the assistance of the xenon and its staff, but the example of one of his successors suggests that Constantine had indeed resorted to the Mangana hospital. When, seventy years later, Alexios I developed a terminal malady, his doctors also transferred him to the Mangana complex. Anna Komnena states that the physicians made this recommendation because they considered the southern exposure of the old palace harmful to the emperor's grave condition. Zonaras, however, adds that the Mangana palace had won the epithet "the healer" because it had access to hospital facilities.[53] The development of the office of *aktouarios*—the emperor's personal physician—provides further evidence that the Mangana Xenon ministered to the emperors.

Scholars have long known that the leading doctor of the imperial court held the title of *aktouarios*, at least from the reign of Alexios I (1081–1118). Thus, the court physician Michael Pantechnes was addressed as *aktouarios* while he served as chief physician to John II Komnenos and his family.[54] Nevertheless, the exact duties of the aktouarios have remained a mystery.[55] A fourteenth-century medical manuscript provides the solution to the problem. Among a collection of remedies in *Vaticanus graecus* 299, one cure bears the name of Abram, the aktouarios of the Mangana Xenon and imperial archiatros. This notice reveals that the aktouarios was essentially a hospital official, a physician on the staff of the Mangana Xenon. Indeed, Abram's prescription appears in a list with several others attributed to doctors at the Mangana.[56] References from earlier centuries support the information in the Vatican manuscript. Michael Pantechnes, the aktouarios at the court of John II Komnenos, had been among the three physicians who had ordered that the old emperor Alexios be transferred to the Mangana palace and the xenon.[57] Moreover, as aktouarios, Michael supervised an instructor of the physicians named Michael Italikos.[58] There is absolutely no evidence that the emperors supported a palace school of medicine as such, but as we shall see shortly, hospitals in Constantinople served as the normal setting for the teaching of medicine. As supervisor of the Mangana Xenon, then, Pantechnes would have been the superior of Italikos, just as the nosokomos at the Pantokrator had charge of the *didaskalos* (teacher of medicine) at his hospital.[59] In addition, there is a seal of Pantechnes as aktouarios which bears the image of Saint George, the patron of the Mangana foundation.[60] The term aktouarios had in its Latin form applied to civilian supply officers who managed the stores for the Late Roman army.[61] As supervisor of the Mangana Xenon the twelfth-century aktouarios would also have been responsible for supplies, in this case for stocking adequate stores of medicines, just as the nosokomos of the Pantokrator had to devote a good part of his time to securing medical supplies.

The emperors surely did not stay in a hospital ward such as those described in the Pantokrator Typikon. Nevertheless, the Byzantine medical profession of the twelfth century must have felt that hospital organization offered the best possible medical treatment and that the emperor should have access to the benefits of such an organization. It would be interesting to know whether or not the poor sick were admitted to a great hall at the Mangana as they were at the Pantokrator, but no sources have survived to indicate what sort of facilities the Mangana Xenon maintained.

While serving citizens of property, Byzantine hospitals did not abandon their commitment to the poor. Justinian, whose reorganization of public medical care raised the professional reputation of hospital staffs, designed his new hospital at Antioch primarily for the poor.[62] From the tenth century comes evidence that xenones in Constantinople actually sent out wandering medics to treat the homeless poor who gathered in the streets and alleys of the city.[63] From the same century, a hagiographical text provides an example of the way in which hospitals kept their facilities open to all in need of medical help. A subdeacon of Hagia Sophia named Sergios quarreled with a mime. As the altercation grew more serious, a fist fight broke out. The mime got the best of poor Sergios, beat him severely about the head, and left him for dead on a manure pile. Here he was later found breathing with difficulty and unable to talk. Despite his wretched condition and apparent poverty, the physicians of the Euboulos Xenon admitted him to a hospital bed, examined him each day, and ordered every kind of medical treatment. After seven days, when no therapy had succeeded, the doctors gave up further treatment. The xenon did not expel Sergios to die in the streets, however. He was moved to a separate building while the xenon staff made preparations for his funeral. Incidentally, Sergios recovered, but only through miraculous intervention.[64]

The Pantokrator *Typikon* also reveals that this famous hospital, endowed by the imperial family with great wealth, admitted some patients so poor that they had only rags for clothing. Moreover, the hospital maintained a cemetery and a special funeral fund for those patients who died while at the xenon and who had absolutely no personal or family resources to pay for burial plots.[65]

These few examples should suffice to demonstrate that Byzantine hospitals continued to serve the poor even after the best practitioners of Greek medicine came to minister to the patients in their wards. As a model of the virtuous hospital physician, Byzantine doctors had before them the legendary Saint Thallelaios, who gladly treated both the rich and the poor at his xenon; some of the destitute he personally carried to the hospital.[66] To the credit of East Roman society, the doors of its xenones always remained open both to the homeless poor of the streets and to solid citizens of property.[67]

That both the poor and those of some wealth resorted to Byzantine xenones distinguished these institutions from the hospitals of the medieval West. As we have seen, Western philanthropic agencies failed to develop the same specialized medical services as the Byzantine xenones did. While the hospitals of Latin Christendom remained refuges for all sorts of suffering humanity—the homeless poor, orphans, the aged, and the maimed—Byzantine xenones focused all their resources on the task of curing the sick. When the physicians of the tenth-century Euboulos Xenon realized that they could not help their patient Sergios by medical means, they ceased treatment; the hospital administration then moved the injured man out of the xenon proper into a separate building in order to free a bed for a person who could benefit from a physician's care.[68] Moreover, Byzantine hospitals were closely linked to the medical profession as a whole. They absorbed the empire's best practitioners; their structure influenced the teaching and practice of Byzantine medicine for centuries, as we shall see. It is thus not surprising that Deacon Stephen—a man holding both a secure post at the richest church in Constantinople and also occupying an office in the Blue Faction—was willing to commit himself to the Sampson Xenon for care while no cleric with a good position in Paris would have even considered visiting the Hôtel-Dieu for medical treatment.[69]

That Byzantine nosokomeia received both the poor and the middle class helped, in turn, to ensure that these institutions continued to provide comfortable wards, proper medical attention, and adequate nursing care for all hospital patients. One can draw a parallel between the Byzantine xenones of the sixth through the twelfth centuries and some of the new hospitals founded by Westerners during the Enlightenment. While most European hospitals were still serving only the poor, the Pennsylvania Hospital, one of the first in the English colonies, admitted both poor and wealthy patients. This no doubt contributed to higher standards of service and medical expertise for all the sick on its wards. As a result, the Pennsylvania Hospital had a much lower death rate among its patients than did all but the very best contemporary hospitals of Europe.[70]

THE STAFF

THE HIERARCHY

To tend their wards, Byzantine hospitals maintained a large and often bewilderingly elaborate staff of doctors and nurses. Historians have often expressed their amazement at the complex organizations of the professional men and women at the Pantokrator Xenon but have usually considered its hierarchy of physicians, assistants, and nurses in isolation. A careful study of the personnel in earlier Byzantine hospitals will emphasize the striking similarities between the Comnenian hospitals and those from the era of Justinian and will indicate how the staff organization at the Pantokrator had evolved from the system used in earlier xenones.

The earliest hospitals of the fourth century do not seem to have had a highly organized cadre of physicans and professional support staff. The accounts of both Basil's hospital at Caesarea and those established by Chrysostom in Constantinople mention only physicians, without distinguishing specific grades.[71] Moreover, these institutions surely did not employ professional nursing staffs. No doubt the monks of Basil's community performed the nursing chores at his hospital just as urban ascetics served the sick in Chrysostom's nosokomeia. The records surviving from the fifth century, when nosokomeia were spreading to many cities of the empire, reveal almost nothing about the medical personnel who treated patients in these institutions. When, in the sixth century, the sources shed more light on the people working in the hospitals of the larger cities, professional physicians and a lay support staff have largely replaced the corps of urban monks who had first manned the wards of Christian hospitals. In Constantinople itself the remnants of the urban monastic movement limited their services in the city's xenones to assisting at the free funerals which the hospitals now supervised.

Again Justinian emerges as the instigator of change in hospital development, this time by reordering the medical personnel. When the emperor transformed the archiatroi from official doctors of the ancient poleis into staff physicians of the church xenones, he introduced all the traditions of the late classical medical profession into the Christian nosokomeia. These doctors no doubt preferred professional assistants to zealous volunteers. Thus, after the beginning of Justinian's reign, references to ascetics waiting on the sick disappear while references to a highly organized lay staff similar to that of the Pantokrator multiply.[72]

In describing the seventh-century Sampson and Christodotes hospitals, the *Miracula Artemii* illumines some interesting features of xenon staff organization after Justinian's changes.[73] According to these descriptions, the Sampson Xenon employed physicians who specialized in surgery, just as the Pantokrator hospital was to do 600 years later.[74] It also provided special facilities for patients with eye problems and perhaps hired physicians expert in treating such cases; so, too, the Pantokrator prepared one of its wards to handle ophthalmic problems.[75] The staff of the Christodotes Xenon included hypourgoi, assistants who were trained in medicine just as were the hypourgoi of the Pantokrator.[76] Moreover, the Christodotes required one of the hypourgoi to be at the hospital at night to supervise the night shift, a practice followed also at the Pantokrator, where five hypourgoi, one for each ward, watched over the patients during the dark hours.[77] The xenodochos who headed the Christodotes Xenon had duties similar to those of the nosokomos at the Pantokrator, though the different legal status of the twelfth-century hospital freed its administrator from the burdensome tasks of representing the institution before the law which had rested on earlier xenon administrators.[78] At the Christodotes Xenon the xenodochos supervised the chief physicians, or archiatroi, who actually treated the patients. The archiatroi, in turn, were divided into monthly shifts so that each chief physician would work only every other month, a system of rotation which the Pantokrator was still using six hundred years later.[79]

Alongside of striking similarities in organization, the Pantokrator *Typikon* reveals features in the staff which are absent in the brief descriptions of earlier hospital personnel. For example, the *Typikon* uses *perissoi* and *embathmoi* to describe ranks of both physicians and medical assistants, terms which do not appear with reference to any of the earlier hospitals. Moreover, the archiatroi, common in descriptions of hospitals after the mid-sixth century, cannot be found on the Pantokrator staff. Nevertheless, a careful examination of the sources from the sixth to the twelfth century reveals a basic continuity in staff organization despite the introduction of new terms and the development of a more complex top echelon of doctors. Regarding the archiatroi, three passages in particular deserve special attention.

By describing one of the head physicians at the Christodotes Xenon as "the archiatros who worked that month," the seventh-century author of the

Miracula Artemii indicated that the physicians of that hospital worked in monthly shifts.[80] His words imply too that the Christodotes had only two archiatroi, each one heading one of the monthly shifts. Thus, these archiatroi seem to correspond in function to the two primmikerioi who alternated each month in supervising the medical staff of the Pantokrator Xenon.[81] By the beginning of the ninth century the archiatroi suffered a reduction in rank, at least at some of the larger hospitals. When Theodore Stoudites referred to a hospital staff, he called the head physicians *protarchoi,* the second rank the *archiatroi,* the regular doctors *mesoi,* and the lowest order *teleutaioi.* Here the protarchoi would seem to correspond to the primmikerioi of the Pantokrator, while the archiatroi parallel the rank of the *protomenitai* at the Comnenian hospital. The mesoi of the ninth-century hospital would correspond to the regular ward doctors at the Pantokrator, and the teleutaioi, to the doctors of the outpatient clinic along with the other physicians described as *perissoi.*[82] Indeed, the title *protomenites* (first of the month) seems to support the conclusion that this office had evolved from that of the archiatros at earlier hospitals, since the *Miracula Artemii* emphasizes that each of the archiatroi at the seventh-century Christodotes Xenon was to lead the medical staff of the hospital for one month.[83] By the tenth century, the new term *protomenites* had replaced the older title *archiatros,* since a physician and author of that century, Romanos, styled himself protomenites of the Myrelaion Xenon.[84] So, too, the ninth-century term *protarchos* was replaced by the synonymous *primmikerios* sometime before John II founded the Pantokrator. Such an evolution of hospital functionaries over several centuries would help to explain the presence of two pairs of top-ranking physicians at the Pantokrator: the primmikerioi, who were by that time responsible for all aspects of medical care at the hospital, and the protomenitai, whose title reflects a position of leadership on the staff but who by the Comnenian period headed only one among several wards. This elaboration of titles and offices among the top-ranking hospital physicians parallels a similar multiplication of high offices in the Byzantine government.[85]

Apparently *archiatros* continued to be used in a general sense for all physicians in high hospital offices. The *Kletorologion of Philotheos,* a ninth-century manual of protocol, used the word with this general meaning in ordering the banquet which the emperor gave on the tenth day after Christmas. According to Philotheos, the emperor was to invite the xenodochoi from the xenones of Constantinople together with the archiatroi— apparently all physicians on hospital staffs.[86] Used in this general sense, *archiatros* survived the introduction of the new titles *primmikerios* and *protomenites.* As late as the end of the fourteenth century a physician of the Mangana Xenon named Stephen called himself an archiatros. Since the Mangana Xenon served the imperial court through the fourteenth century, however, Stephen might have used the title here in its most primitive sense, that of court physician.[87] Lesser hospitals probably never developed a highly articulated staff of physicians. The typikon of the small Lips Xenon, restored in the late thirteenth century, refers to the three medical men simply as *iatroi*.[88]

OUTPATIENT SERVICES

The Pantokrator Xenon and other twelfth-century hospitals in Constantinople also retained physicians specifically to treat outpatients. By the time of the Komnenoi, out-patient services seem to have been the normal channels through which people had access to scientific medical treatment. Thus, when a twelfth-century monk of a small monastery developed a sore foot, he asked his superior for permission to leave the monastery "to go to the xenon and show [his foot] to the doctors."[89] When the historian Kinnamos discusses the new drugs discovered by the emperor Manuel I, he adds that people usually obtained pharmacological products from the public nosokomeia.[90] The people of twelfth-century Thessalonica resorted to the city's xenon not only when they needed hospitalization but also when they required any sort of medication. Once the Latins destroyed the city's hospital in 1185, the seriously ill had no refuge, and those who wanted medicinal liquids or powders had to go elsewhere.[91] The outpatient clinic thus formed an important part of a xenon's work. To staff its dispensary, the Pantokrator *Typikon* assigned four physicians—two generalists and two surgeons—together with four ordained hypourgoi and four extra hypourgoi.[92]

The outpatient clinics continued to serve the people of Constantinople after the twelfth century, although they probably did not dominate the medical practice in later years as they had during the Comnenian period. The fascinating illustration in *Paris. gr.* 2243 (fol. 10ᵛ) provides strong evidence that hospital dispensaries still functioned as late as the first half of the fourteenth century. Besides the furnishings and decorations, this miniature depicts the staff, which, in the clinic pictured, consists of a physician, an assistant (probably a hypourgos), and a pharmacist. In the center of the picture two patients have entered the dispensary: one a man with crutches, the other a crying mother with a sick baby. The hypourgos is standing to the right of the patients holding a tripod, perhaps a portable stove. To the left of the patients upon a great chair sits the physician examining a vial of urine. To the far right of the picture the pharmacist tends his supplies.[93]

The miniature in *Paris. gr.* 2243 offers additional information which no doubt applies to all hospital personnel, not just those assigned to the outpatient clinics. In the illustration each person on the hospital staff has a distinctive gown and conical hat. The physician wears a blue-green gown, a color traditionally assigned to doctors since late antiquity. Over the gown he has a red mantle which matches his red half-boots. His conical hat is violet. The hypourgos wears a violet tunic, red half-boots, and a pale yellow conical hat with a red vertical stripe. The pharmacist wears a variegated red and blue tunic, yellow half-boots, and a red conical hat with a vertical white stripe. The colors of the tunics, boots, and hats clearly denote rank and function, just as the colors and patterns on the costumes of Byzantine officials indicated their title and office in the imperial government.[94] From other sources describing medical men, however, one can verify the significance only of the blue gown as the prescribed uniform of physicians.[95]

Outpatient clinics do not seem to have existed in the early xenones; at least they do not appear anywhere in the sources before the twelfth century. Xenones before 1000 maintained instead a corps of medical men, perhaps apprentice iatroi or hypourgoi, who toured the city's streets. Such a service undoubtedly had formed part of the routine in the earliest hospitals of the fourth and fifth centuries, when urban ascetics would aid any of the poor sick they found in the byways of the town, sometimes carrying the seriously ill back to the hospices or hospitals where they were serving as nurses. In fifth-century Jerusalem, the spoudaioi frequented the baths, taverns, and other places where the poor congregated to offer their help.[96] The *parabalani* and philoponoi of Alexandria also combed the baths and streets of the city in search of the poor stricken with disease and no doubt carried them to hostels or hospitals.[97] The legend of Saint Thallellaios provides a good example of such services directly connected with a xenon. According to one biography Saint Thallelaios opened a hospital somewhere in Lebanon where he treated all the sick who came to his shelter. At the same time he himself made rounds throughout the city in search of the helplessly ill, whom he would carry back to his hospital on his shoulders.[98]

When in the sixth century the professional staffs of physicians, hypourgoi, and nurses replaced urban ascetics as the work force in larger xenones, these lay employees also took over the ambulance duties. No direct evidence of such services survives from Constantinople before the tenth century, but from Visigothic Spain comes a report that a hospital at Merida had just such a corps of physicians (*medici*) who combed the city's streets in search of the sick.[99] In the tenth or early eleventh century, Romanos, a protomenites of the Myrelaion Xenon in Constantinople, wrote a handbook designed especially for these wandering doctors who, as Romanos states in his introduction, went through the streets and neighborhoods of the Byzantine capital to treat the sick.[100] By the time of the Pantokrator hospital, the corps of wandering medics working out of the xenones in Constantinople had disappeared; the walk-in clinics had replaced them.

MEDICAL TRAINING

Besides organizing the hospital staff to ensure the best possible medical care for its patients, the Pantokrator *Typikon* also sought to provide quality medical training so that an adequate number of good physicians would always be available to work in its wards. In pursuit of this goal, the *Typikon* stipulated that the hospital was to hire a respected physician to instruct medical students in the basics of the healing art.[101] This teacher ranked higher than any of the practicing physicians of the staff, including the primmikerioi. In addition, the Pantokrator Xenon maintained some physicians who had not finished all their training—those the *Typikon* describes as *perissoi* (extra). These no doubt assisted the ordained (*embathmoi*) iatroi much as interns do in modern hospitals. The physicians of the dispensary and those of the monastic infirmary were chosen from the ranks of these extra iatroi. The hospital also hired extra hypourgoi; with regard to these the *Typikon* specifies how many were to be assigned to each ward of the xenon. When vacancies occurred, the apprentice doctors and probably the hypourgoi could advance to the positions for ordained professionals if they had obtained sufficient experience in the hospital.[102]

In his study of Byzantine hospitals, Alexandre Philipsborn maintains that teaching medicine in a hospital setting such as the Pantokrator had not been part of the Byzantine xenon tradition before the Pantokrator. He suggests that John II Komnenos had adopted this program of medical instruction from Islamic institutions which Arab sources reveal as teaching hospitals.[103] It is true that no texts refer directly to scholastic programs in Byzantine hospitals before the Pantokrator, but such a practice would be consistent both with the history of Greek medicine from its earliest days in Knidos and Kos as well as with the development of Christian nosokomeia. In the days of Hippocrates, Greek physicians taught medicine to apprentices who worked with them in their iatreia. In referring to a doctor's office in fourth-century (B.C.) Athens, the orator Aeschines described the physician's attendant apprentices.[104] When, eight hundred years later, the future Arian leader Aetios studied medicine, he attended the iatreia at Alexandria together with other medical students.[105] In listing the hallmarks of the physician's profession about the year 400, John Chrysostom ranked as the first, opening a iatreion and as the second, acquiring students.[106] These examples should suffice to demonstrate that Greek physicians had always taught their trade as part of their normal activities. When doctors came to work in Christian hospitals toward the end of the fourth century, their apprentices naturally accompanied them on their rounds.

At the same time, the municipal archiatroi of East Roman cities were assuming an ever greater role in teaching medicine. According to one legend, the doctor-saint Thallelaios boasted that the archiatros Makarios had introduced him to the science of medicine. According to his biography, Saint Theodore of Sykeon always knew exactly how to cure the sick who sought his aid because he had been a prize student of Christ, the true archiatros.[107] In rephrasing a law of Constantine issued in 333, Justinian stated that the city archiatroi especially bore the responsibility for training new medical men.[108]

When that same emperor later forced these chief physicians to join the hospital staffs, it is logical to assume that they maintained their traditional teaching roles in the new environment. Thus, the fully developed xenones of Justinian's day also became theaters for the study of medicine.

Xenon libraries and their manuscripts provide additional evidence that Byzantine hospitals were also teaching institutions. After the sixth century, sources sometimes refer to manuscripts containing medical texts as hospital books (*xenonika biblia*). For example, a medical work attributed to Theophilos Protospatharios contains a collection of prescriptions aimed at restoring a patient's strength, prescriptions which had been collected from different xenon books.[109] From the end of the tenth century comes a richly illustrated codex of surgical works, a manuscript which the copyist and illustrator Niketas had prepared for hospital use.[110] The verse introduction to this collection emphasizes that Niketas had designed his codex as a tool for instruction, although it could also serve as a reference work for experienced staff physicians.[111]

During the last centuries of the empire—the Palaeologan period (1261–1453)—hospitals continued to teach medicine. In a letter from the beginning of the fourteenth century, George Lakapenos recounts how his friend the physician John Zachariah was continuing to train in the healing art at a Constantinopolitan xenon.[112] During the fifteenth century, the Krales Xenon of the capital managed to maintain its library and its courses of instruction. As late as 1415, the nosokomos of this hospital hired John Chortasmenos to rebind a famous manuscript of Dioskorides.[113] In the 1440s the renowned physician and philosopher Argyropoulos was teaching both medicine and natural philosophy in the same institution.[114] In sum, the whole tradition of Greek medicine and of hospital development points to the xenon as the place most suitable for physicians to teach both medical theory and practice. Although only those sources have survived which demonstrate that the twelfth-century Pantokrator Xenon and the fifteenth-century Krales Xenon maintained medical schools, most probably all the large hospitals of Constantinople supported teaching programs.

Sources dealing expressly with xenones offer very little assistance in reconstructing what methods Byzantine hospitals such as the Pantokrator used to train students in medicine. Fortunately, a source unrelated to hospitals helps to elucidate the role xenones played in training medieval Greek physicians. In attempting to describe the priestly profession, the patriarch Leo Stypes (1134–43) drew the familiar analogy between the priests and bishops—the physicians of the soul—and the physicians of the body. The patriarch embellished his metaphor with a detailed account of how one became a doctor in the Byzantine Empire. First, a student had to study the *logos* of medicine, the theories of Galen and Hippocrates. Second, he had to complete a long period of practical experience. Finally, he underwent a test at the hands of a medical officer. Having completed such a course, he received his symbol, his license.[115]

Stypes' system shows some similarity to the course of instruction at the Pantokrator Xenon. The *didaskalos* at the hospital taught the medical *logos* to the apprentices. Thus, his students would represent the apprentices at the first stage of Stypes' program—those learning the theories of Galen and Hippocrates.[116] The physicians who worked as extra doctors (*perissoi*) were still gathering practical experience in the hospital. They would correspond to students at the second stage of Stypes' program, those men studying the *praxis* of medicine.[117] From the ranks of the perissoi doctors, the Pantokrator selected the most advanced to serve the monastic infirmary and the outpatient clinic.[118] Perhaps, these perissoi physicians had to prove their abilities at this stage by passing an exam, the one Stypes describes, although the *Typikon* contains no references to an examination of perissoi doctors or of any regulations regarding licensure before they could assume a permanent post on the medical staff. In general, the *Typikon* provides too little information about perissoi doctors and those described as *embathmoi* (ordained) to reach any conclusions regarding the methods of promotion. Still, it is tempting to suppose that the promotion system at the Pantokrator was linked in some way to the educational plan which Patriarch Stypes, a contemporary of the imperial xenon, outlined, even though the exact relationship escapes us.

PROFESSIONAL SOCIETIES

In discussing the ranks of physicians and medical assistants at the Pantokrator Xenon and the system of teaching medicine, one should consider the similarities between some of the terms which the *Typikon* uses for medical personnel and those which the tenth-century *Book of the Eparch* employs in legislating for the guild of notaries (*taboullarioi*). If a man wanted to become a notary, he had first to have a general education and to have studied the standard law books, the *Procheiros Nomos* and the *Basilika*. He then spent some time as an apprentice and finally took a written test. When he had passed his exam, the notaries received him into their guild. According to the *Book of the Eparch,* the successful student received the rank (*bathmos*) of a notary, an expression very similar to *embathmos,* which the Pantokrator *Typikon* uses to describe the more advanced hypourgoi and the physicians who entered permanent hospital posts.[119] In addition, the *Book of the Eparch* refers to the head of the notary guild as a *primmikerios,* the same title which the *Typikon* applies to the hospital's chief physicians.[120] It is thus possible that the professional hospital staff at the Pantokrator was organized along lines established by rules of a physicians' guild, similar to the notaries' society.

Other sources support such a conclusion. In presenting the steps by which a young student of medicine trained to be a physician, Patriarch Stypes outlined a process very similar to the requirements of entering the notaries' guild—basic education, professional training, some experience, and a passing grade on an exam.[121] A few years later Patriarch Lukas Chrysoberges mentioned that the physicians had to participate in parades on certain occasions, dressed in their traditional blue garments.[122] The notaries also had to participate in imperial processions and other official ceremonies, also in prescribed professional gowns.[123] Since the *Book of the Eparch* does not mention iatroi, we can assume that the city prefect had no jurisdiction over the doctors' society. In his commentary on Stypes' description, Professor Grumel suggested that the highest-ranking court physician, the *aktouarios,* supervised the physicians' guild throughout Constantinople.[124] It is more likely, however, that his authority was limited to the staff doctors of the Mangana Xenon, as we saw above.

What relationship did hospitals have to the guild of physicians? Could they have represented the major divisions of the physicians' professional organization? In support of such an hypothesis is the fact that the first reference to any kind of professional guild in the medical field refers to hospital hypourgoi in seventh-century Alexandria.[125] By that time in the Egyptian metropolis and no doubt in Constantinople itself, the medical assistants who worked in hospitals had formed guilds. Thus, in the twelfth century, the embathmoi medical assistants of the Pantokrator Xenon had full guild membership while the perissoi did not. The physicians, on the other hand, had no guild or *collegium* in the ancient world, nor do the sources reveal clearly any such organization in the Byzantine period before the twelfth century. However, the ancient public physicians and their successors, the archiatroi of the cities, had formed a closed association of the professional elite.[126] In the fourth century the emperor Valentinian ordered that the fourteen archiatroi of Rome should replace retired members of their group by electing new members on the basis of their professional qualifications.[127] A similar system must have functioned in Constantinople and other great cities of the East, although in some of these centers the old curial councils probably retained some role. When Justinian assigned archiatroi to Christian xenones, he introduced a closed group of tested physicians as the top echelon of the medical staff in every hospital. As xenones multiplied in Constantinople, the number of archiatroi also increased to supply new hospitals with expert medical personnel. When in the late ninth century the archiatroi played a role in court ceremonial, they attended in their traditional blue robes organized under the xenodochoi of the city's hospitals.[128] Already they resembled the guild of notaries who had also to participate in imperial ceremonies. One can suppose too that the methods for testing a possible archiatros were expanded to include not only admission to the highest rank among doctors but to any applying for a position as a hospital physician. Thus, by the twelfth century, all xenon iatroi had to pass an exam and receive a license. I hesitate to say that only hospital physicians had passed such tests and thus were the only members of the doctors' guild. Still, I believe that the hospital organization and its archiatroi stimulated the development of a tighter professional organization, just as xenones had played a role in organizing the hypourgoi of Alexandria into a society by the seventh century.[129] That the supervising physicians, the primmikerioi, of the Pantokrator bore the same title as the masters of the notaries guild adds considerable weight to this argument.

SALARIES

By examining carefully a puzzling feature of the Pantokrator *Typikon*—the low salaries paid the staff physicians—it is possible to cast some additional light on the relationship between the Byzantine medical profession and the xenones. The top-ranking physicians of the Pantokrator staff—the primmikerioi—received 8 *noumismata* and forty-five *modioi* of wheat valued at twelve modioi a noumisma for a total yearly salary of 11.75 noumismata. At the other end of the scale, the perissoi doctors of the outpatient clinic were paid annually 6.75 noumismata a year.[130] One hundred and fifty years later, the physicians at the Lips Xenon were collecting a salary of 16 noumismata (or 10.6 noumismata in twelfth-century currency), a stipend only slightly less than that of the primmikerioi at the Pantokrator.[131] George Ostrogorsky has calculated that an annual income of 12 noumismata represented a living wage in the East Roman Empire.[132] Had the physicians at the Pantokrator and Lips depended on their hospital stipends alone for financial support, then all of them, including the primmikerioi, would have been poor men. Of course, xenon service represented only half of a staff doctor's professional activity. During six off-duty months, he could supplement his stipend with the fruits of private practice.

Why were the leading physicians of the East Roman Empire willing to work in hospitals during half the year for such low pay? The professional organization of American doctors in the nineteenth century can offer an analogy for understanding the Byzantine system. First in England and then in the United States, physicians began to set up new hospitals during the eighteenth century. In these institutions the doctors were to treat the patients without collecting any fees.[133] Surprisingly, such hospitals attracted the voluntary services of the leading physicians. Although altruism played a part in stirring doctors to undertake hospital work, such service provided material rewards as well. Treating ward patients offered new opportunities for gaining practical experience and improving a man's medical expertise; it also enabled him to win prestige in the profession and in the community—prestige which translated into a more prosperous private practice. Since staff physicians did not work year-round for hospitals but usually for only four months of the year, they could devote most of their time to the patients who paid them.[134] Gradually, in the course of the nineteenth century, an elaborate hierarchy of hospital positions evolved. Local doctors competed for such jobs, and only the best or most influential attained regular hospital appointments and the concomitant increase in the fruits of private practice.[135]

A similar system seems to have developed in medieval Constantinople and perhaps in some of the other Byzantine towns as well. Physicians were compelled to work in xenones in order to gain experience and to win prestige in the medical profession. In return for their services, xenon doctors were given a small salary; most of their income was to come from private practice. Hospital service, however, greatly enhanced the amount of money they could gain from such practice. A primmikerios or a protomenites of a famous xenon no doubt won the patronage of the wealthy and could demand higher fees than a perissos hospital doctor. Both, however, could charge far more than a physician with no hospital affiliation. The staff doctors of the Pantokrator Xenon had achieved such renown that aristocrats, including the emperor's courtiers, attempted to lure these experts out of Constantinople to treat them at their country estates.[136]

Even the nosokomoi or xenodochoi of Byzantine hospitals earned low salaries. At the Pantokrator the nosokomos collected a yearly salary of 12.5 noumismata, half a noumisma above Ostrogorsky's minimum wage.[137] Unlike the staff doctors, the nosokomoi had to work the whole year and thus had no opportunity to supplement their income. On the other hand, such hospital directors regularly held court titles. The *Kletorologion of Philotheos* ranked them with the *spatharioi,* while lead seals indicate that they could also hold the higher rank of *protospatharios.*[138] Such court titles carried with them substantial yearly salaries. For example, in the eleventh century a protospatharios received an annual salary of 72 noumismata.[139] This plus the stipend paid by the xenon represented a respectable income.

As hospitals exerted increasing influence on the structure of the Byzantine medical profession and on its training, one would expect that physicians would have sought some role in governing them. The sources indeed reveal that doctors gradually came to dominate hospital administrations. As we saw in Chapter Six, episcopal clergy had supervised the early nosokomeia.[140] Even after Justinian's reforms, xenodochoi still came from the ranks of the clergy. In the early seventh century the xenodochos of the Christodotes hospital was an important clerical advisor of the patriarch, not a practicing physician. When he discovered a stricken church singer alone and unattended, he made no attempt to treat him, but handed him over to the archiatroi for medical help.[141] By the twelfth century, however, a physician held the highest administrative post, that of nosokomos, at the Pantokrator Xenon.[142] During the same years, when Theodore Prodromos underwent cautery treatments at a Constantinopolitan xenon, the nosokomos himself performed the operation.[143] Although all our evidence indicating that the top hospital administrators at Constantinople (whether called xenodochoi or nosokomoi) were also medical doctors comes from the twelfth century, it is likely that the physicians' guild had taken over these administrative posts some time earlier as the medical profession had grown more tightly bound to hospital staff organization. In addition, when the emperors of the late ninth century began to manage hospital resources through officials of their private estates, they no doubt facilitated the rise of physicians into the top managerial posts at xenones, since these officials were no longer involved directly in legal and financial matters.[144]

METHODS OF TREATMENT

From the very beginning Christian hospitals had fostered secular Greek medicine to treat the bodily ills of their patients. Both Aetios and Basil, key figures in the development of hospitals, had studied the classical Greek science of medicine and used its principles in fullfilling the corporal works of mercy towards the sick.[145] After Justinian's reorganization, the archiatroi—the leading physicians of the Greek tradition—assumed responsibility for medical care at Christian hospitals throughout the cities of the East. Under the auspices of both the church and the state, the nosokomeia helped to bring good medical care, based on the tenets of Hippocrates, Galen, and the other great Greek physicians, to a much wider circle of the population than had been the case in earlier centuries.[146]

As part of rational Greek medicine, the physician needed first to examine his patients to establish the causes of their maladies. Thus, one of the earliest descriptions of a Christian hospital, found in the letter of Neilos (ca. 400), portrays the physician examining patients. Neilos recounts how the doctor had to observe each sick person with care to determine what treatment was needed.[147] By the sixth century doctors made their rounds each day both to examine new patients and to check on the progress of the others. At the seventh-century Christodotes Xenon, the archiatros made his rounds every morning during the month he was on duty.[148] Although neither the Pantokrator *Typikon* nor any other document describing Byzantine xenones in detail mentions that hospital physicians kept written records of the medical treatments they prescribed and the subsequent progress of patients, there are several indications that they did use such procedures. First, Islamic hospitals maintained patient records.[149] Since the Moslems had adopted their hospitals from Nestorian Christians in Persia, who had in turn brought their medical institutions to the East from Antioch, Edessa, and Nisibis in the fifth century, it is possible that such record-keeping originated in the early Byzantine xenones of Syria.[150] Second, the heading of a treatment list compiled by a Constantinopolitan xenon in the tenth or early eleventh century indicates that this particular hospital routinely collected from its staff physicians therapies which experience had demonstrated as effective.[151] This heading implies, first, that xenon physicians were not bound by the treatments which ancient physicians ordered but were willing to devise new therapies in search of successful remedies. Second, it implies that these doctors kept some record of what they had prescribed and of the patients' responses.[152]

The treatments xenon doctors ordered derived from the principles of Galenic medicine. Their theory of uroscopy in diagnostics and their frequent use of phlebotomy demonstrate this dependence. Nevertheless, the hospital physicians always referred to experience—the success or failure of a particular therapy—as the final judge in approving a prescription. The various xenon treatment lists which hospital staffs collected from the tenth through the fourteenth century all stress that the remedies they have recorded had stood the test of *peira* (experience).[153] So too in the preparation of his handbook for the hospital physicians of the ambulance corps, the protomenites of the Myrelaion Xenon assigned an important role to his personal observations.[154]

Among the approved procedures, these xenon treatment lists mention blood-letting, baths, salves, plasters, sitz baths, and a multitude of medicaments taken orally. For stomach pains one such list recommends bitter honey, mint mixed with wine, and a number of other herbs taken internally. It also suggests several emetics to relieve the discomfort. Finally, it requires two baths followed by external applications of laurel leaves. The ancient theory of humors plays a part here in the diagnosis and therapy of stomach pains. The list recommends different medicines for patients whose stomach pains arise from an excess of the cold humor, phlegm, than it does for those due to an imbalance of the hot humor, yellow bile.[155] Although these treatment lists have absorbed many facets of ancient medical practice, they ignore surgery beyond phlebotomy. The surgical manuscript of Niketas, however, indicates that twelfth-century physicians still had some familiarity with the operations and techniques developed by ancient practitioners and by their successors at Alexandria.[156]

Historians of medicine have debated how far doctors of the Byzantine era departed from the classical physicians in developing new treatments from experience and even in advancing novel theories. To answer this question satisfactorily would require comparing hospital therapies as they have been noted down in xenon treatment lists with the medical wisdom contained in the vast corpus of Galen and Hippocrates and with the epitomes of other ancient medical writers preserved by compilers such as Oribaseios. Such a thorough examination of Greek medicine falls outside the scope of the present study. Nevertheless, the few previous attempts to compare hospital treatment lists and other medical treatises of the Byzantine period with the works of classical physicians have indicated that medieval Greek medicine differed substantially from that of the ancients.[157] The next chapter will explore Byzantine medical literature and its relationship to the classical tradition in more detail.

From the Pantokrator *Typikon* and other sources bearing directly on hospitals, the image of a well-organized institution emerges, an institution which tries to provide its patients with the very best in medical and nursing care. Rows of clean, well-equipped beds surround a great hearth; a large staff of servants, hypourgoi, and physicians of various ranks examine and serve the patients, each member of the staff clothed in his distinctive robe and cap. Above the hospital floor frescos or mosaics decorate the ceiling and walls; icons too hang in the hospital proper and its chapels. Not only the poor but men of standing such as Deacon Stephen from Constantinople seek these hospitals as refuges from their suffering and as places which at least offer them some hope of a cure. Thus, Bishop Eustathios of Thessalonica considered the destruction of the city's xenon a great tragedy for all his people.[158] To correct a too rosy conception of Byzantine nosokomeia, however, it would be well to consider another description of a xenon, this time from an observer who saw the institution on his back, as it were, as a patient. Since his hospital experience was painful and ultimately unsuccessful, his account will provide a different perspective on the Byzantine xenon than have the typika, narrative histories, and saints' lives we have considered thus far.

Theodore Prodromos, a prolific writer of Comnenian Constantinople, suffered from chronic bad health and finally ended his life in a gerokomeion.[159] During one of his bouts with disease he committed himself to a xenon in the capital for treatment. From his hospital bed he addressed a poem to his patroness, the princess Irene—the *Sebastokratorissa*—in which he provides some fascinating details on the xenon. This poem Prodromos describes as an anguished cry to Irene from a fiery furnace, not the furnace of Babylon of old into which the king threw the Hebrew children, but the furnace of Galen and Hippocrates—the hospital. Whereas the children suffered nothing in Babylon, Prodromos must here undergo excruciating torture from the doctors' cautery irons, a pain which pierces his whole being, a pain beyond his strength to bear.[160]

Prodromos then describes one of his cautery sessions. Upon entering the operating room, he is struck with amazement at the size of the fire blazing there. Several assistants—holy executioners, Prodromos refers to them— heat up the irons in the fire while others fan the flames. Some assistants strip off his clothes as though he were a condemned criminal and prepare the cold operating table. Supervising the whole scene stands the physician in charge: at the hospital where Prodromos stayed this was the nosokomos himself. The poet portrays him as a kind man and an excellent physician, the best in his field: "My dear healer of diseases, a healer who charges no fee," Prodromos exclaims. The poet relates how the nosokomos joked with him, smiled, and tried to comfort him with sweet words, a medicine for the coming pains. At the same time the doctor was carefully measuring poor Prodromos. He marked the area for cautery with a surgical pencil and then applied the glowing iron. A screech of pain from the patient, and Prodromos lay ashen-colored, charred like a piece of coal.[161]

Prodromos' account of his bitter sufferings in the hospital provides a valuable addition to the picture of a xenon presented by the Pantokrator *Typikon,* a picture only of the hospital's administrative structure with no reference to the fate of the patients. Prodromos' poem vividly illustrates that the wards and operating rooms of Byzantine hospitals often echoed with the cries and groans of their patients. Many suffered there; some died under treatment. Prodromos himself never fully recovered from his ailments. In the words of one friend, he died young, having been purified by the suffering he underwent.[162] It is impossible to determine what percentage of patients survived a stay in a hospital or how many of them were healed as a result of xenon treatment. Whatever the rate of success, however, no patient, however bitter he might be regarding his sickness and the pain of treatment, has left us an attack on the hospitals themselves. They were, in the words of the fourteenth-century emperor John Kantakouzenos, "the glory of the Romans."[163]

CHAPTER NINE

Hospitals and Medical Literature

The Christian hospitals of the Byzantine Empire employed professional physicians from their earliest days in the fourth century to the declining years of Constantinople under the Palaeologan dynasty. Before 400 Basil of Caesarea and John Chrysostom had both hired physicians, or iatroi, to treat the poor patients in their hospitals.[1] By the mid-sixth century Byzantine physicians considered hospitals essential for practicing their profession properly. Influenced by East Roman doctors, Christian physicians in the service of Shah Khusro I convinced the Persian monarch that they needed a xenon for their work.[2] In the twelfth century, a single imperial institution, the Pantokrator Xenon, offered employment to nineteen accredited physicians and maintained a cadre of interns as well.[3] By that time, if not long before, hospitals had become the usual workplaces for well-trained physicians in large Byzantine cities such as Constantinople and Thessalonica.[4]

Byzantine hospitals surely affected both the practice and the theory of Byzantine medicine, since by the second half of the sixth century these institutions had attained a central place in providing medical care and in training new physicians. To determine the relationship between xenon practice and Byzantine medical science, however, requires a careful survey of professional medical literature from the late fourth century to 1453—an extremely difficult task. For many Byzantine medical texts are either unpublished or available in uncritical editions. Moreover, the manuscript traditions of these texts are so complicated and contain so many different recensions that historians and philologists have been unable to date most of them or to determine their authors.[5] It is possible, therefore, to provide only a brief survey of Byzantine medical literature and of the interaction between the hospital milieu and these works. Pursuing this goal will also introduce wider questions concerning the continuity of Greek medical science during the catastrophic period of the seventh and eighth centuries and concerning the empirical orientation of Byzantine medicine in general.

The very nature of professional medical works further complicates our task, since these rarely include details about the institutional surroundings in which observations were made or treatments administered. Thus, even the xenon treatment lists contain few if any internal references to hospitals, although they clearly are describing therapies used by xenon physicians. The fourteenth-century medical writer John Zachariah—who studied medicine in a Constantinopolitan hospital and later served as *aktouarios* (the emperor's personal physician) in the Mangana Xenon—does mention his xenon experiences within his voluminous writings. Nevertheless, these references are so few that historians had been unaware of Zachariah's hospital duties until Professor Armin Hohlweg recently reexamined his works.[6] Thus, professional medical texts, considered by themselves, have left the impression that hospitals played a limited role in the development of Greek medicine in the medieval period. To evaluate these texts correctly, therefore, we must keep in mind the convincing evidence in nontechnical sources that xenones were at the center of the Byzantine medical profession.

THE EARLY BYZANTINE PERIOD

Historians of medicine usually classify Oribaseios of Pergamon as the first Byzantine physician. During the reign of the emperor Julian (361–63), he published a huge digest of classical medicine in seventy books which summarized the work of ancient physicians from Hippocrates to the doctors of the second century A.D. He designed his compendium to reduce the vast corpus of classical medical literature to its essential core. Selecting material primarily from Galen's writings, but including passages by other physicians as well, Oribaseios tried to offer what was most helpful in curing disease. Subsequent Byzantine physicians would pursue a similar method in organizing the great heritage of Greek medicine.[7] Since Oribaseios wrote just at the time that the first hospitals were forming in Antioch, Constantinople, and the towns of Asia Minor, his work preceded their influence on the practice of medicine.

Sometime after Oribaseios and before the great physicians of the sixth century, a doctor named Theon prepared a practical treatise on medicine which he called *Anthropos.* Though this work has not survived, the patriarch Photios provides us with a brief description of it in his *Bibliotheca.* A man of some medical expertise himself, Photios ranked Theon's *Anthropos* with Oribaseios' compendium by stressing its usefulness in medical practice. Theon organized the *Anthropos* into two parts: the first section discussed diseases, beginning with those afflicting the head and closing with those attacking the limbs and joints; the second section provided a *materia medica.*[8] Theon's arrangement of disease *a capite ad calcem* (from head to foot) had originated with Galen, but it did not gain wide popularity until Theon's time.[9] Byzantine physicians writing after the fifth century, however, used it frequently, probably because it served the working doctor well. Theon himself held the office of archiatros at Alexandria. Though he seems to have flourished before the city physicians had any relationship with the Christian hospitals, Alexandrian archiatroi of a few generations later entered xenon service, bringing with them the same emphasis on practice and indifference to theory which Photios describes as a hallmark of the *Anthropos*.[10]

The sixth-century reign of Justinian saw the emergence of two great medical writers: first Aetios of Amida and a generation later Alexander of Tralleis. Both men practiced and wrote at a time when the archiatroi of the Greek cities were moving into the Christian xenon, the new focus of both their healing and teaching duties, yet neither explicitly refers to hospitals in their works.[11]

Aetios' *Sixteen Books on Medicine* followed closely the pattern set by Oribaseios. As Photios explained, this work concentrated on the task of healing, omitting discussions of human anatomy and medical theory. Aetios' treatise found favor with later Byzantine physicians for its clarity and usefulness in daily practice.[12] Alexander of Tralleis, on the other hand, ventured beyond compiling and clarifying Hippocrates, Galen, and the other ancient physicians. He sometimes relied on his own observations, daring at times to criticize Galen himself when the great physician's views did not seem to reflect what he himself had observed.[13] He also included novel pharmacological treatments in his work.[14]

Living in the reign of Justinian, Alexander surely knew the xenones and their growing influence on the medical profession. Medical historians, however, have found no evidence that he treated hospital patients. Most of his clients were wealthy people who could afford to hire him as a private doctor. Moreover, Alexander did not stay at Tralleis in Asia Minor or in Constantinople but travelled to the Western provinces, where medical hospitals had not taken root.[15] Yet it is certain that Alexander's writings influenced the Christian hospitals even though the author himself was unaffected by them, for later xenon manuscripts reveal the popularity of his treatises among hospital physicians. As late as the fourteenth century, the doctors of the Mangana Xenon prepared a treatment list which included therapies extracted from his writings.[16]

Two aspects of Alexander's work reflect the close relationship between the Greek medical profession as it had evolved by the sixth century and hospital practice. First, Alexander stressed the importance of baths in treating disease. Since the time of Hippocrates, Greek physicians had been elaborating treatment procedures which included bathing in waters of various chemical properties. Oribaseios had preserved these ancient therapies, and Alexander developed them further.[17] The firm belief of Alexander and other leading fifth- and sixth-century physicians in the efficacy of bath regimens no doubt convinced hospital founders to include complete bathing facilities for their patients. Moreover, hospital supervision made it easy for physicians treating many patients to integrate disciplined bathing routines into their therapies.[18] Private doctors, on the other hand, surely found it difficult to monitor effectively such treatments for more than a few patients at a time.

Second, Alexander prepared a monograph on diseases of the eyes.[19] In this, too, he was building upon a tradition within the ancient Greek medical profession—namely, the field of ophthalmology.[20] That Alexander and other leading physicians emphasized eye problems as a distinct field of study convinced hospital builders to include special wards for eye patients. In the seventh century the Sampson Xenon already maintained separate facilities for ophthalmic cases; this practice probably originated a century earlier at the same time Alexander was active.[21]

The last of the early Byzantine physicians, Paul of Aegina, never came to Constantinople. He spent all of his professional life in Alexandria, studying and practicing medicine during the first half of the seventh century.[22] Here he witnessed the Arab invasion of the Eastern provinces and the collapse of Byzantine rule in Egypt. Since Christian hospitals were well-established in Alexandria by the end of the sixth century and Egyptian archiatroi now supervised their patients, Paul undoubtedly knew them well. Nevertheless, in the seven books of his medical treatise, the *Epitome,* he never describes a xenon or a nosokomeion, or even an ancient iatreion, so that it is impossible to determine in what setting he carried out the treatments he recommends.[23]

Despite Paul's silence regarding xenones, there is at least a suggestion that Alexandrian hospitals played a role in his professional life. Later Arab sources link him with obstetrics; they usually refer to him as *alqawabeli* (the birth helper) because he advised midwives in Alexandria.[24] At the same time that Paul was practicing there, the patriarch John (610–19) established a system of seven special institutions, each with forty beds, distributed throughout the Egyptian capital, institutions designed solely to provide poor women a place to bear their children and recuperate for a week thereafter.[25] Perhaps Paul served as a physician advisor in one of these institutions and hence won his sobriquet, the birth helper.

Beyond this suggestion, it is impossible to find evidence that hospitals affected Paul's practice or his professional writing. On the other hand, it is clear that his *Epitome* influenced later hospitals. Paul displayed special interest and skill in preparing chapter 6 of the *Epitome,* a concise treatise on surgery. Medical historians consider this essay the best work on surgical techniques which has survived from the ancient Greek tradition of medical literature. Although Paul's instructions derive from the work of earlier physicians, he was able to describe the procedures in a concise, clear fashion, so that, with regard to several operations, modern scholars have been able to understand correctly the ancient procedures only from Paul's account, although Celsus and Galen also discussed the same operations.[26] In the centuries after Paul, xenon physicians consulted his work for its clear explanations of surgical operations. In the late tenth century the doctor Niketas prepared an illustrated manuscript on surgery which included a section from Paul's chapter 6. Niketas designed his codex for the students and the medical staff of a xenon somewhere in Constantinople. Later, at the end of the twelfth century, the Nosokomeion of the Forty Martyrs acquired this rich codex for its medical staff.[27] I will have more to say about Niketas' codex later.

THE BYZANTINE DARK AGE

From the beginning of the seventh century, Paul's city of Alexandria and the other great urban centers of Greek culture in Syria, Palestine, and Egypt declined rapidly. Factional fighting rent them from within while the Persians and later the Arabs attacked them from without.[28] By Paul's death the East Roman Empire had lost control of Alexandria, Antioch, Caesarea Maritima, and the other Oriental cities. Now Constantinople emerged as the undisputed hub of Greco-Roman civilization. It had been the political capital since 330; from about 600 it became the sole cultural center as well. Along with the other fields of study, Greek medicine now revolved about the city on the Bosporos. But even here, behind the impregnable walls of Constantinople, Greek learning waned during the seventh and eighth centuries—according to some researchers almost to the vanishing point.[29] Historians have called the era following the catastrophes of the late sixth and early seventh centuries the Byzantine Dark Age, a period which saw classical culture reach its lowest ebb. Unassailable in their fortress city, the East Roman emperors reordered Byzantine society to wage defensive warfare against Persians, Avars, Arabs, Bulgars, and Slavs. During these years of constant military emergency, every area of Greek intellectual life declined. No evidence survives that the men of those generations wrote narrative accounts of the events they witnessed, nor that they continued to compose poetry, philosophical works, or rhetorical pieces.[30] Paul Lemerle has emphasized how rare good professors became during the Dark Age. Moreover, he stresses that scriptoria almost ceased producing books. We have today very few manuscripts which were executed during those years and none, preserved in their original state, which contain works from the classical pagan past.[31]

In those difficult days, Byzantine society seems to have consumed most of its energies in self-defense. Moreover, the enemies of East Rome destroyed many of the empire's provincial cities. Some of these in Asia Minor had flourished as centers of Greek learning. After 600 Miletus, a town renowned for its classical culture, ceased to exist as a polis.[32] The rich city of Ephesus survived, but robbed of its former glory.[33] Despite the severe strains of those years, however, Byzantine society managed to train some men of each new generation in ancient Greek and in the elements of the classical heritage. Hagiographical sources of the eighth and ninth centuries reveal the continued existence of schools both in Constantinople and in the provinces where children learned to read and write and where they acquired the rudiments of grammar, rhetoric, and logic as well as music, arithmetic, geometry, and astronomy. In addition, high government officials often trained apprentices in the skills necessary to manage a sophisticated society, skills which included some knowledge of the classical tradition.[34]

In considering centers of instruction and the survival of Greek culture during the Dark Age of the Byzantine Empire, scholars have overlooked the role which the xenones of Constantinople played in transmitting classical civilization to later generations. Several of the great hospitals of the capital kept their doors open from the prosperous days of Justinian through the Dark Age to the Renaissance of the mid-ninth century. When Constantine Porphyrogennitos copied his list of xenon administrators for the Book of Ceremonies in the tenth century, he included xenodochoi of four hospitals which had been founded before the end of the sixth century: the Sampson, the Euboulos, the Irene in Perama, and the Narses dedicated to Saint Panteleemon. Since the particular description incorporating the procession of xenodochoi reflects ceremonies from the ninth-century reign of Michael III, it is reasonable to assume that these four hospitals survived the tumults of the seventh and eighth centuries, preserving a continuous tradition from the days of Justinian I.[35] Although xenones like the Sampson had probably been simple establishments in the late fourth and fifth centuries, they developed into important centers of the medical profession in the sixth century as a result of Justinian's legislation. At these hospitals the archiatroi both taught and practiced medicine.[36] During the three centuries following Justinian's death (565), they continued to instruct medical students at the four city xenones which Constantine VII listed and perhaps at other large hospitals as well.

For the convenience of their staff physicians and their students, hospitals began to collect books containing useful medical works. Gradually they assembled libraries. By the time the anonymous xenon treatment list attributed to Theophilos was composed sometime in the tenth or eleventh century, hospitals normally possessed a collection of books.[37] In later centuries xenones had manuscripts copied and old codices rebound.[38] It is impossible to determine when hospitals first began to organize libraries and sponsor copying efforts. Perhaps, they initiated these programs when the archiatroi took up their teaching duties in the xenon setting. In this connection it is worthwhile to consider the results of Professor Lemerle's research on manuscripts of the Byzantine Dark Age. After searching in major European libraries for Greek manuscripts which had been copied during the seventh or eighth century, he could find only one that included a nonreligious text. *Coislini-*

anus 120 contained four leaves copied probably in the late eighth century. These leaves preserved a list of medical remedies, written in very early minuscule script, a list of remedies which resembles the very kind of medical literature which the Byzantine hospital practice of later centuries generated in abundance—the xenon treatment list. Could Lemerle's four leaves represent the product of a scriptorium in a Constantinopolitan xenon?[39]

At least four hospitals in Constantinople continued to serve the people of the capital by providing medical care and by training new physicians during the turbulent Dark Age of the empire. Perhaps they supported scriptoria as well. They thus contributed to keeping alive the tradition of ancient Greek medicine which had experienced a revival during the sixth century. As Byzantine society trimmed its intellectual establishment after 600, the hospitals which survived assumed an ever more prominent position in the medieval medical profession and in the educational establishment as a whole. Surely, this new prominence had an impact on the medical writing of the seventh century and after. In fact, the few medical works of the Dark Age and especially the more abundant production of the ninth- and tenth-century revival exhibit major changes due primarily to the influence of the Christian xenones.

Very little evidence has survived regarding the doctors of the Dark Age and their professional writing. Through careful study of Latin, Arabic, and Greek manuscripts, however, Professor Owsei Temkin has identified a few Byzantine treatises from this period. He has demonstrated that the anatomical terms *basilic* and *cephalic* originated, not with Moslem medical works as scholars had previously held, but with short Greek manuals for bloodletting which Byzantine surgeons prepared sometime after 600 and before 850— i.e., during the Byzantine Dark Age. Temkin emphasized that the authors of these phlebotomy texts broke with the tradition of classical Greek medicine as it was expressed by leading physicians from Hippocrates to Galen not only by formulating new anatomical terms, but also by ignoring much of the medical theory in the works of their ancient predecessors. Their short essays thus differ sharply from the works of classical physicians and from the earlier Byzantine authors such as Aetios or Alexander, who still incorporated some of the ancient theoretical principles in their writings.[40] It is tempting to see these new treatises as products of xenon instruction and practice, since they employ a terse, telegraphic Greek identical to the style found in later works which manuscripts clearly identify as xenon treatment lists.[41]

The *De pulsibus* of the monk Merkourios also seems to date from the Byzantine Dark Age, and it surely shares the characteristics of the phlebotomy manuals. The author has prepared a simple set of twenty-eight rules for taking a patient's pulse and for using this information in diagnosis, without any discussion of medical theory. Although this short text gives no clue that it was designed for hospital use, it is worth noting, first, that the title describes

Merkourios as a monk.[42] As we have seen, Byzantine monks were assigned to work in xenones and to study medicine from the time of Dorotheos of Gaza until the fourteenth century. Second, short manuals on pulses were popular in xenon codices. As late as the fifteenth century, a medical student or intern at the Krales Xenon composed a short guide to pulses based on the hospital lectures of the famous philosopher and physician John Argyropoulos.[43]

Three medical manuscripts (*Paris. gr.* 2224 and 2236 and *Monac. gr.* 288) contain a medical treatise attributed to the archiatros John which resembles the style of Merkourios' *De pulsibus* and may also date from the Dark Age. It presents a list of more than two hundred remedies arranged according to the ailments against which these were effective. The ailments, in turn, follow a rough *a capite ad calcem* order. Reflecting the methods of other Dark Age texts, John's collection contains no discussion of imperceptible or underlying causes, but simply presents a number of effective remedies. As with Merkourios' *De pulsibus* the text itself never refers to hospitals, but there are several indications that this composition emerged from xenon practice. First, John was an archiatros. After Justinian's reorganization of the city archiatroi, these high-ranking physicians always appear in hospital service. Second, this collection forms the opening section of a later xenon treatment list of the tenth century, a list that had assembled some of its entries from the prescriptions attributed to doctors of previous generations. Apparently, John's collection of remedies represented a valuable deposit of earlier hospital wisdom for the compilers of the later xenon list. Third, the specific therapies which John recommends are different from most of those in the works of classical medicine. Unlike earlier Byzantine physicians such as Aetios or Paul of Aegina, John seems to have depended only on his own observations or the collective experience of his hospital in selecting effective cures. As a result, very few recipes in his list depend on the works of Galen or his epitomizers.[44] The novel conditions of the Byzantine Dark Age were thus stimulating significant changes in the actual practice of medicine.

Outside the sphere of professional literature there is additional evidence that physicians of the Byzantine Dark Age were capable of major innovations. The ninth-century *Vita S. Theophanis* by Nikephoros Skeuophylax includes a remarkable passage describing an operation which Saint Theophanes underwent for kidney stones. The physicians passed instruments up Theophanes' urinary tract, ground down the stones in the bladder, and then allowed the stone fragments to pass out of the body with the flow of urine.[45] No ancient sources mention such a procedure; they all describe operations which involve cutting into the bladder to remove or to grind down the stones.[46] Writing in the early seventh century, even the thorough Paul of Aegina knew only kidney-stone operations involving incisions.[47] The bloodless operation which the early ninth-century physicians performed on Theophanes thus represents a substantial innovation over ancient practice. I shall discuss this operation in detail later.

THE MACEDONIAN RENAISSANCE

By the mid-ninth century the East Roman Empire had begun to recover from the catastrophic shocks of the Dark Age. The year 843 saw the end of the destructive quarrel over images; 863 brought a decisive victory over the Arab armies that had been raiding Asia Minor. Now Byzantine society could devote itself more fully to reexamining and developing its cultural heritage. Historians have called this revival of intellectual life the Macedonian Renaissance.[48] In the medical field the ninth-century reawakening motivated several scholars to produce new treatises. Among these writers were Theophilos Protospatharios and Theophanes "Nonnos." The most innovative of these—Theophilos—surely practiced medicine in the service of a hospital.

Until recently scholars knew very little about Theophilos Protospatharios despite his significance both in Byzantine medicine and in the early development of the Salerno medical school in Italy.[49] They could not even determine the century in which he lived. Through the careful philological work of Leendert Westerink and Ihor Ševčenko, however, it is now clear that Theophilos practiced and wrote sometime in the late ninth or early tenth century—that is, after the dawning of the Macedonian Renaissance.[50]

The manuscripts give Theophilos a variety of titles: *protospatharios, archiatros, monachos,* and *philosophos.*[51] When all these titles are considered together, they indicate that the man who bore them occupied a high post on a hospital staff. First, most of the extant manuscripts describe Theophilos as a protospatharios. According to the precedence manuals of the ninth century, hospital administrators ordinarily held the honorary rank of spatharios.[52] One seal, however, reveals that the ninth-century xenodochos of a hospital in the town of Loupadion had attained the higher rank of protospatharios.[53] Thus, hospital officials could receive the same honorary title as Theophilos held. Second, some of the manuscripts not only mention Theophilos' rank but also list his position, that of archiatros. By the ninth century an archiatros worked either in a hospital or served as one of the emperor's court physicians. In this latter case, however, the manuscripts would have referred to him as an imperial archiatros. Since none of the surviving codices do, he surely held a xenon post.[54] Third, some of the manuscripts state that Theophilos was a monk. Again, a survey of Byzantine xenones has demonstrated that monastic communities had always been closely tied to hospitals since the days of Basil of Caesarea. Although lay physicians came to dominate the xenones by the sixth century, monks continued to support and administer public hospitals and occasionally to serve in them as physicians.[55] Thus, the manuscripts do not necessarily contradict one another when they call Theophilos protospatharios, archiatros, and monachos if he worked in a Christian hospital. His fourth title, philosophos, is ambiguous; it could here mean simply that Theophilos was a learned man, for the Byzantines often called scholars in any field philosophoi. Or it could be a synonym for *monachos*, another frequent use of the word in medieval Greek.[56] In neither case, however, would it argue against the conclusion that can be drawn from the other three titles, namely that Theophilos worked as an archiatros and perhaps as an administrator in a Christian hospital of Constantinople.

Further evidence of Theophilos' association with hospitals comes from a text entitled "Tonics Which Theophilos Collected from Various Xenon Books," a xenon treatment list which is found only in one manuscript, *Laurentianus* 75.19. This short collection of recipes presents a number of chronological problems. First, the *Laurentianus* 75.19 dates from the fourteenth century and thus is too late to provide any argument for assigning the list to Theophilos.[57] Second, the redaction found in the Laurentian manuscript surely dates from a time long after Theophilos' death, since it includes among the prescriptions some attributed to Romanos, a physician who lived in the tenth century, and another prescription supposedly discovered by the emperor Basil II.[58] Although Theophilos surely did not draw up the present redaction of the list, it is significant that the manuscript tradition associates his name with hospital libraries and with a genre of medical literature that emerged from xenon practice.

Other works which the manuscripts ascribe to Theophilos tend to confirm my hypothesis that he worked in the hospitals of Constantinople. The manuscripts attribute five treatises to him besides the xenon treatment list just discussed: essays on the structure of the human body, on urines, on excrement, and on pulses, as well as a commentary to Hippocrates' *Aphorisms*. Although Theophilos based his essay concerning the structure of the human body on Galen's physiological study, *De usu partium,* he introduced Christian concepts into his treatment. So too in his work *De urinis,* he begins with an appeal for aid to "Christ our God."[59] Throughout his writings he frequently invokes the Savior's assistance. The strongly Christian tone of Theophilos' treatises naturally distinguishes his writings from those of the great classical physicians, who were pagans. But they also mark his writings off from the works of Alexander of Tralleis and Paul of Aegina, even though these men were at least nominally Christians.[60] It seems that Theophilos had learned his profession in a new setting—one more thoroughly Christian than that of his predecessors. Such a setting, of course, the Christian xenones would have offered, both for practice and teaching. Although Justinian first realigned classical medicine around the Christian hospitals in the mid-sixth century, the old pagan traditions must have survived for several generations. The xenones and their teaching staffs, however, had succeeded in welding a Christian attitude to the classical science of medicine long before Theophilos had begun his career.

Theophilos won a reputation as a medical writer particularly interested in practice with his two treatises, *De pulsibus* and *De urinis*. His work on pulses relies heavily on Galen. Nevertheless, it presents the intricacies of ancient pulse doctrine in a clearer, more concise fashion than Galen had, and even provides the reader with a diagram of the various pulse classifications.[61] His essay represents a great improvement on the sketchy outline of Merkourios.

Theophilos, however, made his greatest contribution to advancing the medical field in his *De urinis*. As he states in his introduction to this work, the ancient physicians—Hippocrates, Galen, and Magnos—had not offered a coherent teaching regarding urine and uroscopy. Theophilos thus perceived a need to expand on ancient doctrine, since uroscopy could serve so well as a diagnostic tool. Using both the wisdom of ancient physicians and the wealth of his own experience, he set out to compose a manual for employing uroscopy in diagnosing disease.[62] His monograph on this subject stands at the head of a tradition of Byzantine essays on uroscopy which ended with the exhaustive treatise in seven books by the last great Byzantine physician, John Zachariah, himself a xenon doctor of the fourteenth century.[63] It is difficult to say exactly what role hospitals played in advancing uroscopy as a diagnostic tool. Archiatroi had certainly used it at their iatreia before Justinian established them in hospitals. Still, it is likely that xenones made systematic use of uroscopy easier. In a hospital setting, physicians could obtain samples quickly, have at hand the various vials and beakers required for proper study, and keep a record of alterations in urine which dietary or pharmacological treatments could effect. It is perhaps no coincidence then that a physician connected with the xenones of Constantinople emphasized the importance of uroscopy.[64] In support of such a hypothesis, it is interesting to notice that the first clinical teaching program in Western Europe—the course of study organized at Padua during the sixteenth century—offered instruction both on uroscopy and on pulses in the hospital of Saint Francis.[65]

The second well-known medical author of the Macedonian Renaissance, Theophanes "Nonnos," certainly influenced Byzantine hospitals, even if he cannot be directly linked himself to xenon practice. Sometime during the tenth century, Theophanes compiled the most substantial summary of Greek medicine since the days of Paul of Aegina. His *Synopsis* contains some three hundred chapters, arranged *a capite ad calcem;* he also appended a section on medicaments and one on gynecology to the end of his treatise. His summary draws most heavily on the early Byzantine physicians rather than on the short monographs of the Dark Age doctors and surgeons. Very little of the compendium is devoted to surgery.[66]

As with all the other medical treatises studied so far, Theophanes' *Synopsis* contains no internal evidence to link it in any way with xenones. The manuscript tradition, however, associates Theophanes' work with two separate xenon treatment lists. *Vaticanus graecus* 292 (fourteenth century) contains not only the *Synopsis* of Theophanes, but ten folios of the xenon treatment list emanating from the great hospitals of Constantinople—hereafter the Vatican List.[67] Moreover, *Parisinus suppl. graecus* 764 (also fourteenth century) consists of several works of Theophanes including the *Synopsis* together with a xenon treatment list—hereafter the Paris List—prepared by the physicians of a single hospital.[68] In two other manuscripts (*Paris. gr.* 2091 and *Baroc.* 150) the *Synopsis* also appears in close association with the Paris List.[69] While Theophanes probably did not compose his treatise only with the exigencies of hospital practice in mind, the manuscript tradition indicates that his compendium quickly found its way into the codices of xenon libraries, where staff physicians could consult it along with their own treatment lists. In fact, the list of tonics supposedly collected by Theophilos Protospatharios from xenon books includes a chapter copied directly from Theophanes' *Synopsis*.[70]

XENON TREATMENT LISTS

In the tenth century there appears a genre of professional medical literature which the manuscript headings unequivocally attribute to the hospital physicians, a genre I have called xenon treatment lists. Although even these offer very little information on the hospital setting in which the doctors were practicing, they surely preserve the therapies these physicians devised. I shall discuss three of these xenon treatment lists—the Paris List, the Vatican List, and a third remedy collection supposedly composed by a certain Romanos.

The Paris List is preserved in three separate manuscripts.[71] On the basis of terms it shares with Theophanes' *Synopsis,* Edouard Jeanselme has dated it to the tenth century.[72] Indeed, one scholar has suggested the possibility that Theophanes himself compiled it.[73] *Parisinus suppl. graecus* 764 (fol. 84) introduces the Paris List with the following title: "Therapeutic treatments put together by various physicians according to the express custom of the xenon."[74] The text of this short collection itself reveals very little about the hospital where it was drawn up. Following the example of the early Byzantine physicians and Theophanes, it begins by discussing ailments of the head and the organs of sense, proceeds to the vital organs of the body, and then considers the genitals. Thereafter, it retains no particular order.[75] The title itself provides the most interesting information. According to some procedure the particular xenon in which the list originated periodically collected the remedies which the staff physicians had used with success. This would support the evidence in the remedy collection of John the archiatros that the hospital physicians did not simply follow treatments they had learned from the classical or early Byzantine doctors, but innovated from case to case in an effort to find more effective treatments. They also kept some record of what they ordered and eventually committed the successful treatments to a hospital remedy list "according to the express custom of the xenon." In his commentary Jeanselme suggests that the hospital physicians drew up the list for quick consultation by ward doctors and pharmacists. Perhaps the random additions at the end of the collection were added later case by case, following a chronological rather than a logical order.[76]

The Vatican List also emerged from xenon practice, as its title in *Vaticanus graecus* 292 reveals: "Orders and routines of the great xenones which according to experience the students of the doctors order for those who suffer in various ways at the xenones."[77] At present no evidence has been found to date the Vatican List exactly. The two manuscripts which preserve the text—*Vaticanus graecus* 292 the whole text and *Vindobonensis med. gr.* 37 a fragment—were executed during the fourteenth century and are surely copies of an older original.[78] The title of the Vatican List, however, offers a clue to the date of the archetype when it mentions the great xenones of Constantinople. As we shall see in the next chapter, the Latin conquest of 1204 severely diminished many of the hospitals of Constantinople and reduced some of them to ruins. Thus it is probable that the Vatican List was prepared sometime before 1204 and certainly after Theophanes completed the *Synopsis*.[79]

As with the Paris List, the title of the Vatican List indicates that the hospital physicians developed these remedies in the course of their daily practice. It also suggests that the collection represents a further stage in assembling and editing the records of successful treatments, since it claims to be a digest of remedy lists from the great xenones, not just a collection of procedures at a single hospital. Only after careful editing of the Vatican List and comparison with other xenon treatment lists will it be possible to determine the place of this text in the evolution of hospital medicine in Constantinople.

The Vatican List contains fifteen sections, clearly marked by headings or marginal notes. The first section discusses therapies for fevers, the second for headaches; the succeeding sections follow roughly the usual order *a capite ad calcem,* the final entry dealing with treatments for kidney problems. The recommended therapies consist primarily of medicines taken internally or external compresses. Some procedures call for baths followed by rubdowns with specific herbs.[80] Some require the patient to inhale certain vapors.[81] One of the remedies for bowel problems includes a hot sitzbath.[82] Outside of phlebotomy, the treatment list does not mention any surgical procedures. The section dealing with lumbago or hip pains refers to a hip instrument of some sort, although the passage does not explain how the physician was to use this device.[83] Since ancient authors do not mention a hip instrument, this tool may represent an invention of Byzantine physicians.[84]

Two qualities of the Vatican List link it with the manuals on uroscopy, pulses, and phlebotomy from earlier centuries. First, the list ignores much of the classical theory of humors and their balance, referring to the humors rarely and then only as means to categorize treatment procedures.[85] Second, the list uses a very terse, simple Greek style—a form of expression which is first found in medical literature written after Paul of Aegina's time.

The third medical text which surely comes from a xenon is the tenth-century *De acutis et diurnis morbis* compiled by the physician Romanos.[86] Again the title of the treatise and the author's short introduction, not the text itself, reveal the hospital origin of this work.[87] The manuscript headings identify the author as Romanos Koubouklisios of the Holy Church of God and Protomenites of the Imperial Xenon of the Myrelaion,—i.e., one of the senior staff physicians at the Myrelaion hospital. Since the office of koubouklisios at Hagia Sophia existed only during the tenth and eleventh centuries, scholars have been able to determine the time frame of Romanos' treatise.[88] In his introduction, Romanos states that he prepared his manual with a specific purpose in mind. He had observed how the medics—physicians of *perissos* (extra) status or perhaps *hypourgoi* (medical assistants)—had to travel through the alleys and backways of Constantinople. Since in performing these duties they could not carry heavy medical books around with them, Romanos had composed this short summary of medical wisdom for the medics to take with them on their rounds. Romanos states that his digest relies both on the teaching of the ancients and on his own observations. His discussion of symptoms follows the same order found in the Vatican List. He begins with fevers in general and then proceeds to problems of the head, thereafter following the order *a capite ad calcem*. Toward the end of the manual, however, this arrangement breaks down, and a number of random entries appear. An explanation of this feature and of other aspects of the manual must await a critical edition and careful comparison with Theophanes' *Synopsis* and surviving xenon treatment lists.

XENON CODICES

Although Romanos' manual and the treatment lists provide the most direct evidence of hospital methods and the system the physicians used to expand their collective experience, it is also possible to gain insights into xenon medicine by examining individual codices prepared for hospital libraries. Most of these contain works of ancient physicians or early Byzantine writers who flourished before the Christian xenones had emerged as prominent centers of Greek medicine. Still, these manuscripts offer some information on xenones because the men who executed them had in mind the needs of hospital practice in selecting and editing the texts for the new books.

One of the most famous of the xenon codices is *Laurentianus* 74.7, Niketas' surgical manuscript. It contains excerpts from Hippocrates, Helidorus, Archigenes, Galen, Oribaseios, Paul of Aegina, and others—all men of the ancient or early Byzantine period. Niketas selected the excerpts because they dealt with a common subject—surgery. Among the selections one of the longest is from the celebrated chapter 6 on surgical operations from the *Epitome* of Paul of Aegina. Alongside the texts, Niketas furnished many illustrations to clarify the operations described by the accompanying treatises.[89] Folio 7ᵛ of the codex contains three epigrams praising Niketas' efforts. They state that indeed Niketas had copied and illustrated the manuscript. They emphasize that the codex and its pictures served as a valuable reference tool for both young and more experienced physicians as well as for the hypourgoi authorized to use the knife.[90] Finally, they praise the manuscript as an excellent teaching aid; Niketas' illustrations and diagrams provided a key for understanding how to set bones or to use surgical instruments. In the words of the poet, Niketas helped *praxis* keep pace with *logos;* through his pictures he taught theory in action.[91]

All the evidence from the epigrams indicates that Niketas had prepared *Laurentianus* 74.7 for a xenon library. He added the illustrations to aid the medical students at the hospital and to provide a convenient reference tool for the hospital staff—the iatroi and archiatroi as well as the advanced hypourgoi. Indeed, a marginal note at the end of the manuscript mentions that the Nosokomeion of the Forty Martyrs acquired the codex in the late twelfth century.[92] *Laurentianus* 74.7 thus represents a medical codex which a copyist prepared expressly for a hospital library. In the tradition of the medical texts which emerged from xenon practice, Niketas designed this codex to meet practical needs. Thus, he chose not to reproduce a single classical author in a careful edition. Rather, he assembled bits and pieces from the Greek medical tradition, all dealing with a single subject, so that the physicians and students would have a convenient reference work on surgery. In copying his archetypes Niketas was not concerned with the exact reproduction of the original. He designed the codex to communicate through word and picture how a physician was to carry out a given surgical procedure. As a result, Niketas' manuscript contains what philologists class as corruptions of the ancient texts it has copied.[93]

Laurentianus 74.7 does not include surgical excerpts by Byzantine physicians after Paul's time. Curiously, medical texts composed after Paul of Aegina's *Epitome* seldom mention surgery. Only the ninth-century physician Leo included substantial sections on surgery in his concise treatise on medicine, referring to over forty operations and mentioning approximately fifteen surgical instruments.[94] He describes these operations, however, in far less detail than Paul of Aegina had. Other medical writers, such as Theophanes and Theophilos, as well as the xenon treatment lists practically ignore surgical remedies. This silence is puzzling, for hospitals certainly maintained surgeons and operating rooms through the twelfth century at least.[95]

How can one explain this almost total silence regarding surgery on the part of Byzantine physicians? First, the accidents of manuscript survival could account for the lack of surgical treatises from the great days of the xenones in the tenth, eleventh, and twelfth centuries. Second, it is possible that surgical skills deteriorated in the fourteenth century and that the xenones and private physicians of that era chose to copy only remedy lists and diagnostic manuals from the earlier Byzantine medical works and ignored those which dealt with surgery. In support of this hypothesis one should bear in mind that most of the xenon treatment lists and other Byzantine medical essays written after 600 survive only in very late Byzantine manuscripts.[96] Finally, it is possible that Byzantine physicians, organized as they were into a guild, did not want to commit their surgical techniques to writing for the benefit of unlicensed practitioners. Legitimate physicians perhaps considered that the medical wisdom of classical and early Byzantine doctors represented an integral part of the Hellenic cultural achievement, but more recent technical advances belonged to the guild in which xenon doctors represented a central element. The Vatican List presents some evidence of this attitude. In the section on pains of the hip it recommends that the attending physician have recourse to a hip instrument, without indicating how to use such a tool.[97] As an apprentice, a medical student would have learned the procedure.

Despite the lack of Byzantine surgical treatises as such, a second surgical codex, *Laurentianus* 74.2, roughly contemporary with the Niketas manuscript, offers some indication that hospital physicians still performed a variety of operations in the eleventh and twelfth centuries, some of which were perhaps unknown to their ancient predecessors. On folio 281 this manuscript contains a list of surgical instruments, probably a checklist for a hospital employee such as the one who maintained the surgical tools at the Pantokrator Xenon.[98] The list mentions eighty-eight instruments; twenty-eight of these do not appear in any classical work on surgery.[99] Although Byzantine physicians might well have employed some new terms for old instruments and extant ancient sources surely omit to mention every tool which doctors had at their disposal, still some of these new names probably refer to instruments needed for innovative procedures such as the bloodless operation for stones. As with the instrument for hips, however, no Byzantine source explains how physicians used any of these novel tools.

THE LATE EMPIRE

Despite the catastrophes of the Latin occupation during the thirteenth century and the ever-growing menace of the Turks during the fourteenth, Byzantine hospitals managed to survive and to exercise a strong influence on medical writing during the late period of the empire. In fact, all of the extant copies of the xenon treatment lists I have discussed in connection with the hospital practice of earlier centuries—the Vatican List, the Paris List, Romanos' work, and the collection of tonics attributed to Theophilos—as well as the phlebotomy texts studied by Temkin have survived only in codices produced during the Palaeologan period.[100] This alone suggests that xenones continued to promote medical libraries and to finance the production of manuscripts useful for hospital work even in the fourteenth and fifteenth centuries. Moreover, it also suggests that the original codices containing such xenon treatment lists had simply worn out by the fourteenth century as a result of constant use and had to be replaced.[101]

In addition to recopying older remedy collections, Palaeologan xenones also sponsored new compilations of classical texts and new collections of xenon treatments. For example, in 1323 a hospital physician named George finished a codex dealing with internal medicine (*Scorialensis* III.Y.14). It included book 7 of Paul of Aegina's *Epitome* (the section which discussed the qualities of herbs and the compounds obtained from combining them), some Galenic remedies, and several handy tables of weights and measures and of medical symbols.[102] The copyist of this manuscript has adopted the same method as Niketas did in preparing the surgical codex; he has attempted to combine in a single codex works by different authors on the same subject. There are sections from the great medical works of the past which treat of pharmaceuticals and their properties and also tables to aid the doctor or pharmacist in measuring ingredients and in writing prescriptions—in short, a useful reference work for the hospital staff. Toward the end of the fourteenth century a copyist and perhaps also a physician, John Staphides, finished a codex which he dedicated to the philanthropic and divine Xenon of St. Panteleemon. John included in his book a treatment list which he himself probably composed.[103]

From the late fourteenth century comes the most useful Palaeologan medical text for the study both of Byzantine hospitals and also of the medical profession in general, the xenon treatment list prepared by the staff of the Mangana hospital.[104] The compilation limits its field to therapies for ailments of the stomach, spleen, liver, and kidneys. It includes some entries under the names of individual physicians working at the Mangana such as Stephen, the archiatros, or Abram, the aktouarios of the hospital.[105] Others it simply introduces as the remedies used at the Mangana.[106] Still others it condenses from the works of classical or early Byzantine physicians. As noted above, it frequently quotes from works attributed to Alexander of Tralleis.[107]

Among xenon treatment lists and other medieval treatises on medicine which I have studied, the Mangana list alone contains a possible reference to the urinary-tract operations for kidney stones in the bladder. Curiously, it attributes this entry to the ancient scientist Demokritos of Abdera.[108] The section begins by describing the symptoms which indicate that a patient is suffering from stones in the bladder—sandy urine and a constant erection of the penis in male patients. Under such circumstances the doctor should use a catheter or administer an oral potion to dissolve the stone in the bladder. As a last resort the physician can turn to the knife and perform a lithotomy—the ancient operation which Paul of Aegina describes in detail.[109] It is perfectly clear what the text is saying when it recommends either a potion for the patient or a lithotomy. But what does it mean by the extremely terse order "in such cases [of stone] use a catheter"? Perhaps this refers to a simple catheter to drain the bladder or to introduce into it some liquid to break up the stone, but it could also refer here to the instrument that Dark Age physicians had developed to grind down stones in the bladder by using the urinary tract. To perform such an operation a physician would first have needed to introduce a catheter into the bladder; then using this as a flange, he could insert another instrument through the urinary tract to begin the grinding process.[110]

Whatever the meaning of this entry in the Mangana treatment list, it seems to provide another example of the guild mentality among physicians in Byzantine hospitals. Here, as in the Vatican List, the compiler does not commit to writing how an instrument is used—in this case the mysterious catheter. The remedy list simply reminds the physician of his options and of the pharmacological components he needs if he chooses to treat the stones with internal medicines. The actual procedure involving the catheter, however, he had to have learned as an apprentice.[111]

In addition to the copying and compiling which hospitals promoted, the Late Byzantine Empire also saw two distinguished Byzantine physicians complete substantial medical treatises. In the late thirteenth century Nicholas Myrepsos finished his pharmacopoeia of 2,600 entries, and by the middle of the fourteenth century John Zachariah had composed his extensive writings, including the most detailed Byzantine monograph on uroscopy ever undertaken.[112]

Nicholas Myrepsos held the office of aktouarios under the emperor John III Vatatzes.[113] Before 1204 the aktouarios had directed the Mangana Xenon, and it is probable that the post was resurrected, with similar hospital responsibilities, once the Nicaean emperors had established some order in Asia Minor.[114] Moreover, Myrepsos' *materia medica*—the *Dynameron*—was just the sort of practical handbook which xenon practice had fostered since the Byzantine Dark Age. Hospital books are full of short, anonymous pharmacological lists arranged in alphabetical order: the xenon codex *Baroccianus* 150 contains an alphabetical list of drugs and their therapeutic uses on folios 41^v–47^v; immediately following a collection of xenon tonics, *Laurentianus* 75.19 preserves a collection of herbs arranged from alpha to omega together with their curative properties. Finally, a section of the *Dynameron* itself was copied into the Mangana Xenon codex (*Vat. gr.* 299, fols. 131–153). It is interesting to notice that *materiae medicae* were also associated with hospital practice in the Arab world. Sabur-ibn-Sahl, the director of the famous hospital at Gondeshapur, had prepared an extensive alphabetical *materia medica* in 869 which later won such acclaim that Moslem hospitals were required by law to have it on hand.[115] In view of the close relationship between pharmacological lists and hospital practice both in the Byzantine Empire and in Islamic society, it is no mystery why *Parisinus graecus* 2243 introduces Myrepsos' *Dynameron* with an illustration of a xenon dispensary.

Like Myrepsos, John Zachariah also held the post of aktouarios. Since Zachariah served the emperor Andronikos III (1328–41), long after the East Roman government had regained control of Constantinople, he probably was working at the old Mangana Xenon.[116] This seems all the more likely since the Mangana treatment list confirms that the aktouarios Abram was associated with the Mangana hospital later in the fourteenth century.[117] Moreover, in his *De urinis* Zachariah specifically mentions that he had made some of his observations on his hospital rounds.[118] Given his close association with hospitals and his practice in them, his seven-book treatise on urology reflects aspects of xenon medicine. His style, however, breaks with the terse Greek of Theophilos and the telegraphic jargon of demotic words and ungrammatical structures which characterize the xenon treatment lists and similar compilations, and is instead written in a polished Greek.[119] In this his work represents a return to the style of Oribaseios, Aetios of Amida, and Alexander of Tralleis.

THE IMPACT OF HOSPITALS ON THE PRACTICE OF BYZANTINE MEDICINE

The works of Nicholas and John close the list of major Byzantine medical treatises which began with the compendium of Oribaseios in the fourth century. From Oribaseios to John Zachariah, Byzantine physicians rarely mentioned the normal surroundings of their examinations and their treatments. Even xenon treatment lists are silent regarding the institutions in which they were compiled. Thus, professional medical writing can be of only limited value in the study of Byzantine hospitals. Nevertheless, this survey of Byzantine medical literature proves that xenon practice influenced medieval Greek medicine in specific ways. First, the Christian hospitals generated a novel genre of medical literature—the xenon treatment lists. Second, the xenon lists evolved out of the new tradition of professional writing which began with the reign of Herakleios and the Byzantine Dark Age, a tradition which no doubt the teaching and practice of xenon physicians helped to create. Third, hospital physicians often broke with the tradition of classical and early Byzantine medicine to develop their own therapies. Fourth, xenon exigencies promoted the reproduction of classical texts in manuscripts that radically changed the organization of the ancient heritage of medicine. Finally, even in a case such as the *Synopsis* of Theophanes "Nonnos," where no evidence exists that the author intended his work for hospital use, the xenon libraries quickly acquired copies. Through their libraries and copying activities, the xenones performed their greatest service to posterity: they preserved the Greek tradition of medicine through the Byzantine Dark Age of the seventh and eighth centuries and through the time of troubles which descended on the empire after the fall of Constantinople to the Crusaders. The heritage of Greek medical wisdom would have been meager, had the Christian xenones not devoted some of their resources to maintaining their own libraries.

In addition to these specific contributions, however, it is possible that xenones exercised a more profound influence on Byzantine medicine. Did they in fact shape the whole perspective of medical science in the East Roman Empire? Did they contribute to advances in medieval Greek medicine just as hospitals were to do in France, England, and Austria during the late eighteenth and early nineteenth centuries? In sum, did Byzantine hospitals produce a movement similar to the Clinical medicine of modern Europe?[120]

When in the mid-sixth century Christian physicians at the Persian court asked the shah to build them a xenon, these doctors and their confreres within the East Roman Empire had already come to see hospitals as the optimum setting for the healing art.[121] This hospital-based medicine continued to flourish at least until 1204, and probably through the thirteenth and fourteenth centuries as well. By contrast, hospitals did not play a major role in Western medicine until much later. First at Padua in the sixteenth century and then slowly in other areas of Western Europe, hospital practice gained in importance both as a means of instruction and as a method of treating disease.[122] Finally in Paris at the turn of the nineteenth century, this hospital-based medicine—the Clinical movement—came to dominate the medical profession and stimulated new discoveries. Since the hospital was so important both to the Byzantine profession and to the Clinical movement in Paris, it is especially interesting to compare the healing art of the East Roman Empire with the enlightened medicine of the French clinicians.[123]

The clinicians of Paris rejected the ancient Greek medical doctrines as they had received them in the works of Galen and in medieval scholastic texts, and emphasized a return to simple observation.[124] Once the French Revolution had succeeded, the clinicians secured the suppression of the old medical faculty of the University of Paris and the foundation of new medical schools, the *écoles du santé*. Here students concentrated on observation and practice and abandoned much of the professional literature of the past. Medical students were now to spend the first day of study observing patients on the hospital wards. The clinicians adopted the motto "Read little, but see and do much."[125]

Our survey of Byzantine hospitals has revealed some intriguing similarities between Clinical medicine as it developed at Paris and the medieval

Greek profession. First, Byzantine physicians began to deemphasize the ancient medical theories as early as the fifth century, when Theon of Alexandria composed his *Anthropos*. Owsei Temkin noted the total absence of theoretical concepts in the Dark Age phlebotomy texts and their Latin and Arabic paraphrases. Second, Byzantine physicians received practical training on the hospital wards, as did the students of the *écoles du santé*. Third, Byzantine xenon tradition limited the number of patients so that the sick would receive the best possible care: the Pantokrator Xenon, with its fifty beds, probably represents the standard size of a great xenon. The Lips Xenon, with only twelve female patients, was no doubt a small institution. Hospitals in the West, however, were far larger than even the Pantokrator. They often sheltered several hundred patients at a time.[126] Like the earlier Byzantine xenon physicians, the leaders of the Clinical movement in Paris promoted smaller hospitals of approximately thirty patients each.[127] Fourth, the terse, telegraphic style of Byzantine medical literature, its ungrammatical sentence structure, and its tendency to boil down the works of classical physicians into meager summaries might easily spring from a policy of reading little, while seeing and doing much.

In one significant area, however, the clinicians of modern Europe seem to have introduced a field of study which profoundly deepened the scope of their observations. As early as the sixteenth century, the forefathers of the Clinical movement emphasized autopsies. At the hospital of Saint Francis in Padua, the instructors gave lectures on urines and on pulses—a practice perfectly in accord with what we have learned about Byzantine teaching methods—but they also conducted autopsies.[128] The practice continued to grow in importance during the next two hundred years. Paris clinicians of the Revolutionary period, such as Xavier Bichat and François Broussais, raised autopsy to a central place in the new medicine. Through autopsies physicians were able to develop penetrating powers of observation. By opening up the corpses of deceased hospital patients they could observe the effects of disease on the body's organs and could correlate internal lesions and inflammations with the external symptoms they had recorded while the patients were still living. They were therefore no longer practicing dissection simply to study anatomy, but to observe the course of diseases within the human body; they had begun to practice pathological anatomy.[129]

With their emphasis on autopsies the Clinical physicians of the modern West had apparently leapt far ahead of the xenon doctors in the Byzantine Empire. Professors Alexander Kazhdan and Lawrence Bliquez, however, have collected evidence which demonstrates conclusively that East Roman physicians also performed autopsies.[130] Moreover, the descriptions of these autopsies indicate that Byzantine doctors were also interested in pathological anatomy, not simply in determining the location of organs in the human body.

As early as the Byzantine Dark Age, physicians were conducting autopsies. According to the chronicle of Theophanes, the emperor Constantine V (741–75) handed a prisoner over to doctors of Constantinople for vivisection.[131] Theophanes, an ardent iconophile, detested the arch-iconoclast Constantine, and had reason to emphasize the heretic's cruelty. That Constantine permitted a vivisection is probably an exaggerated tale which Theophanes incorporated into his history to demonstrate the iconoclastic emperor's inhumanity. In view of later accounts describing autopsies, the truth behind the rumor was probably that Constantine allowed physicians to conduct an autopsy on the body of a deceased prisoner, as Theophanes reports "to learn the structure of man." Theophanes' account does not indicate that these Dark Age physicians were interested in anything more than studying anatomy. Two later sources, however, reveal Byzantine doctors concentrating on pathological anatomy.

Expanding on the traditional image of the spiritual doctor in one of his celebrated tracts, the eleventh-century monastic leader Symeon the New Theologian alluded to the autopsies conducted by contemporary physicians. Holy men studied closely the spiritual diseases of the soul to learn the active forces of these disorders and to determine their causes. They did this in order to help others by discovering effective remedies for the illnesses of the soul. In this they resembled physicians, who cut open the bodies of the dead so that they could discover the unseen causes of disease and thus develop more successful medicines for those who were still living.[132]

A century later, the court orator George Tornikes again described medical autopsies, this time in a eulogy in honor of the empress Anna Komnena, sister of the emperor who founded the Pantokrator Xenon. Tornikes records how the physicians studied where each organ of the human body was located and the structure of each. He also relates how the doctors observed the relationship of the organs to one another, how when one was healthy so was its neighbor. Conversely, they observed how the disease of one organ could affect the condition and structure of its neighbors and how it could even destroy them.[133] Here, again, the physicians have progressed beyond simple anatomy and are gazing at the effects of disease on the internal organs and are mapping the spread of these diseases within the body.

The revelations of Kazhdan and Bliquez, thus, prove that Byzantine physicians were conducting autopsies until the twelfth century at least and that they developed a form of pathological anatomy remarkably similar to the hospital dissections conducted by Bichat and Broussais. Although the Byzantine references to autopsies do not mention that these were performed in xenones, such institutions would have been the natural locations for such study. Only in a hospital could the physicians have ready a corpse for dissection and at the same time have a record of the dead person's illness and of his external symptoms before his death. Moreover, only in a hospital could doctors begin to dissect before corruption set in and obscured the internal symptoms proper to the disease.[134] Finally, xenones were the major schools of medicine, and such dissections would have aided in teaching simple anatomy as well as pathology.

In the field of surgery also, the Paris clinicians made advances along the lines which Byzantine doctors had pursued. Without antiseptic techniques or anesthesia, physicians of the Clinical movement were usually unable to employ surgical therapies successfully. For treating kidney stones, however, they developed a revolutionary new technique. They designed instruments which they could introduce into the bladder through the urethral canal, and then use to grind down the stones so that the small fragments could pass out of the bladder in the urine flow. Jean Civiale first performed this bloodless operation for the stone on 13 January 1824.[135] It quickly became the standard therapy for kidney calculi. As we saw above, Byzantine physicians had performed this very operation on Saint Theophanes 1,000 years earlier at the beginning of the ninth century.[136] Is this merely a coincidence or had similar circumstances led Byzantine physicians down the same paths which the Paris clinicians were to follow in the early nineteenth century? Lack of effective antiseptics and anesthetics surely encouraged Byzantine surgeons to develop bloodless operations just as it did the Paris doctors. But is it not possible that the xenones of Constantinople offered the same opportunities for instruction, careful observation, and autopsies as did the Paris hospitals of the 1820s and that these medical institutions of the East Roman Empire encouraged similar advances in the healing art?

CHAPTER TEN

After 1204

On 13 April 1204 the Latin army of the Fourth Crusade poured over the seawalls of Constantinople and began a fearful plunder which was to last three days.[1] During the pillaging a group of knights broke into the ancient Sampson Xenon and ravaged its treasures, desecrating even its hallowed iconostasis.[2] During their subsequent occupation of Constantinople the Latins also destroyed the Panteleemon Xenon; it lay in ruins until the mid-fourteenth century.[3] Many other hospitals of the capital suffered a similar fate, for only two of the pre-1204 xenones can be found in operation during the final centuries of the empire's history.[4]

The conquest of Constantinople in 1204 dramatically ended the great days of the East Roman Empire. The almost superhuman efforts of the Laskarid emperors saved a remnant of the old Byzantine state in western Asia Minor. They were also able to forge an army sufficiently powerful to push back the Latin invaders and finally to regain Constantinople in 1261.[5] But neither the Laskarids nor their successors, the Palaeologan emperors, could ever restore the Byzantine society which had flourished before 1204. The conquest of Constantinople and the fifty-seven years of Latin occupation had not only altered the political, economic, and social structure of the ancient East Roman state, but had also changed the habits and world view of the empire's people.[6]

Thus, the 250 years from the sack of Constantinople in 1204 to the Turkish conquest in 1453 mark a new phase in the evolution of the Byzantine state and society. It therefore seems appropriate to consider in a separate chapter the hospitals which served the empire during its final two centuries and the features which distinguished them. Such a study must begin by tracing the survival of Byzantine xenones in the western provinces of Asia Minor under the Laskarids. It must then examine the new or restored hospitals of Constantinople which opened up once the East Roman government regained control of the ancient capital in 1261 and compare the relative prosperity of these institutions with the fate of xenones in the provincial towns. It must also explore the relationship of the Late Byzantine or Palaeologan xenones with the groups in society which had traditionally supported such philanthropic institutions—the emperors, the aristocracy, the episcopal church, the monks, and the physicians. Finally, it will attempt to evaluate the quality of these late hospitals in light of the excellent care offered by the great xenones of earlier centuries.

PROVINCIAL HOSPITALS UNDER THE LASKARIDS

In the anarchy which followed the Latin conquest of Constantinople, Theodore Laskaris succeeded in organizing a new Byzantine state in Asia Minor with Nicaea as its capital. In 1208 he was crowned emperor; in 1211 he stopped the westward advance of the Seljuk Turks; and in 1214 he signed a treaty with the Latin government of Constantinople.[7] His military and diplomatic skills thus secured the new state from external threat. His successors, John III Vatatzes (1222–54) and Theodore II (1254–58), inherited a more stable situation; they therefore could devote some of their energies to restoring Byzantine culture and learning. Both of these emperors supported libraries in the towns of Asia Minor and helped to reorganize schools.[8] John Vatatzes hired the most brilliant scholar in his dominions, Nikephoros Blemmydes, to travel in Asia Minor and Thrace in search of ancient manuscripts for the cabinets of these new libraries. Blemmydes also taught a number of children from the leading families of the Nicaean state, including Vatatzes' own son and heir, the future emperor Theodore.[9]

As part of their effort to restore the old fabric of Byzantine society, the Laskarids patronized a number of hospitals. John III and his wife Irene constructed both ptochotropheia and nosokomeia with revenues from the imperial estates.[10] Theodore Metochites indicates that the Laskarid emperors and their Palaeologan successors helped to maintain several hospitals in his beloved city of Nicaea.[11] Theodore II not only continued his father's support of imperial xenones, but he also encouraged local bishops such as Phokas of Philadelphia in their efforts to build hospitals for their towns.[12] The medical institutions of the Nicaean Empire no doubt served a propaganda purpose for the new regime as well. As a patron of xenones in Nicaea and in the other towns of western Asia Minor, John III inherited the mantle of the great imperial philanthropists from Romanos I to Isaak II Angelos, who had financed two new hospitals for Constantinople not long before the Latin conquest of the capital.[13]

These Laskarid xenones also had a place in the intellectual revival which John III and his son Theodore fostered. The chief architect of their cultural program, Nikephoros Blemmydes, had himself studied and practiced medicine in Ephesus and Smyrna before he took up a monastic vocation.[14] As a former physician, his efforts to save the intellectual inheritance of the Byzantine Empire surely encompassed the science of medicine. Thus, by mid-century Theodore II described citizens of Nicaea studying all branches of

Greek learning, including the physician's art.[15] Since xenones had traditionally trained the doctors of Constantinople and housed the specialized medical
libraries of the capital, it is probable that the hospitals which the Laskarids
supported in Asia Minor not only formed part of the empire's philanthropic
program but also contributed to the intellectual revival of the thirteenth
century. Moreover, the Laskarid court restored the office of aktouarios; the
holder of this post had been linked to the great hospital at the Mangana
Palace in Constantinople and had supervised the teaching of medicine at this
institution. It is reasonable to suppose that such an official took up the same
duties at a xenon attached to one of the Laskarid palaces either in Nicaea or
outside of Ephesus, especially since the aktouarioi resumed their duties at
the palace hospital in Constantinople once the East Roman government regained control of the capital in 1261.[16] Indeed, as we have already seen, the
aktouarious under John III Vatatzes, Nicholas Myrepsos, wrote a treatise on
pharmacology ideally suited to serve as a reference work both for hospital
physicians and for medical students.

HOSPITALS AFTER THE RECONQUEST OF CONSTANTINOPLE

After the Nicaean government regained control of Constantinople in 1261, it
began the laborious process of restoring the hospital facilities of the capital.
The fifty-seven years of Latin rule in Constantinople had been more destructive to the Byzantine xenones than the initial conquest of the city. Since the
Crusaders had failed to conquer all of the Eastern Empire's provinces, their
control of Constantinople severed the capital's hospitals from the rich estates
in Asia Minor and Thrace that had largely supported their operations. Moreover, the Latin government assigned the more important xenones of Constantinople to the jurisdiction of Western religious orders. Thus, the Sampson
fell to the Templars, while the Knights of Saint John took over the Mangana.[17]
Under these Latin administrations, the great xenones of Constantinople either
ceased functioning or came to resemble the hospitals of Western Europe
more than they did the medical facilities of former Byzantine days. Jacques
de Vitry, a man trained at Paris and widely travelled in the regions of the
eastern Mediterranean, classed the thirteenth-century Sampson together with
Western institutions such as the Hôtel-Dieu at Paris.[18] In the final analysis,
the disruption which the Latin regime brought to the hospital system of
Constantinople was so severe that neither the old city xenones nor the more
recent imperial foundations survived. Not a trace of the Euboulos, the
Sampson, or the Markianos can be found in Palaeologan sources. So, too,
the Pantokrator Xenon, the Myrelaion, and the Petrion had vanished. The
Panteleemon survived only because the monk Niphon restored it about
1340.[19] When the emperor Michael VIII entered the queen of cities on 15
August 1261, he must have found both its splendid churches and its hospitals
in ruins.

During Michael's reign, he and his wife restored a number of hospitals. The patriarch Gregory of Cyprus praised the emperor for establishing medical centers for the sick and for assigning them sufficient revenue to treat patients with the proper methods.[20] Sometime after Michael's death, his widow, Theodora, used her estates to refurbish the old Lips monastery. The detailed typikon which she drafted for the nuns of her new community required them to maintain a xenon for women patients.[21] During the fourteenth century several additional hospitals were set up in Constantinople. At the beginning of the fifteenth century the satirist Mazaris testified to the survival of a number of xenones in the capital.[22] Fifty years later Andronikos Kallistos lamented the destruction of Constantinople's wonders when the Turks finally conquered the city. Among these he listed harbors, stoas, piers, palaces, and the city's hospitals for the sick.[23] One of these fifteenth-century institutions—the Krales Xenon—still fostered the teaching traditions of earlier Byzantine hospitals as late as the 1440s.[24]

Once the Byzantine government again ruled from Constantinople, the city gradually acquired new xenones for its sick. But what of the provincial towns during the years after 1204? Byzantinists have long known that the political fragmentation of the old East Roman state after the Fourth Crusade broke Constantinople's iron grip on Greek cultural life.[25] Of necessity, the Laskarids had to promote their cultural renaissance in the towns of Asia Minor, not in the old Byzantine capital. Thessalonica, too, became a thriving center of Hellenic civilization during the late thirteenth century.[26] In the following century, Mistra began to flourish as a cultural hub, when it became the political capital of a nearly independent Byzantine province in the Peloponnese. As Robert Browning has observed, several provincial cities challenged Constantinople as the sole capital of medieval Greek culture in the years after 1204.[27] This new local vitality should also have stimulated the development of hospitals in provincial cities, not only under the Laskarids in thirteenth-century Asia Minor, but also in the European towns under the Palaeologan emperors. The sources, however, paint a much different picture. The evidence suggests that xenones almost vanished outside Constantinople in the fourteenth and fifteenth centuries.

The last evidence of hospitals in the cities of Asia Minor is found in Theodore Metochites' paean to his town of Nicaea, composed around 1290.[28] Once Nicaea and the other Asian cities fell under the Turks in the early fourteenth century, all traces of hospitals or indeed of professional medical care of any sort disappeared. When Matthew of Ephesus travelled to Turkish Ephesus in 1339, he fell sick just outside the town. He had to suffer on the threshold of death without the aid of a physician or of any medical remedy, for in Matthew's words, "the city was so far removed from the Romans [Byzantines], or rather from God Himself, that it was lacking both in the care of the soul and of the body."[29]

One would expect that the Turkish invasions had destroyed the Byzantine hospitals of Asia Minor, but even in Thrace a similar picture emerges. In 1322 this same Matthew had received an appointment as metropolitan of Brysis, a town in the Balkan (Haemus) Mountains, east of Adrianople. Matthew described his new home as rustic. Moreover, it had no medical facilities at all, not even the ministrations of a physician in private practice. Rather, all the townspeople expected their new bishop, Matthew, to treat their physical ailments and provide them with medicines as well as carry out his spiritual duties.[30] In a town such as Byrsis without a well-established medical profession, the traditional Byzantine hospital with a staff of lay physicians and hypourgoi (medical assistants) could not possibly have functioned. In the Catalan dominions of central Greece, one finds a similar lack of trained physicians. In 1356 King Frederick III of Sicily dispatched Western-trained doctors to his city of Thebes because there were so few men adequately trained in surgery or general medicine.[31] As for the great metropolis of northern Greece, Thessalonica, it too seems to have lacked xenones by the end of the fourteenth century although it surely supported physicians in private practice. Whereas the invading Normans of 1185 ransacked the city's xenon and scattered the patients, the Turks who captured the town in 1387 found only churches and monasteries to pillage.[32] Of course, this is only an argument *ex silentio,* and it is certainly possible that xenones were still functioning in Palaeologan Thessalonica, but so far no sources have been presented which describe such institutions.

So, too, the vibrant culture of Mistra should have supported some xenones, but none of the documents analyzed by Denis Zakythinos mention hospital facilities there.[33] Once again, however, the case against xenones at Mistra must rest on an argument *ex silentio.* Indeed, it is possible that some monasteries in the Peloponnese were financing hospitals for the general public or even allowing their monks to serve in them, for the harsh critic of Byzantine monasticism George Gemistos Plethon admitted that some fifteenth-century ascetic houses still were performing the liturgies of *agape* for the benefit of the commonweal, a category which could include the support of the traditional Byzantine xenon.[34] Since Plethon made these observations in connection with the Peloponnese, he probably had in mind monasteries in or around Mistra.[35]

SUPPORT FOR HOSPITALS AFTER 1204

It is thus possible that a few xenones still operated in provincial cities during the Palaeologan period; a number of them certainly served the people of Constantinople throughout these years. But who provided these institutions with sufficient resources to offer free medical care during the bleak era of the declining Byzantine state? And who provided the skills to treat the sick in the hospital wards? Was it the same balance of imperial, aristocratic, episcopal, and monastic patronage that had guaranteed the survival of the hospitals in the past? To answer these questions it is necessary to look more closely at the xenones which were still admitting patients after 1261.

FINANCIAL UNDERPINNINGS

As in earlier, more prosperous times, the emperors continued to finance hospitals even though their resources were constantly shrinking. Thus, as we have already seen, Michael VIII, the first of the new dynasty, restored several hospitals (although his panegyrist, Gregory of Cyprus, does not specify which ones), and Michael's wife, Theodora, rebuilt the Lips Xenon. During the fourteenth century the Mangana Xenon was again functioning with the imperial aktouarioi at its head.[36] Michael VIII probably renovated this hospital when he reestablished the imperial court together with the aktouarios in Constantinople.

Most of the other hospitals that opened after 1261, however, owed their existence, not to imperial philanthropia, but to private donations. During the reign of Andronikos II (1281–1327) the general Michael Glabas established a xenon, probably near the Church of the Theotokos Pammakaristos.[37] Shortly after 1341, the wealthy monk Niphon used a good portion of his personal property to repair the ancient Panteleemon Xenon and allotted it sufficient funds to treat the sick. An imperial chrysobull states that this new Panteleemon surpassed the ancient hospital of Narses in size and beauty. If this is not mere rhetoric, then Niphon's hospital was probably the biggest xenon in Palaeologan Constantinople. Niphon retained personal control over the hospital and its property, as had private founders since the ninth century. Because he had no legal heirs, the Panteleemon probably became an independent legal entity upon his death.[38] It was still thriving in 1384 when the copyist John Staphidas prepared a xenon treatment list and codex for the hospital library.[39] At the beginning of the fifteenth century a leading figure in the government of Manuel II, George Goudeles, converted one of his palaces in Constantinople into a nosokomeion. John Chortasmenos praised Goudeles' hospital as the crowning deed of philanthropia in a life devoted to charity. Unfortunately, Chortasmenos' letter describing this hospital gives no details about its size or location.[40]

One of the wealthiest hospitals in Constantinople owed its existence to an unusual property owner, the Serbian king Uroš II Milutin (1281–1321). Sometime after 1308, Milutin purchased villages within Byzantine territory from the imperial government. Acting as a wealthy landowner, Milutin then assigned this private property of his to restore the Monastery of John Prodromos in the Petra district of Constantinople and to build there a new xenon. He also provided an endowment to secure the services of experienced physicians for the xenon patients.[41] Milutin's hospital, called the Krales Xenon, must have been one of the most prominent in the late empire. In the fifteenth century, it was still rich enough to rebind a manuscript and to hire for its school the famous philosopher and physician John Argyropoulos.[42] Although Milutin's biographer praised the king's hospital as an expression of pure philanthropia, the Serbian ruler and rival of the Byzantine emperor Andronikos II doubtless saw the propaganda value of such a foundation. At a time when the legitimate East Roman ruler could restore only some of the capital's hospitals—the famous Panteleemon Xenon had lain in ruins throughout the long reign of Andronikos II—the Serbian king was wealthy enough to endow an impressive facility for the sick in the emperor's very capital and thereby enhance his image as a leader among the Eastern Christians. In the fourteenth century, the Serbian royal house, not the Palaiologoi, were imitating the magnanimity of the great Byzantine dynasties.

Thus, the share of imperial patronage in maintaining Constantinopolitan hospitals seems to have declined in the years after 1261. Whereas government subsidies to independent xenones of Constantinople and land grants for imperial hospitals financed the illustrious medical facilities of the Comnenian period and before, private donors such as Niphon and Milutin of Serbia now shouldered more of this responsibility. As in other areas of Byzantine life, so in the maintenance of hospitals, private patronage was expanding as imperial resources available for philanthropic projects declined. As Robert Browning has observed, some of the leading aristocrats now could draw on greater resources than the emperors could for subsidizing a whole range of activities.[43]

But was the private patronage of the Palaeologan period sufficient to maintain an adequate number of hospitals for Constantinople? At least one source from the fourteenth century suggests that it was not. In his dialogue between the rich and the poor, Alexios Makrembolites attacked the wealthy of the empire for their indifference to the suffering of others. In ancient days the rich could not endure to see the pain of the unfortunate in their cities. Thus, they financed xenones, gerokomeia, orphanotropheia, and similar institutions to succor those in distress. Now, the rich had abandoned such philanthropia.[44] Evidence from other writers indicates that Makrembolites' accusations were not completely accurate regarding the capital, for some aristocrats such as Michael Glabas and George Goudeles did finance hospitals, but his comments might indicate that the efforts of the rich to benefit the poor and lower middle class of Constantinople were insufficient to meet the needs. His complaint, however, surely fits the conditions in provincial cities. Despite the warnings of their bishop, Philotheos, the wealthy citizens of fourteenth-century Herakleia sought to despoil the poor rather than to assist them in any way.[45] At the end of the same century, Thessalonica's leaders were busy seizing what goods the poor still possessed.[46] In a world of shrinking resources, the rich and powerful of this city had little interest in endowing philanthropic agencies of any kind.[47] It is therefore not surprising to find that hospitals had disappeared from the list of important buildings there. Although some of the aristocrats in the capital kept alive the ancient virtue of benefactions for the polis and chose to express it by constructing xenones for the people, the sources reflect that such civic munificence had all but evaporated in the provinces.

Acting both as religious leaders and as civic officials, the bishops had financed hospitals during the prosperous days of the empire, especially in the cities outside Constantinople, where imperial support was less prevalent. The last example of such episcopal patronage comes from thirteenth-century Philadelphia in Asia Minor when Bishop Phokas constructed a xenon for his city during the reign of Theodore II. Local civic patriotism must still have played a role in motivating Phokas' action, for his hospital promoted the fame of his city and aroused the jealousy of the neighboring bishop of Sardis.[48] Philadelphia in fact managed to foster a spirit of local loyalty and to preserve harmony among its citizens in the face of constant emergency. The people of this city fiercely resisted the Turkish invasions long after the imperial government had abandoned any attempt to regain control of Asia Minor.[49] It is indeed interesting that a city which still felt the need to possess a xenon in the thirteenth century also held out most successfully against foreign invasion in the fourteenth century.

Since the days of Basil of Caesarea, monks and their monasteries rivaled and even surpassed the bishops in supporting hospitals for the general public. In Constantinople, they continued this ancient tradition during the fourteenth and fifteenth centuries. Although the nuns of the Lips Monastery were not to mix with the world and thus could not serve personally the sick of their hospital, their typikon bound them to maintain a xenon and to ensure its proper functioning.[50] So, too, King Milutin organized his xenon as part of the ascetic community he restored at the Monastery of John Prodromos in Petra.[51] Moreover, at Milutin's xenon the monks apparently took part in the labors of the hospital, for the nosokomos of the Krales Xenon who hired John Chortasmenos in 1406 was also a member of the monastic community there.[52] Monks served in other hospitals as well. For example, the monk George who copied the second section of the Escorial manuscript (III.Y.14) worked as a physician for an imperial xenon somewhere in Constantinople.[53] The monk and spiritual advisor to Andronikos III, Niphon, restored the ancient Panteleemon Xenon for the people of the capital.[54]

While these examples prove that some monks still accepted the old notions about active philanthropia as an essential element in the monastic life, other sources suggest that ascetics were abandoning Christian *praxis* and thereby any interest in xenones. Monks of the Orthodox tradition had always felt a tension between the life of Christian charity and that of withdrawal and total absorption in prayer. A radical, contemplative movement gained strength during the late thirteenth century and came to dominate both the monastic world and the official church during the course of the following century.[55] The proponents of the new asceticism adopted the old term *hesychasm* (devotion to silence) to describe their life of total prayer. The hesychasts emphasized the role of silent contemplation aided by certain physical exercises as the sole path to personal salvation. Since they viewed this *theoria* as the essential element in a Christian life, they felt very uncomfortable with any worldy duties, even with service for the church. When the monk and hesychast Philotheos received the episcopal chair of Herakleia, he constantly yearned for a return to the contemplation and solitude of his former life. While bishop he never ceased agonizing over his proper vocation. Should he remain to pastor the wicked citizens of Herakleia or should he follow the path to the Lord in contemplation?[56] If hesychasts had reservations about the propriety of serving in the episcopal office, they surely shied away from any role in public hospitals. In this regard, it is revealing to read a new version of the life of Saint Sampson composed by Constantine Akropolites probably at the beginning of the fourteenth century.[57] Akropolites does not change any of the essential elements of the ancient story concerning the doctor-saint, but he inserts a section describing the anargyros' confusion regarding his proper vocation. According to Akropolites, Sampson yearned to follow John the Baptist into the desert; only his desire to help the sick restrained him. Often he felt as though he stood on the beam of an evenly balanced scale; sometimes he inclined one way, sometimes the other, as first one group of advisors urged him to flee the world, and then another to continue in his philanthropic medicine. Sampson's final decision to serve the sick came only after a long struggle.[58] The early vitae of the saint contained no hint of such a struggle over the proper Christian life.[59] Akropolites surely inserted this section to reflect the confusion among monks of the late thirteenth and early fourteenth centuries regarding the relative merits of the life of practical charity and the life of total *theoria,* now called hesychasm.

Outside of Constantinople, the monasteries seem to have abandoned their public charities including their hospitals, probably as a result of the ever-growing enthusiasm and influence of the hesychasts. When Niphon restored the nosokomeion at the Lavra Monastery on Mount Athos around 1340, it was intended to serve only sick monks. No trace survived of the baths, hostels, and hospitals for those from outside the monastery—facilities which Athanasios, the founder, had included in his monastic complex in the tenth century.[60] At the beginning of the fifteenth century George Gemistos Plethon attacked the monks for their refusal to perform any tasks for the good of society. He claimed that most of them were simply drones. They lived from the precious resources of the community while they withdrew totally from the world to pray by themselves, since they cared only for the salvation of their own souls.[61] This emphasis on private prayer that Plethon condemns so vehemently reflects the theology and ascetic practices of the hesychasts. Plethon contrasts the ascetics who performed no useful services with the few monks who still did benefit the commonweal through charitable labors.

PROFESSIONAL CARE

When the fortunes of the East Roman state had been rising, emperors, aristocrats, bishops, and monks had patronized the great xenones of the empire primarily by funding their services with the fruits of the land. Physicians, on the other hand, had contributed their knowledge and labor in support of the hospitals. During the Palaeologan period Byzantine doctors continued to treat xenon patients although such hospital service no longer seems to have dominated the profession in the same way as it had before 1204. Nevertheless, xenones were still important institutions in the medical profession. John Zachariah, the most eminent physician of the fourteenth century, studied medicine at a hospital in Constantinople and later served as aktouarios of the Mangana Xenon, as we saw in the preceding chapter. King Milutin hired a number of senior physicians for the Krales Xenon.[62] According to a satirical letter of Mazaris written in the early fifteenth century, the physician Malakes listed among his principal sources of income, first, the salaries he collected from several hospitals in Constantinople, and second, the fees he charged the Genoese officials at Galata.[63] Finally, the famous physician John Argyropoulos was teaching a number of doctors at the Krales Xenon only a few years before the Turks finally extinguished the empire's independence.[64]

On the other hand, under the Laskarids and the Palaiologoi, doctors apparently spent more time in private practice. After the collapse of xenones and their system of training in 1204, Michael Choniates advised his friend the physician Nicholas Kalodoukes to keep his fees low and to offer very poor patients free care.[65] At that time Kalodoukes must not have been treating the poor sick in a xenon setting, but, rather, was seeing them as private patients. In the reign of Manuel II (1391–1425), the writer Mazaris expected physicians to come to his home when he fell sick, rather than his having to go to the xenon as Deacon Stephen had done in the seventh century or the monk of the Pseudo-Prodromos poems had done in the twelfth.[66] Although John Chortasmenos considered himself a poor man in the fifteenth century, he did not visit the hospital when he was stricken with a severe illness. He stayed at home in his own bed; the doctor finally came to him on the fourth day of his illness to let some blood.[67]

These few references indicate that middle-class patients no longer visited physicians at the hospitals as many had done before 1204. Indeed, Theodore Metochites described the late-thirteenth-century hospitals of Nicaea as institutions for those who suffered both from disease and poverty.[68] Even in Constantinople Goudeles designed his nosokomeion with only the poor in mind.[69] On the other hand, the poet Manuel Philes was treated in the Glabas Xenon at the end of the thirteenth century; although constantly begging for money, Philes was not one of the desperately poor.[70] Although no clear statement of the shift in emphasis survives, the impression emerges that the new xenones of the Palaeologan era were no longer the principal theaters for the practice of medicine. They still offered employment to a number of doctors in Constantinople and still taught medical students, but they ceased to provide most of the population with access to trained physicians. Now, these facilities aimed their services only at the very poor. If the Lips Xenon with its twelve beds reflects the size of most imperial and private hospitals founded after 1261, then it would have been impossible for the Palaeologan facilities to have treated the large number of sick from many classes as the great Constantinopolitan xenones of earlier centuries had done. Private practice must have expanded to fill the gap.

The restricted role of xenones and the expanded scope of private practice after 1204 could reflect the influence of the West, where physicians had never viewed hospital service as an important part of their professional service. It could also reflect the nature of traditional Byzantine practice in the provinces. Although hospitals were surely functioning in other cities of the Byzantine Empire before 1204, there is no evidence that they dominated the medical profession in such towns as they had in Constantinople. When Michael VIII entered Constantinople, the comprehensive hospital system of earlier years had collapsed. Probably Michael and his successors tried to establish a more modest system similar to that of Nicaea or other provincial towns. The change could also be due simply to the impoverishment of the Byzantine government, which could no longer afford to support enough hospital beds in Constantinople to treat the sick of both the lower and the middle class.

THE QUALITY OF XENON CARE AFTER 1261

When one considers that the few surviving references to Palaeologan hospitals indicate that they were modest institutions, that imperial patronage radically declined, and that physicians expanded considerably their private practice, it seems safe to conclude that fewer hospital beds were available in Constantinople in 1300 than in 1150. Granted that xenones were smaller and fewer in the Palaeologan period, did they maintain the same high-quality care which distinguished the Pantokrator Xenon of the twelfth century and the other great hospitals of earlier periods? Unfortunately, no sources surviving from the years after 1261 present as complete a picture of xenon operations as does the Pantokrator *Typikon*. When the empress Theodora drafted the Lips *Typikon* around 1281, however, she included enough information concerning her small xenon to offer some basis for comparison with the Pantokrator.[71]

At first glance the Lips Xenon appears to differ radically from the Pantokrator hospital on account of its small size. The Lips received only twelve patients, compared to fifty at the Pantokrator. The Lips hired only three physicians; the Pantokrator, nineteen. Remember, however, that the empress Theodora designed her hospital exclusively for women; if, therefore, we compare it only with the *ordinos* for female patients at the Pantokrator, we soon find that the two institutions resembled each other very closely. First, the Lips maintained twelve beds, probably arranged in four rows of three beds each around a central hearth. The Pantokrator also had twelve beds for women arranged around a fireplace.[72] Second, the Lips equipped its beds with mattresses, sheets, and covers, following closely the rules at the Pantokrator.[73] Finally, the Lips medical staff corresponded almost exactly to that which the Pantokrator assigned to its women's ward. Three physicians, six hypourgoi, and three servants cared for the twelve patients in both institutions.[74] The medical staffs differed, however, in that no women were working at the Lips, whereas all but the two head physicians were women at the Pantokrator. Apparently females had been forced out of hospital careers between 1136 and 1282, perhaps by the spread of Western customs. The Lips *Typikon* also does not refer to any monthly shifts among the three physicians nor to the two classes (ordained and extra) among the hypourgoi, two features of staff organization which the Pantokrator *Typikon* mentions several times. Since private practice was more important by 1281 than it had been earlier, the Lips physicians also must have had some shift system so that they had adequate time to treat paying patients. In her brief hospital section (25 lines compared to the 442 in the Pantokrator *Typikon*), Theodora simply did not trouble herself about standard professional practice. Because the Lips had three male physicians instead of two, it is possible that each of the three worked only four months a year at the xenon, a system which would have allowed more time for private practice. The twelfth-century distinction between the two classes of hypourgoi, on the other hand, seems to have died out, since the Lips *Typikon* assigned all medical assistants the same yearly salary—10 *hyperpera*.

The administrative staff at the Lips Xenon also paralleled closely that of the Pantokrator, though of course it was smaller. A nosokomos governed both the Lips hospital and the Pantokrator. He was assisted by a man called the *epistekōn* (supervisor), who matches the *meizoteros* at the Pantokrator. In addition, one accountant advised the nosokomos of the Lips, compared to the two who worked at the Pantokrator.[75] Finally, the mother superior of the Lips Monastery, assisted by her oikonomos, supervised the xenon's material resources, just as the abbot and oikonomoi of the Pantokrator community had governed the finances of their public hospital.[76] The administrations of the two xenones differ only in that the Lips did not maintain a set of primmikerioi to govern all the medical procedures of the institution. Since the Lips Xenon only had one ward and apparently no out-patient clinic, it dispensed with a top echelon of medical supervisors above the ward doctors. The absence of the title *primmikerios* at the Lips might also reflect the breakdown of the traditional physicians' guild after 1204.

The support staff at the Lips Xenon also resembled closely that at the Pantokrator although it was much smaller. Theodora hired two pharmacists, one cook, and one washerwoman for the twelve patients. Her typikon does not mention any of the other auxiliary employees—porters, tool sharpeners, latrine cleaners, provisioners, etc.—which appear in the rules governing the Comnenian hospital.[77] The work force which the Lips *Typikon* did list, however, reveals a patient-staff ratio very close to that mandated by the Pantokrator *Typikon*. Thus, one laundress served twelve patients at the Lips, while five worked for fifty at the Pantokrator, roughly one laundress to ten patients at both institutions. Two pharmacists at the Lips provided medicine for twelve (1 to 6), compared to six who served fifty patients at the Pantokrator (1 to 8). Finally, one cook at the Lips prepared meals for the twelve patients (1 to 12), while two cooks and two bakers performed the same chores for fifty sick at the Pantokrator (roughly 1 to 12). The ratio of patients to medical staff at the Lips Xenon was exactly the same as that in the women's ward at the Comnenian hospital, and its support staff was proportionally very close to the same strength as that maintained at the bigger institution. Obviously, the empress Theodora reduced the expenses of her hospital by limiting the number of wards in it to one for female patients. But, she did not want to sacrifice the quality of care for each patient by reducing the patient-doctor ratio or the number of necessary auxiliary personnel relative to each sick woman.

What quality of physicians, hypourgoi, and support staff could Theodora hire for the Lips Xenon? Here the empress could only maintain traditional xenon salaries to hire dependable people. She could not regulate the overall standards of the medical profession or the quality of laborers available. The Lips *Typikon* proves that Theodora took the one step within her power to maintain the standards of her hospital staff; she not only paid the Lips employees at the same rate which John II had established for the men and women who worked at the Pantokrator Xenon, but she increased the salaries across the board.

The three physicians at the Lips Xenon all received a salary of 16 hyperpera a year with no annona allotments. The physicians of the women's ward at the Pantokrator had been paid 6⅓ hyperpera with an annona allotment of 36 *modioi* of wheat, probably valued at one hyperperon per 12 modioi. Thus, their total income would have been worth 9⅓ Comnenian hyperpera, which represented 14.1 hyperpera in the coins of 1281.[78] Granted that the Pantokrator *Typikon* also authorized special donatives for the staff, still the Lips physicians seem to have earned a little more than their predecessors of the twelfth century. Indeed, all ranks of employees at the Lips with

Table 1. Comparison of salaries at the Lips Xenon and at the Pantokrator (in 1281 hyperpera)

Staff Position	Lips	Pantokrator
Medical assistant	10	7.1
Servant	10	10.2
Pharmacist	12	8.3
Cook	10	8.3
Laundress	5	3.8
Nosokomos	14	19.2
Administrative assistant	12	11.0

the exception of the nosokomos received salaries higher than or equal to those of their counterparts at the Pantokrator, as Table 1 indicates. The salary scale at the Lips Xenon thus does not reflect diminishing standards. The nosokomos alone received a significantly lower salary than had the director of the Pantokrator hospital; in fact he earned even less than the three ward doctors under his supervision. Presumably, he was not a physician, as the nosokomos at the Pantokrator had been. It is possible that as private practice grew in significance after 1204, physicians were no longer willing to hold hospital management positions, since these were full-time posts and did not allow free months to devote to paying patients. Thus, either lawyers or monks took over the responsibilities of hospital management. The nosokomos who hired John Chortasmenos in 1406 was in fact a monk.[79]

The Lips *Typikon* gives no indication of the range of treatments its physicians administered. But it does mention the expenditures for the food served the patients. Although there is a certain ambiguity in the text, Theodora seems to have allotted each of the sick 30 modioi of wheat a year—which would mean a ration of 1.1 kilograms of bread a day, considerably more than the 850 grams which the patients at the Pantokrator had received.[80] The typikon also provided 70 hyperpera for wine, 60 for legumes and fresh vegetables, 6 for salt and flax oil, and 3 for barley. In view of the uncertainty regarding food prices under the Palaiologoi, it is impossible to determine these rations for comparison with those of the Pantokrator. But since Theodora strove to equal or surpass the Comnenian hospital in so many other areas, here too she probably followed closely the standards set by John II. It is interesting to note as well that the daily menu served at the Lips matched that prescribed for patients at the Pantokrator. It consisted of a large amount of bread, supplemented with two vegetable dishes served with olive oil. Wine was the standard beverage. Neither hospital offered its patients any meat or fish.[81]

The Lips *Typikon* suggests that the new hospitals of the Palaeologan period were consciously patterned on the great xenones of the past even if they might have been smaller in scale. Theodora's institution reveals so many characteristics common in medical facilities before 1204 as to banish any suspicion that the Byzantine hospital tradition did not survive the Latin conquest and the difficult years afterwards. On the other hand, other sources from the fourteenth and fifteenth centuries indicate that in practice the quality of hospital care was declining to some extent.

In a poem commemorating the new xenon of Michael Glabas, the poet Manuel Philes prays that no lazy or dishonest man would ever plague the institution, nor that any bold and unfeeling person would attack those paralyzed with disease. Otherwise, the hospital could not continue to offer free care, but would cease to function as it had originally been conceived.[82] Here Philes issues a much stronger warning against wrongdoing on the part of the staff than had John II Komnenos in organizing the Pantokrator Xenon. John had advised the physicians and other staff members always to remember the ever-watchful eye of Christ, the Ruler of All, who would certainly punish those who harmed or neglected the patients, his beloved brothers and sisters.[83] John also included a prohibition against accepting tips from patients but without any hint that such practices were a major threat to his institution's survival.[84] Philes' strident warning, on the other hand, suggests that dishonest and greedy personnel were destroying the very nature of Byzantine xenones and thereby undermining the system of free medical care. His remarks indicate that at some hospitals staff members were either despoiling the xenones' resources so that these philanthropic institutions could no longer operate, or that they were insisting upon receiving various tips before they would assist the patients. In the first instance, the directors and their associates would have been involved; in the second, the doctors, hypourgoi, and some of the auxiliary personnel.

Mazaris, the early-fifteenth-century satirist, describes the income of the wealthy physician Malakes as consisting of salaries from several xenones in Constantinople and of fees from private practice at Galata.[85] His description of Malakes implies that it was not unusual for such a physician to collect salaries from several hospitals at the same time. The system at the Pantokrator had required that hospital doctors devote every working hour of every day to the xenon during the six months that they were assigned hospital duty.[86] During the other six months, they might have held down a post at another hospital, but granted the low salaries in xenon service, they probably used these months to develop their private practice. Under the strict rules which had governed the Pantokrator, it would not have been possible for a doctor like Malakes to have worked in more than one hospital at a time and to have pursued a lucrative private practice as well. Mazaris' letter suggests that in practice fifteenth-century physicians were no longer devoting half of their work effort to the patients of a single hospital. As a consequence, either more physicians were being hired for the patients at each hospital so that the staff physicians could have shorter duty shifts, or the doctors were simply spending less working time in each hospital. Given the declining prosperity of the Byzantine Empire, it seems more likely that most hospitals could not have hired more physicians. Thus, Byzantine doctors must have reduced their time commitment to each xenon in which they held a post.

At the beginning of the fifteenth century, John Chortasmenos composed a short stanza concerning the time he spent working in a Constantinopolitan hospital. He was probably referring to the Krales Xenon, where he rebound the famous manuscript of Dioskorides, now known as the Vienna Dioskorides. His poem expressed contempt for the workers in this institution, men whom he considered ignorant and dangerous, at least to his intellectual life. Chortasmenos' remarks are not easy to interpret.[87] They might refer to the cooks, laundresses, and other auxiliary help, but they were more probably aimed at the physicians and hypourgoi with whom Chortasmenos would have come in contact while working in the xenon's library. If they were directed against the medical staff, they could simply reflect the prejudice of a literary man toward ordinary physicians, a prejudice which John Zachariah mentions briefly in the introduction to his *De urinis*.[88] On the other hand, they might indicate a deterioration in the education of physicians and their assistants.

None of these passages regarding hospitals proves conclusively that the physicians, hypourgoi, or other xenon employees of the Palaeologan period were inferior to their predecessors. When considered together, however, they do create the suspicion that care was not as thorough by the fifteenth century as it had been under the Komnenoi. Moreover, other sources describing the Byzantine medical profession in general strengthen this impression. The monk Joseph Bryennios maintained that the East Romans of his day (late fourteenth century) were entrusting themselves to Jewish physicians in violation of the church canons.[89] Since we know from other sources that Byzantine physicians were numerous at this time, this preference for Jewish doctors must have sprung from a distrust in the quality of Christian physicians. So, too, one of the aktouarioi who directed the Mangana Xenon sometime during the fourteenth century was selected not from among the leading East Roman physicians, but from among Moslem doctors. Apparently, the xenones of Constantinople had not produced a sufficiently expert medical man to serve in the emperor's own hospital.[90] Moreover, Mazaris' *Journey to Hades* never ceases to ridicule physicians for their lack of knowledge despite their political and economic successes. One of the characters in the satire claims that many doctors could not even read Galen or Hippocrates, let alone understand them.[91] Finally, the continuous stream of Byzantine medical literature ceases about 1350. After John Zachariah finished his works, no Greek physician undertook to compose a significant treatise on medicine.[92] As in other areas of Byzantine cultural life, so in medicine the second half of the fourteenth century was a period of decline, primarily because the struggle simply to survive absorbed society's resources.[93]

Several sources describing xenon personnel as well as some discussing the medical profession in general paint a picture of deteriorating care in hospitals, if not after the recovery of Constantinople in 1261, surely by the middle of the fourteenth century. Nevertheless, xenones continued both to provide the poor with access to trained physicians and to teach Greek medical science. While John Argyropoulos was lecturing at the Krales Xenon between 1444 and 1451, this hospital was considered one of the leading educational institutions of Constantinople. Students from all over Greece and Italy flocked to its lecture hall to pursue both medicine and Aristotelian philosophy. A manuscript containing a collection of Aristotle's works (*Baroccianus* 87) preserves a sketch on folio 35 of Argyropoulos teaching from a high cathedra. Behind him rise the cupola and auxiliary buildings of the Krales Xenon, even on the eve of the Turkish conquest still an important institution in the Byzantine capital.[94]

The Turkish conquest of Constantinople in 1453 finally brought an end to the phenomenally resilient East Roman state and extinguished its culture forever. No succeeding government was able to keep alive the ancient empire as the Laskarids had done after 1204. Learned Greek scholars managed to export Byzantine humanism to Italy; monastic retreats such as Athos and the Meteora preserved Orthodox spirituality; the Greek peasants kept alive the folk life of the empire; but the integrated whole of Byzantine culture had been destroyed. With it, too, Byzantine xenones vanished. Although the Ottoman conqueror soon turned his attention to establishing a new hospital for Turkish Constantinople, his institution represented a late stage in Islamic medical facilities rather than a revival of the Byzantine-Christian tradition. Hospitals were also functioning in the cities of Latin Christendom, but the philanthropic agencies of the West differed considerably from xenones even though they had borrowed much from the Byzantine hospitals. Thus, the Krales Xenon, where John Argyropoulos taught in the 1440s, represents the last example of an institution which had been born at the close of the fourth century and matured during the late antique era, an institution which had been at the very center of medieval Greek medicine since the reign of Justinian.

CHAPTER ELEVEN

Epilogue

This survey of Byzantine hospitals has stressed the central position of the xenon in Byzantine society, at the intersection of state, ecclesiastical, and professional interests. Indeed, it ranked after church buildings as a hallmark of a true Christian polis. As a result, the hospital drew on almost every facet of East Roman life for financial and spiritual support—from the imperial government, the bishops, the monastic movement, the aristocracy, and the medical profession itself. In fact, it occupied a place in the Byzantine world similar to that of hospitals in twentieth-century society and especially to the place of health-care centers maintained by modern Christian churches.[1]

Byzantine xenones resemble more closely modern hospitals than they do any of the institutions of pagan antiquity or any of the houses of charity in the Latin West during the Middle Ages. Therefore, a careful consideration of their birth in the fourth century, their increasing role in providing secular medical services in subsequent centuries, and finally their decline in the years after the Latin conquest of Constantinople should give some new perspectives on modern hospitals in general and on the role of Christian churches in such institutions. Moreover, since the xenones were institutions thoroughly integrated into their own society, unraveling their history has also brought to light a number of significant threads in the fabric of East Roman civilization as a whole—threads which certainly warrant further study. It is appropriate, then, to close this study by restating some aspects of xenones which might have some relevance to modern hospitals and by directing attention to the broader questions which Byzantine medical centers have raised about East Roman government and society in general.

Byzantine hospitals clearly developed out of Christian institutions for the poor and homeless. Philanthropia provided the initial impulse to create hospices (xenodocheia) and to expand these institutions into specialized medical centers (xenones). Later, the same impulse motivated bishops to maintain old hospitals and open new ones. It inspired the emperors to patronize xenones as an expression of imperial beneficence. It also served as the leaven of the Byzantine ascetic movement, constantly inspiring new generations of monastic leaders to support hospitals despite their strong desire to flee the world and dedicate themselves to pure *theoria*—prayer and the contemplation of God. In their typika, founders always stressed that philanthropia should motivate the physicians and other hospital employees to provide each patient with the best possible care. Liturgical celebrations involving all the staff served to reinforce the Christian dimension of hospital service.

Despite the central role of philanthropia in creating and sustaining the Byzantine hospital, it would be naive to suppose that no other factors helped to generate these institutions and to maintain them for so many centuries. Some bishops built xenones and other charitable foundations to win political influence for themselves or their ecclesiastical faction. A few of the less virtuous urban monks might have chosen hospital work in order to mix with the world in sin, while some strict cenobitic leaders might have agreed to finance hospitals because these popular institutions could win for their communities greater wealth and power. Physicians, too, joined hospital staffs for more than simply charitable purposes. After Justinian incorporated the city archiatroi into the Christian hospital system, xenon physicians received both government stipends and great prestige in the profession; such prestige could win them wealthy private patients and substantial fees. Since the Pantokrator Typikon had to warn all staff members, including physicians, to recall the all-watchful eye of the Lord in fulfilling their hospital duties, some doctors must have failed in carrying out even the letter of their responsibilities, not to mention achieving the philanthropic ideal of the xenon. Nevertheless, the overriding standard of philanthropia—a concept which included not simply kindness, but also self-sacrifice for man in the image of Christ's sacrifice— surely inspired some of the hospital employees.

Christianity and its cardinal virtue of charity shaped the rules and customs of the xenones. Thus, staff physicians were never permitted to collect fees from patients. In the twelfth century, the poet Theodore Prodromos praised the nosokomos who was to operate on him as a virtuous man who collected no fee. The Pantokrator *Typikon* barred its doctors from taking tips even from wealthier patients. Physicians had to be content with the stipends hospitals assigned them and with the opportunities for better training and a more lucrative private practice which xenon service offered. That philanthropia dominated medical practice in the hospitals is indeed remarkable since these institutions were not simply hospices to serve as the last resort for the destitute sick, like those of the medieval West, but were the chief institutions of the medical profession, employing the leading physicians and accepting some patients who could have afforded to pay.

Philanthropia also required Byzantine hospitals to provide each patient with shelter, a bed, and proper nourishment free of charge. Poor patients, of course, never paid for their needs, but there is no evidence that men of standing such as Deacon Stephen were ever expected to pay either. The founders established xenones with sufficient endowments to cover all costs. It is possible that wealthier patients might have donated a sum of money or left property as a legacy to hospitals in thanksgiving for the care they had received while patients, but I have been unable to find any certain evidence of this.[2]

Granted that Christian philanthropia underlay the entire hospital system in the East Roman Empire, what effects did this have on the xenones and on the medical professionals practicing in them? First, it made the hospitals very popular, so popular that they entered ecclesiastical and secular politics. During the fourth century Christianity as a whole captured the hearts of many people in the Eastern cities by supporting philanthropic agencies such as the emerging hospitals. During the same years, bishops representing specific doctrinal formulations used hospitals to build support for their creeds. During the fifth and sixth centuries wealthy Christians founded hospitals to win renown and no doubt political influence in their native cities. Finally, the emperors themselves saw the importance of hospital support in gaining the affections of the people. It was no accident that imperial houses from the Lekapenoi to the Palaiologoi wanted to associate their families with prominent xenones in Constantinople. In a similar manner, church leaders in the nineteenth and early twentieth centuries financed hospitals where they believed that they were competing with other religious groups and felt the need to protect or extend their influence. There is some evidence that Christian denominations are again turning to hospitals in a contest of virtue just as the various Arian and Nicaean factions did in the second half of the fourth century.[3]

The philanthropia of hospitals also added to the prestige of the medical profession. While as early as the writings of the Fathers, physicians were respected for their active charity, Christian literature still expressed some reservations about secular medicine through the sixth century. Indeed, the anargyroi tales of the sixth and seventh centuries contain bitter attacks on the medical profession. These hostile passages usually emphasized the greed of physicians in charging for their services. As hospitals superseded the older system of public physicians and probably encroached substantially on private practice, such charges lost their sting. The oldest vita of Saint Sampson emphasized the role of its hero's hospital in teaching physicians Gospel philanthropia.[4] Infused as they were with Christianity, the xenones also blunted the other major criticism of physicians—their pagan roots. Once the hospitals had replaced the private iatreia of the public physicians in training doctors, the ancient pagan connections of medicine were severed, and a new, Christian tone appeared in the medical writing of men like Theophilos Protospatharios. As a result, Byzantine Christians ceased to suspect their doctors of paganism.

The philanthropia of Byzantine hospitals also limited the scope of private enterprise in the practice of medicine. While working at the xenon, physicians received salaries, not fees. During the months they were not on duty, however, they could treat private patients. Thus, the Byzantine system resembled that of some modern states, where doctors see both patients covered by the state health plan and those who are willing and capable of paying for private care.

It is difficult to determine the extent to which the philanthropic medicine of the hospital system diminished the wealth of physicians compared to other classes in society. Or to approach the question from another angle, were Byzantine physicians significantly less prosperous than had been their ancient predecessors who operated in a completely free market? (The classical city and the Roman imperial government did not even impose a licensing system before the conversion of Constantine.)[5] Hellenistic and Roman inscriptions indicate that some ancient physicians grew fabulously wealthy in the cities of Asia Minor. There is no comparable evidence that Byzantine doctors amassed large personal fortunes, although some of them wielded considerable political influence, especially in the fourteenth century.[6] Moreover, xenon stipends for staff physicians were much lower than had been imperial stipends for archiatroi before Justinian's introduction of the hospital system. For example, the chief physician at the twelfth-century Pantokrator Xenon received a salary valued at only 11.75 *noumismata* a year, while in 534 the senior archiatros in a city of the African prefecture was to be paid 99 *solidi* (*noumismata*) in addition to grants in kind.[7] We do not know, however, what Byzantine physicians were able to collect as private fees.

Given the philanthropic nature of Byzantine hospitals, what quality of health care did these institutions offer patients, especially in comparison with other health-care systems? Certainly, Byzantine xenones far surpassed the philanthropic hospitals of the medieval and early modern West. Simply comparing the Pantokrator Xenon with the Hôtel-Dieu of Paris should demonstrate the superiority of the East Roman hospitals. The Pantokrator rules guaranteed patients private beds, required physicians to wash their hands after each examination, and arranged the physical plant to keep all the sick warm.[8] The Hôtel-Dieu did not take similar measures for the comfort and hygiene of patients until the French Revolution; introducing these measures at that time halved the mortality rate in Paris hospitals.[9] Moreover, if the Pantokrator and Lips hospitals were typical, Byzantine xenones offered far better doctor-patient ratios than do even modern hospitals in Europe and America.

Yet the high quality of patient care in Byzantine hospitals could not compensate for the inadequacies of secular medicine in the ancient and medieval world. Even when xenon doctors carefully examined patients, prescribed proven treatments, and monitored these with attention, their success rate surely did not approach that of modern facilities. Bishop Phokas' concern to secure an adequate cemetery for his xenon in Philadelphia vividly reflects the limitations of hospital care.[10] It is not at all clear, however, that the philanthropic nature of hospitals had anything to do with retarding the initiative of Byzantine doctors in developing more effective remedies or more advanced technology. The decline of hospitals and the rise of private practice in East Roman society which followed the Latin conquest of Constantinople did not stimulate any great forward movement in medical science. If anything, the healing art declined in the last two centuries of the empire as hospitals became less important to the profession.

It is perhaps more fruitful to compare Byzantine hospital care with the treatment of the sick in the ancient world, since both of these systems operated in societies of similar technological development. Did the free-market system of the classical profession provide better health care than the bureaucratic hospital medicine of the East Roman system? Such a comparison demonstrates, first, that the xenones provided poor patients with far superior care than did any of the classical institutions. They not only offered the destitute access to secular medicine's best practitioners, but also guaranteed them warm beds, sufficient food, and continuous nursing care. Even the most altruistic public physicians of the ancient world had not the facilities in their private iatreia to offer such care.

Comparing the quality of medicine which ancient archiatroi dispensed with that of the xenon physicians yields no positive answers. On the one hand, the individual physicians of the hospital era never displayed the vast scope of a Galen or the experimental brilliance of the Alexandrian physicians. On the other hand, over the centuries Byzantine doctors added new elements to the ancient arsenal of medicaments by borrowing from Arab, Persian, and Indian *materiae medicae*. With so many new drugs, they were no doubt able to develop some better therapies. Moreover, in the field of surgery, they made one spectacular improvement on ancient procedure—the bloodless operation for kidney stones in the bladder. This was indeed a great achievement: Western surgeons were not able to perform a similar operation before the nineteenth century. The final verdict on Byzantine surgery, however, must await the discovery or identification of medieval surgical instruments or at least some explanation why none have been found to date.[11] Moreover, given the vast number of unedited and unstudied Byzantine medical treatises, it is impossible to draw up a final balance sheet on the contributions of Byzantine physicians and their hospital practice to advancing surgery or any other field of medical science beyond the achievements of their ancient Greek ancestors. It is intriguing, however, to consider the advances which the Clinical medicine of France, England, and Austria made during the eighteenth and early nineteenth centuries as a result of careful observations in the hospital wards. In a similar fashion, xenon practice may have enabled Byzantine doctors to expand their field of experience and to discover more effective therapies. That medieval Greek physicians conducted autopsies to study the internal symptoms of disease, as the Paris clinicians were to do some seven hundred years later, suggests that they did.[12] As yet, however, we have no written evidence of scientific progress resulting from Byzantine interest in pathological anatomy.

In setting professional standards of competence, the hospital medicine of the medieval era certainly surpassed the free-market practice of ancient physicians. Outside of the closed collegia of public physicians, citizens of ancient Greek poleis and their posterity of the Hellenistic and Roman periods had no guarantee of the quality of their doctors other than the reports and rumors about their past successes and failures. By the twelfth century, on the other hand, Byzantine society had developed a professional medical guild which required that future doctors complete courses on theoretical medicine, receive adequate practical experience, and pass an exam before they received a license to practice. This guild system was closely tied to the xenon staffs, at least in Constantinople. It is even possible that service as a hospital intern (*perissos iatros*) provided the only forum for the directed experience which the guild system mandated.

Consideration of the physicians' guild introduces another fascinating question concerning Byzantine hospitals. Who actually determined hospital policy? Since we know most about the Pantokrator Xenon, it must again serve as an example. First, the emperor exercised authority over this hospital not only as the executive of the state, but as its owner, since he had established it as a private, imperial foundation. Second, the Pantokrator *Typikon* expressly granted the superior of the Pantokrator monastery authority over the hospital's finances. Third, the nosokomos and his assistants, the hospital administration, supervised the daily functioning of the institution and its proper provisioning. Finally, the primmikerioi headed the medical staff, monitored treatment of all patients, and made the final decisions on admitting new patients; they apparently represented the physician's guild and its standards in the hospital. Because the Pantokrator was a privately endowed foundation, the patriarch of Constantinople had no jurisdiction over it. In sum, several interest groups shared authority over this hospital. Since the imperial founder delegated most of his authority to the superior of the monastery, we can reduce the groups to three. The superior represented the entirety of rights and resources which the Pantokrator complex entailed and also symbolized the Christian presence in the whole institution;[13] the nosokomos kept the hospital functioning; and the primmikerioi guaranteed the best possible medical care. There is no reason to believe that the Pantokrator Xenon differed from other imperial hospitals. The old polis xenones such as the Sampson probably resembled the Pantokrator, except that the patriarch would have retained some influence over the hospital director in such institutions.

That the church, the state, a separate hospital administration, and the medical profession all exercised some jurisdiction over a single xenon illustrates the striking similarity between Byzantine hospitals and modern medical centers, which also are governed on one level by professional hospital administrators, on another by church representatives or a board of trustees, and on a third by representatives of the medical profession.[14] Moreover, Byzantine hospitals allowed employees beneath the physicians—the hypourgoi, or medical assistants—to organize a guild of some sort. Unlike modern hospitals, however, they did not permit the income of the top echelon of employees—the physicians—to rise at a faster rate than that of other workers. For example, the Lips Xenon of the late thirteenth century paid its doctors only slightly more than the Pantokrator had 150 years earlier, while the salaries of hypourgoi and manual laborers rose more substantially in comparison to those of their twelfth-century predecessors. Neither the physicians' guild nor the xenon managers seem to have taken advantage of economic difficulties, political upheavals, or military catastrophes to change what both parties considered fair remuneration for hospital doctors.

Since Byzantine society considered hospitals Christian institutions and therefore agents of Christian morality—indeed, they were always classified with monasteries and other pious houses—hospitals probably confronted problems of medical ethics just as their modern counterparts do. The extant sources, however, reveal only a few glimpses of the ethical issues faced by the Christian xenones. One source, the tenth-century *Vita S. Lucae Stylitae,* describes how the physicians of the Euboulos Xenon treated what they considered to be a very difficult case for seven days. At the end of that time, the doctors decided that the patient could not recover. Following the norms of the Hippocratic tradition, they ceased treatment and had the patient removed from the xenon proper to a nearby hostel so that a new patient could be admitted.[15] These xenon physicians were not practicing a form of passive euthanasia, since they had no special means to keep the patient alive. Their ethical concern here was to make another bed available as soon as possible so that they could concentrate their efforts on a person they could help. By removing the hopeless case from the hospital ward, the physicians were following the professional and ultimately pagan guidelines of their profession, but the xenon observed Christian philanthropia by continuing to feed and house the dying man in a separate facility.

The eleventh-century surgical manuscript *Laurentianus* 74.2 might provide evidence that xenones performed some abortions. Two of the instruments listed on folio 281 were used for abortions by ancient physicians. On the other hand, since the exact nature of this list is not yet clear, it is not certain that xenon surgeons employed all the instruments mentioned. Until archaeology and a better knowledge of Byzantine medical texts clarifies the state of medieval Greek surgery, this list offers no conclusive proof that Christian hospitals permitted abortions.

A final issue—the place of women in Byzantine xenones—cannot properly be limited to a consideration of hospitals only. It is the sort of question which requires a study of women in the society beyond the xenon gate. Despite the growing interest in women's history in the past fifteen years, no one has attempted a thorough evaluation of their role in the East Roman world. Within the limits of a study on hospitals it has, of course, been impossible to treat this vast subject. Nevertheless, the sources permit a few observations based solely on the conditions within the xenones.

Both the Pantokrator *Typikon* and the Lips *Typikon* paint an apparently contradictory picture of women's status in Byzantine hospitals. On the one hand, female employees of the Pantokrator Xenon received the same salaries as their male counterparts at all levels of the staff with the exception of the woman physician (*iatraina*). Moreover, women could hold jobs which required some professional training. The Pantokrator Xenon included six salaried positions for female medical assistants and one place for a female physician.[16] Both the assistants and the physician would have had some medical training. In a society which supposedly restricted women's freedom and their access to public life, it is surprising that the xenones offered them established careers outside the home. Were the hospitals the only places where women could pursue a respectable profession, or were there perhaps other career opportunities? On the other hand, the Pantokrator *Typikon* assigned the women's section the lowest status within the hospital proper; its two male physicians ranked below all other ward physicians in the staff hierarchy. Moreover, the woman doctor in this ward received a salary less than half that of her male counterparts, even though she was on call all twelve months of the year while the male doctors worked for only six months of the year. It is, of course, possible that the female physician did not have to be present for all examinations and worked only when needed. Perhaps this explains her much lower salary.

While the Pantokrator hospital did not focus its best efforts on its female patients, the Lips Xenon admitted only women. Here the empress Theodora organized a staff of three male physicians, six medical assistants, and one nosokomos to treat twelve sick women. Although the Lips was a far smaller institution than the Pantokrator, it offered its female patients just as favorable a doctor-patient ratio as the Comnenian hospital provided and seems to have paid its physicians slightly more. On the other hand, the Lips Xenon no longer included women on the professional staff. Whereas one woman physician and six trained nurses (*hypourgissai*) worked in the women's ward at the Pantokrator, only men performed these skilled jobs at the Lips.[17] It is possible that increased Western influence during the twelfth century and after the conquest of 1204 had closed professional careers to women.

The history of Byzantine hospitals touches on several other issues besides the place of women which raise major questions about Byzantine society and government as a whole. In order to unfold a coherent history of hospitals, it has been necessary to skirt these issues or treat them only very briefly, although discussing them might be of great importance in readjusting present ideas about the East Roman Empire. Here follows a summary of these issues with a few comments on their significance.

A careful review of the fourth-century sources has indicated that the Arian controversy and the ecclesiastical turmoil which it generated were closely linked to the development of hospitals and other philanthropic agencies. Factions within local Christian communities combined a characteristic stance regarding the central theological questions raised by Areios with propaganda efforts, including conspicuous patronage of philanthropic programs, to establish control of the episcopal offices in their cities. Very few studies of the Arian controversy within the Roman Empire have included any discussion of factors other than doctrinal which might have shaped the nature and direction of the conflict. Perhaps this study has uncovered enough evidence regarding the local politics of the dispute to interest ecclesiastical historians in reexamining the church turmoil of the fourth century from a perspective which would integrate both the doctrinal and the local forces at work in each polis. So, too, the contrast between the highly professional hospitals of the Chalcedonian church and the volunteer diakoniai sponsored by the Monophysites might offer some new insight into the church unrest of the sixth century. The philoponoi and other lay associations which manned the diakoniai must have formed a powerful block within local churches of the East. When these groups were hostile to the episcopal establishment, they might well have adopted the Monophysite creed to widen a political battle into a doctrinal one. Further research on the philoponoi would surely aid in establishing a clearer pattern in the confusing battles over the Chalcedonian creed.

Hospitals can also offer new perspectives on the vexing question of Byzantine cities. Historians have been unable to determine whether the polis in its late ancient form survived the Persian and Arab invasions of the seventh century. Some researchers have argued against the continuity of urban life outside of Constantinople by emphasizing the collapse of ancient amenities such as theaters, racetracks, and other sumptuous buildings. But the importance of these ancient pagan facilities had been waning since the fourth century, when bishops like Gregory of Nazianz, Basil, and John Chrysostom set forth the vision of a new Christian city based on philanthropia. Churches and hospitals, not temples and theaters, would mark the City of God. The emperors of the next two centuries made a noble attempt to implement the ideals of the Fathers and the ecumenical councils. Thus, churches, hospitals, and other charitable agencies were no doubt more important to the Greek city on the eve of the Persian invasions than were the ancient amenities of a dying pagan society. If archaeologists could establish that ninth-century Ephesus supported a flourishing xenon, this would be significant in demonstrating the continuity of a Christian polis there after the catastrophes of the seventh century. Unfortunately, archaeologists have not yet identified any distinct features of xenon construction, nor have they uncovered any deposits of Byzantine surgical tools to help in identifying hospitals.

Since East Roman xenones also served as teaching institutions, their survival through the Byzantine Dark Age helped to preserve the culture of the ancient world, at least in Constantinople. The xenones of the capital certainly provided medical instruction, and they might have included some general courses in Greek language and culture as well. Hospitals and other philanthropic foundations might also provide a clue to the form which education in general assumed in the sixth century and the troubled years of the Byzantine Dark Age. Professor Paul Lemerle has shown that the seventh-century polymath Tychikos taught at a *martyrion* in Trebizond.[18] Perhaps the founder of this shrine had included a school as part of his institution, just as the fifth-century Paulinos had linked his church of Cosmas and Damian outside Constantinople to a hospital. In the tenth century, a boy from Cappadocia named Niketas arrived in Constantinople to attend a school founded by a certain Mosellos. Here, the school formed part of a private monastic complex, just as the contemporary Myrelaion Xenon did.[19] Further research on philanthropic institutions in general and on the nature of private foundations in the Byzantine Empire might help to solve some of the issues regarding the educational system both in Constantinople and in other East Roman cities, a system which was strong enough to save Hellenic culture from the disruptions of the seventh and eighth centuries.

The history of hospitals has also dealt with the legal status of private foundations in the Byzantine Empire. Such institutions and the forces which supported them exercised enough power inside East Roman society to alter the standard interpretations of both Roman law and the conciliar decrees. By the twelfth century, private monasteries and philanthropic houses such as xenones and gerokomeia had restricted the role of the bishop in local Christian affairs and had even limited the competence of the imperial bureaucracy. A careful consideration of private foundations and their impact on Roman law might compel medieval and Byzantine historians to alter their conception of the East Roman Empire as a state where the rights of private property had little effect in limiting the power of the emperor and his officials.

Hospitals also furnish a new perspective on Byzantine monasticism. In the fourth century, xenones emerged in close association with monastic movements in many urban areas of the East. Both monasteries and hospitals drew financial support from the same patrons of Christian virtue—the bishops, the emperors, and the aristocracy. Nevertheless, this survey has emphasized that some monastic leaders viewed the xenones as a threat, as an open window to the world through which disturbances, temptations, and sin itself could penetrate the *hesychia* (silence) of the ascetic life. Hospitals thus posed a basic challenge to the monks of the East. Was the perfect Christian life one of philanthropic service or of mystical prayer? Generation after generation, this question surfaced in the writings of monastic thinkers. Modern historians of Byzantine monasticism have not sufficiently explored this basic dichotomy in Orthodox asceticism, especially in analyzing the many reform movements and schisms which monasticism generated during the 1,100 years from 300 to 1400. A careful study of the question might be especially useful in sharpening our understanding of the Hesychast Controversy of the fourteenth century, which not only divided the Orthodox monastic establishment, but also rocked the Byzantine state to its very foundations. So far, I have been unable to find any clear evidence that the Hesychasts attacked monastic participation in and support of philanthropic institutions, but I have only touched the surface of the vast literature dealing with the controversy. Such a position on the part of the Hesychasts would certainly be consistent with other aspects of their thought and would help to explain why the movement met with such hostile reactions in some quarters of both the church and the state.

Examining hospitals has revealed new facets of Byzantine society. Further research on xenones and on other kinds of philanthropic agencies should offer even more fascinating information about the East Roman Empire, for these institutions moved in a milieu outside of the imperial court and the highest circles of the bureaucracy. The hospitals served the very poorest people of the empire and some of the middle class. The old-age homes and orphanages also touched the lives of simple people. In examining such agencies, Byzantine institutional history has the rare opportunity of moving beyond the organization of the bureaucracy to consider currents in the daily lives of middle-class physicians, the lower clergy, and the destitute poor of the streets. Exploring xenones, gerokomeia, and orphanotropheia of the East Roman Empire thus helps to shift the focus of Byzantine studies from the realm of emperors and great officials to that of *homo byzantinus,* a shift which both Byzantinists and medievalists have urged.[20]

Notes

CHAPTER ONE: INTRODUCTION

1. Henry Sigerist, "An outline of the development of the hospital," *Bull. Hist. Med.*, 1936, *4:* 579. For abbreviations and short titles used throughout consult the section Abbreviations and Bibliography, following the Notes.

2. Starr, p. 145.

3. For example Kenneth J. Williams, *Encyclopedia of Bioethics*, s.v. "Hospitals," has considered only hospitals after 1800 as institutions closely tied to the medical profession. He discusses only hospital administration after 1950 as relevant to contemporary ethical questions in hospital administration. Ivan Belknap and John Steinle state that "the changes occurring during this transition [medieval to modern period] have been so great that it hardly seems appropriate to use the same word for the early and modern forms of the hospital." *The Community and Its Hospitals* (Syracuse: Syracuse University Press, 1963), p. 3. John D. Thompson and Grace Goldin in their architectural history *The Hospital: A Social and Architectural History* (New Haven: Yale University Press, 1975), pp. 6–8, discuss an East Roman (Syrian) hospital-hospice, and include one paragraph on the Pantokrator hospital in Constantinople, but in the remaining medieval sections (pp. 10–79) they base their generalizations on the lack of practical, treatment-oriented hospital facilities solely on Western models. Foucault pursues his discussion of hospital observation and clinical teaching with no reference to the teaching at either Byzantine or Moslem hospitals.

4. For example, the old, standard history of Byzantine medicine—Bloch, "Byzantinische Medizin"—views the developments of Greek medicine after the fourth century (A.D.) as all negative with the exception of the hospital, but the extent to which the hospital affected Byzantine medical science is not discussed. Starr, pp. 147–48, suggests that institutions based on philanthropy cannot at the same time be institutions of medical science and professionalism. In this regard, see Chap. 2.

5. Sigerist, "Development of the hospital" (see n. 1 above), p. 577; Karl Sudhoff, "Aus der Geschichte des Krankenhauswesens im früheren Mittelalter in Morgenland und Abendland," *Sudhoffs Archiv,* 1929, *21:* 166–83; Schreiber, "Hospital," pp. 3–10; Uhlhorn, *Liebestätigkeit,* 1:319–20; Reicke, 1:3–5.

6. Jerome, *ep.* 60(3:177), describes the hospice which Pammachius built in Rome as a transplant from the East; see Reicke, 1:3–5.

7. Miller, "Knights," pp. 709–33.

8. *Encyclopedia of Islam,* 2:1120. Sami Hamarneh, "Development of hospitals in Islam," *Journal of the History of Medicine and Allied Sciences,* 1962, *17:* 366–68. See the recent article by Friedrun Hau, "Gondeschapur: Eine Medizinschule aus dem 6. Jahrhundert," *Gesnerus,* 1979, *36:* 98–115 and esp. 112–15, which provides references to other secondary sources.

9. The *New Encyclopedia Britannica* (1978), Micropaedia, 5:147, defines a hospital as "an institution staffed and equipped for the diagnosis and treatment of the sick or injured, for their housing during treatment, for health examinations, and for the management of childbirth."

10. Thompson and Goldin, *The Hospital* (see n. 3 above), p. 6; Belknap and Steinle *The Community and Its Hospitals* (see n. 3 above), pp. 3–4; Starr, pp. 145–62.

11. *MGH Conc.* 1:105.

12. *MGH Poet.* 1:554.

13. *Statuta domus Dei Pariensis,* chap. 22, *Statuts,* 46.

14. *Regula ordinis Sancti Spiritus in Saxia,* capp. 40, 42, and 43, PL, 217:1145–46.

15. Miller, "Knights," pp. 709–23.

16. Edward Kealey, *Medieval Medicus: A Social History of Anglo-Norman Medicine* (Baltimore: Johns Hopkins University Press, 1981), pp. 82–106.

17. *Statuta domus Dei Pariensis,* in *Statuts,* 43–53, do not once refer to physicians. For the absence of staff physicians before the fourteenth century see Miller, "Knights," p. 722.

18. John H. Knowles, "The teaching hospital: Historical perspective and a contemporary view," in *Hospitals, Doctors, and the Public Interest,* ed. John H. Knowles (Cambridge: Harvard University Press, 1965), p. 1, states that the hospitals had no relationship to physicians or the medical profession before the modern era.

19. *Statuts de l'Hôtel-Dieu de Saint-Pol,* in *Statuts,* 119–20.

20. For the evidence that the Hôtel-Dieu assigned more than one patient to a bed see E. Coyecque, *L'Hôtel-Dieu de Paris au Moyen Age: Histoire et documents,* 2 vols. (Paris, 1891), 1:72–76. Coyecque bases his assertion on iconographic evidence in the *Livre de vie active* and on scattered references in the sources to the number of patients and the number of beds in the Hôtel-Dieu during the fifteenth century. For the early modern period see Ackerknecht, p. 16.

21. Charles Coury, *L'Hôtel-Dieu de Paris: Treize siècles de soins, d'enseignement, et de recherche* (Paris: L'Expansion, 1969), pp. 31–33, describes the poor conditions of the premodern wards of the hospital.

22. See Miller, "Knights," p. 719.

23. Thus the Hôtel-Dieu at Paris paid physicians to treat its patients and finally hired staff doctors (Ibid., p. 722). See also *Statuta domus Dei Pariensis,* cap. 21, *Statuts,* 46: the sick are to be served "donec sanitati restituatur."

24. Wolfgang H. Hein and Kurt Sappert, *Die Medizinalordnung Friedrichs II: Eine pharmaziehistorische Studie* (Holstein: Internationale Gesellschaft für Geschichte der Pharmazie, 1957), have assembled all of Frederick's regulations regarding the practice of medicine. Nowhere do they mention hospitals.

25. *Regula ordinis Sancti Spiritus in Saxia,* PL, 217:1137–56.

26. Reicke, 2:115–16.

27. Abel-Smith, p. 7.

28. Miller, "Knights," pp. 713–23.

29. The most thorough political history of Byzantium is Ostrogorsky, *History.* Browning, *Empire* offers a brief but excellent account of both political and cultural history.

30. *Theophanis chronographia,* 29.

31. Theodoretos, *Hist. eccl.* 5.19.2–5.

32. *Monodia de Constantinopoli capta,* PG, 161:1135.

33. Soz. 6.31.7–8.

34. *Vie de Théodore de Sykéôn,* chap. 161, pp. 138–45.

35. "Diataxis Attaliate," pp. 25–26; Lemerle, *Cinq études,* p. 103.

36. *Typikon Kosmosoteiras,* chap. 70, p. 53.

37. Charles D. Du Cange, *Historia Byzantina, II: Constantinopolis Christiana* ... (Paris, 1680), bk. 4, no. 9, pp. 163–66.

38. Edward Gibbon, *The History of the Decline and Fall of the Roman Empire,* introduction and notes by John B. Bury, 7 vols. (London: Methuen and Co., 1897), 3:27 (chap. 25), 3:375 (chap. 32), and 4:218 (chap. 40).

39. *Vita Sampsonis,* PG, 115:281.

CHAPTER TWO: THE PANTOKRATOR XENON

1. *Bildlexikon*, pp. 209–15; see map E-5, no. 6, for location of the Zeyrek Kilisi Cami. Ann W. Epstein, "Formulas for salvation: A comparison of two Byzantine monasteries and their founders," *Church History*, 1981, *50:* 394 provides a good description of the Zeyrek Kilisi Cami and its surroundings.

2. Janin, *Eglises,* pp. 515–23.

3. The document which John II issued to regulate this institution and all its constituent parts has survived and has been edited by Paul Gautier, *PantTyp,* pp. 27–145. See also the report on the buildings still standing by Arthur H. S. Megaw, "Notes on recent work of the Byzantine Institute in Istanbul, Zeyrek, Camii," *DOP,* 1963, *17:* 335–65.

4. Hunger, *Reich,* p. 180.

5. *Bildlexikon*, pp. 209–15, esp. illustration 237 (p. 210). See also the poem describing the Pantokrator complex most recently published by Volk, *Klostertypika,* pp. 189–90.

6. See the ms. descriptions and the history of earlier editions of the Pantokrator Typikon by Gautier (*PantTyp,* intro., pp. 5–8).

7. Philipsborn, "Krankenhauswesen," p. 355. Schreiber, "Hospital," pp. 3–79, is essentially a commentary on the Pantokrator Typikon and does not attempt to trace the development of the xenon from earlier institutions. Charles Diehl, *La société byzantine à l'époque des Comnènes* (Paris: Gamber, 1929), pp. 50–57, discusses the Pantokrator as an institution of the twelfth century. Hunger, however (*Reich,* pp. 173–81) includes the Pantokrator Xenon in a general discussion of philanthropic institutions, as do Edouard Jeanselme and Lysimachos Oeconomos, *Les oeuvres d'assistance et les hôpitaux byzantins au siècle des Comnènes,* Communication faite au premier congrès de l'histoire de l'art de guérir, Anvers, 7–8 août 1920 (Anvers: Imp. de Vlijt, 1921).

8. Constantelos, *Philanthropy,* pp. 171–84.

9. Cf. the *Typikon Kosmosoteiras* and the *Typikon Libos.*

10. *PantTyp,* 83.904–85.924. Numbers refer to page and line.

11. *PantTyp,* 85.916–20, describes the five extra beds, one in each ordinos. These were to be used if the regular beds were full. It was not the normal practice to assign more than one patient to a bed. Moreover, *PantTyp,* 83.904–6, states that the xenon was designed for 50 patients. Temkin, "Byzantine Medicine," p. 218, apparently did not notice these statements and focused on the large number of hospital physicians. Thus, he has postulated that the Pantokrator assigned more than one patient to a bed as Western hosptials did.

12. *PantTyp,* \85.930–36.

13. For hearths, *PantTyp,* 99.1152–54; for latrines, 93.1088–89; and for cleaning latrines, 89.1006.

14. *PantTyp,* 93.1057–60.

15. *PantTyp,* 91.1035–50. See also Gautier's commentary, ibid., intro., pp. 18–19. For the value of the Comnenian noumisma, see Chap. 10, n. 78.

16. On the xenon staff, *PantTyp,* 85.937–87.954; on doctors for the monks, 93.1063–68. See Chap. 8 below regarding *embathmos* and *perissos.*

17. The hierarchy is revealed in the salary list, *PantTyp,* 101.1182–94; also by the statement ἀπὸ δὲ τῶν τοιούτων ἰατρῶν τῶν εἰς ὀρδίνους κατατεταγμένων οἱ μὲν δύο οἱ πρῶτοι καὶ πρωτομηνῖται ὀνομασθήσονται (*PantTyp,* 85.944–45). The promotion system is mentioned again at *PantTyp,* 93.1067–73.

18. *PantTyp,* 87.965–79; ibid., 91.1022–24.

19. *PantTyp,* 87.955–58.

20. *PantTyp,* 85.939–41.

21. *PantTyp,* 87.957–64.

22. Kantakouzenos, *Historia,* 1.13 (1:62–63).

23. List of staff members, *PantTyp,* 89.996–1006; the salary list (105.1271–82) mentions two additional employees.

24. *PantTyp*, 113.1414–115.1443.
25. *PantTyp*, 87.980–84 and 93.1074–99.1151.
26. *PantTyp*, 87.983–984: οὗτοι [nosokomos and meizoteros] δὲ καὶ ἀλογαρίαστοι ὑπὲρ τούτων [hospital allotments] ἔσονται πρὸς τὸ ποιεῖν ἀνελλιπῆ τὴν πρόνοιαν ἁπάντων.
27. *PantTyp*, 101.1195–97, 1202–4.
28. *PantTyp*, 93.1082–95.1098.
29. *PantTyp*, 97.1120–22.
30. Tzetzes, *ep.* 81, p. 121.
31. Prodromos, *Gedichte*, poem 46, p. 432.
32. Cf. the job description of the nosokomos (*PantTyp*, 93.1074–97.1119) with that of the meizoteros (97.1120–99.1151).
33. *PantTyp*, 93.1058–62.
34. *PantTyp*, 91.1051–93.1056.
35. *PantTyp*, 93.1082–97.1119. See also nn. 26–30 (ibid., p. 94) and notice esp. 95.1114–16: ὑπὲρ ἐξωνήσεως τῶν ἰατρικῶν εἰδῶν, τῶν βοηθημάτων, τῶν ἐμπλάστρων καὶ τῶν λοιπῶν σκευασιῶν τοῦ ξενῶνος . . . λίτρας ὑπερπύρους δύο.
36. *PantTyp*, 105.1071–79.
37. *PantTyp*, intro., pp. 18–19. See also Jeanselme and Oeconomos, *Les oeuvres d'assistance* (see n. 7 above), p. 13.
38. *PantTyp*, 99.1154–58; 89.1001 (the two chapels).
39. *PantTyp*, 89.1002–5.
40. *PantTyp*, 89.1007–19.
41. *PantTyp*, 29.32–31.44.
42. *PantTyp*, 85.925–30.
43. *PantTyp*, 107.1305–12; see also Gautier's n. 59 (p. 106).
44. *PantTyp*, 109.1347–111.1385.
45. *PantTyp*, 111.1370–77.
46. Eusebios, *Hist. eccl.* 7.22.1–11.
47. *Cod. Theo.* 16.2.10. This law has been dated to 320 by Clyde Pharr et al., *The Theodosian Code and Novels* (Nashville: Vanderbilt University Press, 1952). See also Hunger, *Reich*, p. 174.
48. *Theophanis chronographia*, p. 29.
49. See below in this chapter, in the discussion of terminology.
50. *Chronicon paschale*, 1:535–36, uses both *xenodocheion* and *xenon* to describe these philanthropic houses. See also Devreesse, p. 111, n. 11.
51. Soz. 3.16.12–16.
52. *Ad Stagirium a daemone vexatum*, 3, PG, 47:490.
53. Theodoretos, *Hist. eccl.* 5.19.2–5.
54. *Palladii dialogus*, p. 32.
55. *Ep.* 110, PG, 79:248 (see Chap. 5, n. 2, for the passage in full).
56. Ibid. emphasizes that the physician adjusted his prescriptions to each patient; this implies the desire to restore health.
57. *Miracula Artemii*, mir. 21, pp. 25–26: mir. 22, p. 30.
58. Ibid., mir. 22, p. 31.
59. See the section on *archiatroi* under Justinian in Chap. 3 below.
60. See Chap. 10.
61. Loren C. MacKinney, *Early Medieval Medicine with Special Reference to France and Chartres* (Baltimore: Johns Hopkins Press, 1937), pp. 176–77; Miller, "Knights," p. 710. For the early nineteenth century see Ackerknecht, pp. 16–17.
62. See those mentioned by Charles D. Du Cange, *Historia Byzantina, II: Constantinopolis Christiana* . . . (Paris, 1680), bk. 4, no. 9, pp. 163–66, or the categories in Janin, *Eglises*, pp. 551–69.
63. For example, *JNov.* 131.15.
64. Dagron, *Naissance*, pp. 511–12; *Epit. Theo. Ana.* 106.9; Evagrios, *Hist. eccl.* 2.11 (p. 63).

65. Janin, *Eglises*, p. 569. See also *JNov*, 7 proem.

66. *Vita Ioannis Hesychastis*, ed. Eduard Schwartz, *TU*, 1939, *49*.2: 204; *Vita Euthymii*, p. 53. See also the Palestinian inscription in *Revue Biblique*, 1892, *1*: 583. The Latin name, Verina, of one of the founders indicates that this inscription comes from the fifth century.

67. Dagron, *Naissance*, p. 512; Janin, *Églises*, pp. 553–54, mentions two gerokomeia from the first half of the fifth century.

68. *Typikon Kosmosoteiras*, 61 (pp. 48–49) and 94 (p. 65).

69. Ibid., 70 (p. 55).

70. For νοσοκομέω see Diodorus Siculus 14.71; for νοσοκομία see Arrianos, *Epicteti dissertationes*, 3.22.70.

71. *Palladii dialogus*, 32.

72. Cf. *JNov*, 120 and 131 passim.

73. *Iuliani epitome*, cap. 32: "Nosocomium, id est locus venerabilis in quo aegroti homines curantur."

74. *Suda:* Νοσοκομεῖον· ὁ ξενών. ἵνα ᾖ τὸ νόσον ἔχειν ἀντὶ τοῦ πάθος ἢ ἔθος τι ἔχειν· νοουμένης τῆς νόσου ἀντὶ οὐδετέρου τοῦδέ τινος.

75. *PantTyp*, 93.1065.

76. *Poenae in monachos delinquentes*, capp. 54–55, PG, 31:1313.

77. Dmitrievskij, *Opisanie*, 1:651–52. New edition by Paul Gautier, *REB*, 1982, *40*: 87, lines 1247–68.

78. For example, the chrysobull of John V (no. 123, *Actes de Lavra*, 23–26) always refers to the public hospital of St. Panteleemon as a *xenon* and the infirmary for monks of the Lavra as a *nosokomeion*.

79. See the sermon by Gregory of Nyssa, Greg. Nys., *Pauperibus, oratio prima*, 3–18.

80. Basil, *ep.* 94 and 150 (Loeb, 2:150 and 366).

81. *Concilii Chalcedonensis actio XII, ACO*, 2.1.3 (p. 405).

82. *Iuliani epitome*, cap. 32: "Ptochotrophium . . . in quo pauperes et infirmi homines pascuntur."

83. See "Diataxis Attaliate," p. 17, lines 3–4, and pp. 17–130 passim.

84. *Artemidori Daldiani onirocriticon*, 1.4, ed. Roger A. Pack (Leipzig: Teubner, 1963), p. 13.

85. *Theophanis chronographia*, 29.

86. *Regulae brevius tractatae*, PG, 31:1284; cf. *Poenae in monachos delinquentes*, capp. 54 and 55, PG, 31:1313.

87. *Panegyrica Rabulae*, 202–3 (Ger. trans. [Bickell], pp. 205–6); *Syriac Chronicle*, 12.7 (pp. 331–32).

88. *Iuliani epitome*, cap. 32: "Xenodochium, id est locus venerabilis in quo peregrini suscipiuntur."

89. *Suda:* Ξενοδοχεῖον· τὸ τοὺς ξένους ὑποδεχόμενον. καὶ Ξενοδόχος ὁμοίως.

90. *Theo. Cont.*, 430.

91. *Kypriaka Typika*, ed. Ioannes Tsiknopoulos (Levkosia: Kentron Epistemonikōn Meletōn, 1969), p. 51.

92. Euripides, *Alcestes*, vv. 543–48.

93. Josephus, *Bellum Judaicum*, 5.177–78 (4, 4).

94. Waddington, *Inscriptions*, no. 2524.

95. *Hesychii Alexandrini Lexicon*, ed. Ioannis Albert and Mauricius Schmidt (Jena, 1858; rep. Amsterdam: Hakkert, 1965), s.v.

96. *Vita Porphyrii*, chaps. 53 and 94 (pp. 44 and 72).

97. *Ad Stagirium a daemone vexatum III*, PG, 47:490; Theodoretos, *Hist. eccl.* 5.19.2–5.

98. Prokopios, *De aedif.* 1.2.14–17; *JNov*, 131.15.

99. The inscription is incorrectly transcribed in J. Milik, "Topographie de Jérusalem vers la fin de l'époque byzantine," *Mélanges de l'Université Saint Joseph*, 1961, *37*: 149.

100. The legend of Saint Sampson is recorded in two quite different versions; both, however,

describe how the saint converted his house into a hospital. *Vita Sampsonis* (antiquior), p. 10, and *Vita Sampsonis*, PG, 115:281. See Pohl, p. 61, and Meyer-Steineg, pp. 10–12.

101. Prokopios, *De aedif.* 1.11.23–27.

102. *Suda:* Ξενῶνες: δόμου τοῦ ὑποδεχομένου τοὺς ξενοὺς καὶ ἀρρωστοῦντας. See also n. 74 above.

103. *Vita Andreae*, p. 176.

104. *Pollucis onomasticon* 1.79, ed. Erich Bethe, 3 vols. (Stuttgart: Teubner, 1967), 1:24 scolium ad lin. 13.

CHAPTER THREE: HOSPITALS AND THE ANCIENT WORLD

1. Tzetzes, *ep.* 81, p. 121.

2. See Chap. 2 above.

3. Uhlhorn, *Liebestätigkeit*, 1:193–202; Philipsborn, "Krankenhauswesen," pp. 338–65; Gask and Todd, pp. 122–30; Paul Diepgen, *Geschichte der Medizin: Die historische Entwicklung der Heilkunde und des ärztlichen Lebens*, 3 vols. (Berlin: De Gruyter, 1949), 1:137; Harig, "Krankenhaus," pp. 179–95; Hunger, *Literatur*, 2:287, 315–16.

4. Harig, "Krankenhaus," pp. 179–95.

5. Meyer-Steineg, p. 3. See also the following works: Karl Sudhoff, "Die geschichtliche Ent-wicklung der Beziehungen zwischen ärztlichem Beruf und dem Krankenhaus," *Nosokomeion*, 1931, *2.1:* 1–19; Henry E. Sigerist, "An outline of the development of the hospital," *Bull. Hist. Med.,* 1936, *4:* 576; Charles Singer, "Science," in *The Legacy of Rome*, ed. Cyril Bailey (Oxford: Clarendon Press, 1923), pp. 293ff.; H. Wildegans, "Ärzte und Krankenanstalten des klassischen Altertums," *Zeitschrift für ärztliche Fortbildung*, 1964, *53:* 158ff.; Franz Bauer, *Geschichte der Krankenpflege* (Kulmbach: E. C. Baumann, 1965), p. 52. See also the longer list of such works in Harig, "Krankenhaus," p. 179, n. 1.

6. Harig and Kollesch, "Krankenpflege," pp. 258–59. See also Henry E. Sigerist, *A History of Medicine*, 2 vols. (New York: Oxford University Press, 1951), 2:16–43.

7. Diepgen, *Geschichte der Medizin* (see n. 3 above), 1:141; *RAC,* 1:720, 795. See Aristides, *Opera* (Keil), *or.* 38.6 (2:314), and the collection of passages in Edelstein, *Asclepius*, 1:T.348–T.381.

8. Pohl, p. 12; *RAC,* 1:720; for example, Plato, *Rep.* 3.14 (406A).

9. Writing in the fifteenth century, the Byzantine satirist Mazaris still referred to physicians as Asklepiads (Mazaris, p. 90, line 6).

10. Pseudo-Hippocrates, *Presbeutikos*, ed. Émil Littré, *Oeuvres complètes d'Hippocrate*, 9 vols. (Paris, 1861; rep. Amsterdam, 1973), 9:410–12. Wesley D. Smith, *The Hippocratic Tradition* (Ithaca: Cornell University Press, 1979), p. 217, believes this portion of the *Presbeutikos* is based on an accurate tradition.

11. *Suda,* s.v. "Hippokrates." The tradition is also found in Stephanos of Byzantion, *Ethnika,* s.v. "Kōs" (6th cent.); in the Pseudo-Soranos, *Vita Hippocratis* 1–4, CMG, 4, p. 175 (2nd cent.); and in the Pseudo-Hippocratic *ep.* 2, Littré (see above), 9:314 (Hellenistic).

12. Nutton, "Archiatri," p. 200; *Dictionnaire des antiquités grecques et romaines*, ed. Charles Daremberg et al., 5 vols. (Paris: Librairie Hachette, 1877–1919), 3.2:1673. See the inscriptions listed by Pohl, pp. 36–39.

13. *RE*, s.v. "Galen"; Galen, *De admin. anat., Opera* (Kühn), 2:280–82.

14. *Damascii vitae Isidorii reliquiae*, ed. Clemens Zintzen (Hildesheim: Georg Olms, 1967), pp. 162–63. For Alexander's family see Hunger, *Literatur*, 2:297 and n. 31.

15. Blemmydes, *Curriculum*, pp. 2–3.

16. *PantTyp*, 107.1313–23. See especially Hohlweg, "Aktuarios," p. 307 and n. 38.

17. Herodotus 3.131; *Suda*, s.v. "Demokedes."

18. Cohn-Haft, doc. 8, p. 76; commentary, p. 11.

19. Susan M. Sherwin-White, *Ancient Cos: An Historical Study from the Dorian Settlement*

to the Imperial Period, Hypomnemata, 51 (Göttingen: Vandenhoeck und Ruprecht, 1978), pp. 283–84.

20. Nutton, "Archiatri," p. 192; Pohl, pp. 15–16.

21. Harig and Kollesch, "Krankenpflege," pp. 259–61; Amundsen and Ferngren, pp. 73–75; Sigerist, *A History of Medicine* (see n. 6 above), 2:84–115.

22. Sigerist, *A History of Medicine,* 2:274–95.

23. Hippocrates, *On the Sacred Disease,* 21. See Owsei Temkin, *The Falling Sickness: A History of Epilepsy from the Greeks to the Beginnings of Modern Neurology* (Baltimore: Johns Hopkins Press, 1945), pp. 3–80.

24. For a full discussion of the relationship between Greek medicine and religion see Ludwig Edelstein, "Greek medicine in its relation to religion and magic," in *Ancient Medicine: Selected Papers of Ludwig Edelstein,* ed. Owsei Temkin and C. Lilian Temkin (Baltimore: Johns Hopkins Press, 1967), pp. 205–46. See also Amundsen and Ferngren, pp. 70–81.

25. For an outline of Theodosius' steps against pagans see Jones, *LRE,* 1:167–69.

26. For a short description of the *anargyroi* cult see Kötting, pp. 215–19. It is significant that only after Theodosius' order to close all pagan temples, including the asklepieia, do the anargyroi saints appear (early fifth century). The sources first mention the Cosmas and Damian cult shortly after 400 (*Kosmas und Damianos,* pp. 44, 82).

27. For the churches of Cosmas and Damian in Constantinople see Janin, *Eglises,* pp. 284–89; see also the *Miracula Artemii,* pp. 1–75, with reference to the cult of Saint Artemios.

28. *Miraculum* 30, *Kosmas und Damianos,* p. 174; for Saint Sampson see *Vita Sampsonis,* PG 115:292–307.

29. *PantTyp,* 99.1154–55 and 89.1002–5. For the anargyroi see Chap. 4 below.

30. Geoffrey Lloyd, "The Hippocratic question," *Classical Quarterly,* 1975, n.s. *25:* 171–92; Smith, *The Hippocratic Tradition* (see n. 10 above), pp. 199–204.

31. Peter M. Fraser, *Ptolemaic Alexandria,* 3 vols. (Oxford: Clarendon Press, 1972), 1:338–69; Scarborough, pp. 34–35.

32. Temkin, "Greek medicine as science and craft," *Janus,* p. 137; Scarborough, pp. 43–44.

33. For Galen's life and work, see the bibliography in Owsei Temkin, *Galenism: Rise and Decline of a Medical Philosophy* (Ithaca: Cornell University Press, 1973), p. 2, n. 2.

34. Ed. Ioannis Müller, in *Galeni scripta minora,* 3 vols. (Leipzig: Teubner, 1884–93), 2:1–8; Hunger, *Literatur,* 2:287–88.

35. Temkin, "Byzantine Medicine," pp. 203–9; idem, *Galenism* (see n. 33 above), pp. 51–94.

36. Dietz, *Scholia,* 2:157.

37. *Miracula Artemii,* mir. 24, p. 34.

38. Tzetzes, *ep.* 81, p. 121.

39. Mazaris, p. 10, line 34–p. 12, line 2.

40. Temkin, "Byzantine Medicine," pp. 202–22, stresses the continuity between ancient and Byzantine medicine while emphasizing that many new elements were added. Hunger, *Literatur,* 2:287, also states that ancient medicine had a tremendous impact on Byzantine physicians, but he too stresses that these later doctors developed some new techniques and treatments. Still Galenic medicine was the frame upon which all Byzantine physicians built. Even Symeon Seth (eleventh century), who ventured to criticize Galen, did not reject Galen's system but only a slavish following of his every statement. Temkin, "Byzantine Medicine," pp. 214–15.

41. Pliny, *Naturalis historia,* 29.6.

42. Ibid.; Scarborough, pp. 38–40.

43. Pliny, *Naturalis historia,* 29.7.

44. Cicero, *De officiis,* 1.42.

45. Pliny, *Naturalis historia,* 29.8.

46. Ibid.: "Solam hanc artium Graecorum nondum exercet Romana gravitas." See also *DACL,* 11.1:113.

47. Vivian Nutton, "Five inscriptions of doctors," *Papers of the British School at Rome*, 1969, *37*: 96–97.

48. Jeanne Robert and Louis Robert, in *Bulletin Épigraphique*, 1953, *66*: 201.

49. Celsus, *De medicina,* ed. Walter G. Spencer, Loeb Classical Library (Cambridge: Harvard University Press, 1935), intro., pp. vii–xii.

50. *Scribonii Largi compositiones*, ed. Georgius Helmreich (Leipzig, 1887); Karl Deichgräber, *Professio medici: Zum Vorwort des Scribonius Largus,* Akademie der Wissenschaften und der Literatur, Abhandlungen der Geistes- und Sozialwissenschaftlichen Klasse, 9 (Mainz, 1950).

51. Owsei Temkin, "History of Hippocratism in late antiquity," *Janus,* pp. 167–77.

52. Harig, "Krankenhaus," p. 185.

53. Hippocrates, *Decorum,* 11: Ἐπὴν δὲ ἐσίῃς πρὸς τὸν νοσέοντα τούτων σοι ἀπηρτισμένων ἵνα μὴ ἀπορῇς, εὐθέτως ἔχων ἕκαστα πρὸς τὸ ποιησόμενον. . . .

54. Ibid., 13–14, 17.

55. Plutarch, "Quomodo quis suos in virtute sentiat profectus," *Moralia,* 81F–82A.

56. Pseudo-Chrysostom, PG, 64:31.

57. *Miracula Artemii,* mir. 21, p. 26 (seventh-century Constantinople); Eustathios, *Espugnazione,* 146 (twelfth-century Thessalonica).

58. Gask and Todd list four pagan institutions—the *asklepieia,* the *iatreia,* the slave *valetudinaria,* and the military infirmaries—that some scholars have offered as examples of ancient hospitals. I have added the *demosieuontes iatroi* (see Pohl, pp. 58–61). By the fifth century A.D. public physicians did offer some free medical care. See Darrel W. Amundsen, "Visigothic medical legislation," *Bull. Hist. Med.,* 1971, *45*: 556–57 and n. 15.

59. Gask and Todd, pp. 123–25.

60. Columella, *Rei rusticae,* 11.1.18. Celsus, *De medicina, prooemium* 65.

61. Harig, "Krankenhaus," p. 188. Concerning the order of Alexander Severus see Aelius Lampridius, *Alexander Severus* 47, in *Scriptores historiae Augustae,* ed. Ernest Hohl, 1 (Leipzig: Teubner, 1965): 288, line 23–289, line 2.

62. Jerome, *Epistolae, ep.* 77 (4:45).

63. Meyer-Steineg, pp. 20–28. His view has been abandoned by scholars who have carefully studied the purely supernatural healing of the asklepieia. Nevertheless, standard reference works still reflect Meyer-Steineg's belief. For example, *Der Kleine Pauly,* ed. Konrad Ziegler et al., 5 vols. (Munich: Alfred Druckenmüller, 1964–75), 5:1119, s.v. "Valetudinarium."

64. *RE,* s.v. "Asklepios."

65. Meyer-Steineg, pp. 20–28; Pohl, pp. 10–16.

66. *RE,* s.v. "Aristides"; Behr, pp. 1–115.

67. Aristides, *Sacra,* 2.34–35.

68. Pausanias 2 (Corinth).27.1–6 (Edelstein, *Asclepius,* 1:T.739).

69. Pausanias 10 (Phocis, Ozolian Locri).32.12 (Edelstein, *Asclepius,* 1:T.719).

70. Edelstein, *Asclepius,* 2:176–77, believes that the asklepieia of the Roman period did house and care for the poor among their suppliants, but he can cite only Pausanias 10.32.12, as evidence for such a practice.

71. Behr, pp. 26–32; see also Edelstein, *Asclepius,* 2:181–213.

72. Behr, pp. 30–35; Edelstein, *Asclepius,* 2:148–50.

73. Behr, pp. 35–37; Edelstein, *Asclepius,* 2:150–54.

74. Behr, p. 32.

75. Aristides, *Sacra,* 1.62–64.

76. Ibid., 2.20.

77. Aristides, *Opera* (Keil), *or.* 28.132 (2:183); cf. Edelstein, *Asclepius,* 1:T.464b).

78. Aristides, *Sacra,* 1.73.

79. Galen, *Hippocratis epidem. VI et Galeni in illum commentarius,* 4.4, *Opera* (Kühn), 17.2:137.

80. See Edelstein, *Asclepius,* 2:139–45.

81. Julian, *Contra Galilaeos*, 200.A–B, Julian (Loeb), 3:374.

82. H. Hepding, "Rouphinion Alsos," *Philologus*, 1933, *88*: 90–91.

83. George Kedrenos, *Historiarum compendium*, ed. Immanuel Bekker, 2 vols., CSHB (1838), 1:299.

84. Kötting, pp. 218–19; see esp. Saints Cyrros and John, ibid., pp. 201–11.

85. Aeschines, *Contra Timarchum*, 40.

86. Meyer-Steineg, pp. 7–18.

87. Plautus, *Menaechmi*, vv. 946–60.

88. Constitution of Claudius quoted in *JCod*, 7.6.1.3; Meyer-Steineg, pp. 17–18. The word *xenon* in this law, however, is surely a sixth-century (A.D.) interpolation. Cf. this same constitution described by Suetonius, *Claudius*, 25.2.

89. Hippocrates, *De officiniis*, 2–6; sections 7–25 deal with bandaging.

90. Galen, *Commentarius ad de officiniis*, *Opera* (Kühn), 18.2:629–718.

91. Harig, "Krankenhaus," p. 185.

92. Galen, *De alim. fac.*, *Opera* (Kühn), 6:598.

93. Plutarch, "Quomodo quis suos in virtute sentiat profectus," *Moralia*, 81F–82A.

94. Chrysostom, *Ad populum Antiochenum*, 12, PG, 49:130.

95. Chrysostom, *In epistulam secundam ad Cor. VII*, PG, 61:455.

96. Chrysostom, *Contra Anomoeos XII*, PG, 48:804.

97. Chrysostom, *Adversus oppugnatores eorum qui ad monasticam vitam inducunt*, PG, 47:322.

98. This version of *Vita Sampsonis*, edited by Symeon Metaphrastes, is found in PG, 115:277–308. See especially 281: καὶ μὴ μόνον ἐπιμελείας ἀξιῶν πάσης, ὥσπερ οἱ τῆς τέχνης βούλονται νόμοι, ἀλλὰ καὶ τροφῆς κοινωνῶν καὶ στρωμνῆς ἀκολούθως ταῖς τοῦ Χριστοῦ ἐντολαῖς.

99. Procopius, *De aedif.* 1.2.15.

100. See Chap. 5 below.

101. *Vita Theophylacti*, p. 75.

102. *PantTyp*, 93.1070, 99.1167, 89.1000.

103. Pohl, esp. pp. 58–61; see also the recent work of Nutton, "Archiatri," pp. 191–226.

104. For the early seventh century see *Miracula Artemii*, mir. 22, pp. 28 and 31; for the fourteenth century see *Vat. gr.* 299, fol. 368ᵛ (*Codices vaticani graeci*, 429).

105. Herodotus 3.131.

106. Aristophanes, *Acharnenses*, vv. 1030ff.

107. Ibid., vv. 1922ff. and 1222–23.

108. Xenophon, *Institutio Cyri*, 1.6.15.

109. Cohn-Haft, doc. 51, p. 84; see also commentary, ibid., p. 37 and n. 20.

110. Cohn-Haft, pp. 32–45; Amundsen, "Visigothic medical legislation" (see n. 58 above), pp. 556–57 and n. 15.

111. Cohn-Haft, pp. 33–38; p. 37 and n. 20 include a discussion of *CIG*, no. 1145.

112. Cohn-Haft, pp. 46–67.

113. Vivian Nutton, "Continuity or rediscovery? The city physician in classical antiquity and medieval Italy," in *The Town and State Physician in Europe from the Middle Ages to the Enlightenment*, ed. Andrew W. Russell (Wolfenbüttel: Herzog August Bibliothek, 1981), p. 13. For Kos, see Sherwin-White, *Ancient Kos* (see n. 19 above), pp. 272–74.

114. Cohn-Haft, pp. 56–67; Pohl, pp. 48–49.

115. *JDigest*, 50.9.1.

116. Pohl, pp. 71–72.

117. *Cod. Theo.* 13.3.8.

118. Nutton, "Archiatri," pp. 199–200; Pohl, pp. 76–77.

119. *Fontes iuris Romani anteiustiniani*, ed. Salvatore Riccobono, 3 vols. (Florence: Barbèra, 1940–43), no. 73, 1:420–22.

120. *JDigest*, 27.1.6.8
121. *JDigest*, 27.1.6.2. See Nutton, "Archiatri," pp. 199–204, for his interpretation of Antoninus' regulations.
122. Nutton, "Archiatri," pp. 193–94 and 201.
123. The personal physician of Leo I (457–74), Iakobos, was called *archiatros*. See also *Cod. Theo.* 13.3.14–16.
124. Origen, *In Lucam XIII*, PG, 13:1831.
125. Aelius Lampridius, *Alexander Severus* 42 (see n. 61 above), p. 284.
126. *Cod. Theo.*, 13.3.8.
127. *Cod. Theo.*, 13.3.9.
128. Chrysostom, *In paralyticum demissum per tectum*, PG, 51:55–56.
129. This scholion is found together with a discussion of its date in Amundsen, "Visigothic medical legislation" (see n. 58 above), p. 556, n. 15: οἱ δημοσίᾳ χειροτονούμενοι ἰατροὶ ὡς δημόσιοι προῖκα ἐθεράπευον.
130. Aristophanes, *Acharnenses*, vv. 1030–32.
131. *Ägyptische Urkunden aus den königlichen Museen zur Berlin, Griechische Urkunden*, vol. 2 (Berlin, 1898), no. 647.
132. Galen, *Commentarius ad de officiniis*, *Opera* (Kühn), 18.2:678.
133. *Vita Sampsonis*, PG, 115:281.
134. Papyrus (Maspero), no. 67151.
135. *Miracula Artemii*, mir. 22, pp. 28 and 30.
136. Theodore Stoudites, PG, 99:1509: ἀλλὰ καὶ πρώταρχοι καὶ ἀρχιατροὶ καὶ μέσοι καὶ τελευταῖοι. . . .
137. *Kletorologion of Philotheos*, p. 183.
138. Daremberg, *Notices*, pp. 22–30.
139. *PantTyp*, 107.1305–7.
140. Prokopios, *Anecdota*, 26.5.
141. Nutton, "Archiatri," p. 211.

CHAPTER FOUR: EASTERN CHRISTIANITY

1. Cf. Matt. 8:3–4, 16–17, 9:27–30, 12:13; Mk. 7:31–37; Lk. 13:10–17, 14:2–5; Jn. 9:6–7.
2. *Const. Apost.* 4.2–3 (pp. 219–21).
3. *Lettre aux Philippines*, 6:1, in *Ignace d'Antioche, Polycarpe de Smyrne: Lettres, Martyre de Polycarpe*, ed. Thomas Camelot, SC, 10 (Paris, 1969), p. 184.
4. Hyppolyte de Rome, *La tradition apostolique*, ed. Bernard Botte, SC, 11 (Paris, 1968), no. 34, p. 117.
5. Eusebios, *Hist. eccl.*, 7.22.1–11.
6. *La doctrine des douze apôtres (didachè)*, ed. Willy Rordorf and Andrè Tuilier, SC, 248 (Paris, 1978), no. 12, p. 188.
7. For commendatory letters see *A Dictionary of Christian Antiquities*, ed. William Smith, 2 vols. (London: John Murray, 1908), 1:407–8, and Uhlhorn, *Liebestätigkeit*, 1:194.
8. Eusebios, *De martyribus Palestinae*, 11.20–22, in Eusebios, *Hist. eccl.* (GCS, 9.2).
9. Greg. Nys., *Pauperibus, oratio* 1, pp. 7–8.
10. Ibid., *oratio* 2, pp. 23–25.
11. Ibid., p. 35.
12. Ibid., pp. 31–32: οὐκοῦν ὅλον τὸ πλήρωμα τῶν ἐντολῶν ἐν τούτοις ἔχεις πληρούμενον καὶ αὐτὸν τὸν τῶν ὅλων κύριον ὑπόχρεών σοι διὰ τῆς εἰς τοῦτον [the sick poor person] φιλανθρωπίας γενόμενον.
13. Greg. Naz., *De pauperum amando*, PG, 35:865.
14. Ibid., 868.
15. Ibid., 864.

16. *In laudem Basilii,* chap. 63.6 (PG, 36:580).

17. Quasten, 1:220–23.

18. Tatian, *Adversus Graecos,* PG, 6:845.

19. Ibid., 852.

20. Quasten, 2:383.

21. Arnobius, *Adversus gentes,* PL, 5:780–81.

22. Cyril, *Catechesis X: de uno domino Jesu Christo,* 13, PG, 33:677–80.

23. Quasten, 3:161–64; *Die fünfzig geistlichen Homilien des Makarios,* ed. Hermann Dörries et al., Patristische Texte und Studien, 4 (Berlin: De Gruyter, 1964), intro., pp. ix–xi.

24. *Homilien des Makarios, or.* 48, pp. 314–15.

25. *S. Isaiae abbatis orationes,* PG, 40:1140, 1144. For Isaiah see *Dict. Spirit.,* 7.2:2083–95.

26. Quasten, 1:220–23.

27. For Makarios see Quasten, 3:161–64; for Isaiah see *Dict. Spirit.,* 7.2:2083–84.

28. Origen, *Homilia I in psalmam XXXVII,* PG, 12:1369.

29. Origen, *Contra Celsum,* 8.60. See also Darrel Amundsen, "Medicine and faith in early Christianity," *Bull. Hist. Med.,* 1982, *56:* 338.

30. Hunger, *Reich,* p. 309; Quasten, 2:75–100.

31. Greg. Nys., *De virginitate, Opera* (Jaeger), 8.1:335–37 (PG, 46:408).

32. Greg. Nys., *Pauperibus,* p. 12.

33. Basil, *Hexaemeron* V, PG, 29:101, 116.

34. Basil, *Regulae fusius tractatae, interogatio* 55, PG, *31:1044–52.*

35. Ibid., 1048.

36. Ibid., 1052.

37. *Dict. Spirit.,* 8:339–40.

38. Chrysostom, *De perfecta caritate,* PG, 56:279–80; idem, *In epistolam ad Philippenses homilia X,* PG, 62:262.

39. Chrysostom, *epp.* 11 and 12, PG, 52:609.

40. Origin, *Contra Celsum,* 8.60.

41. Basil, *Regulae fusius tractatae, interogatio* 55, PG, 31:1049. Amundsen, ("Medicine and faith" see n. 29 above), pp. 326–50, stresses that the orthodox writers did not sanction the use of secular medicine in all cases.

42. Greg. Nys., *De sancta trinitate, Opera* (Jaeger), 3.1:3 (PG, 32:684).

43. *Vita Sampsonis,* PG, 115:281.

44. For George Tornikes' biography see the introduction in *Tornikès,* pp. 25–32. For refer-ences to philanthropic aspects of the medical profession, ibid., ep. 24, p. 164, and *Eloge d'Anne Comnène,* see ibid., p. 293.

45. *Eloge d'Anne Comnène,* p. 307.

46. *Michaelis Acominati (Choniatis) opera,* ed. Spyridon Lampros, 2 vols. (Athens, 1880), 2:264.

47. This tradition is based on Col. 4:14, where Paul refers to a physician named Luke among his companions. See Adolf Harnack, *Medicinisches aus der ältesten Kirchengeschichte* (Leipzig, 1892), pp. 1–2.

48. Harnack, *Medicinisches,* p. 5, based on Eusebios, *Hist. eccl.* 5.1.49ff.

49. *DACL,* 11.1:165.

50. Eusebios, *Hist. eccl.* 8.13.

51. Ibid., 7.32.23.

52. Jerome, *De viris inlustribus,* cap. 89, p. 45. Since there is no corroborating evidence for Jerome's statement, a number of scholars have reservations. See Johannes Schladebach, *Basilius von Ancyra* (Leipzig, 1898), p. 8.

53. Eusebios, *Hist. Eccl.* 8.13.

54. Soz. 8.6.3–9: Dagron, *Naissance,* p. 462.

55. Greg. Naz., *In laudem Caesarii,* PG, 35:761–68.

56. Greg. Naz., *In laudem Basilii,* chaps. 23.6, 81.4, and esp. 63.6 (PG, 36:528, 604, and 580).

57. Greg. Nys., *De sancta trinitate, Opera* (Jaeger), 3.1:3–4 (PG, 32:684–85).

58. Gregory of Nyssa praised the practice of medicine as the epitome of charity and praised his friend the physician Eustathios for healing both the body and the soul—the latter primarily the duty of the clergy (ibid., 3–4). Gregory of Nazianz (*In laudem Caesarii*, PG, 35:768) describes how his brother Kaisarios, the physician, never forgot his Christian faith even in the midst of great secular fame and wealth.

59. See esp. *Photii epistolae, ep.* 230, pp. 543–44. See also Warren Treadgold, *The Nature of the Bibliotheca of Photius* (Washington, D.C.: Dumbarton Oaks, 1980), p. 103.

60. Hunger, *Literatur*, 2:310.

61. See Balsamon's commentary on Canon 16 of the Council of Carthage, RP, 3:344. Balsamon implies that the practice of medicine was considered among the sordid professions, but Chrysoberges' canon only states that deacons and priests should not be members of a lay professional organization.

62. *Matthaios von Ephesos, ep.* 64, p. 199.

63. Origen, *Homilia I in psalmam XXXVII*, PG, 12:1369.

64. Eusebios, *Hist. eccl.* 10.4.11; cf. Hippocrates, *De flatibus*, 1.

65. Greg. Nys. *De oratione dominica*, 4, PG, 44:1161.

66. *Vie de Théodore de Sykéôn*, 146, p. 115.

67. Rudolph Arbesmann, "The concept of 'Christus Medicus' in St. Augustine," *Traditio*, 1954, *10*: 1–28, esp. 4–5.

68. Edelstein, *Asclepius*, 2:252–53.

69. Ibid., p. 257, n. 9. For the cult of Asklepios at Rome, see Scarborough, pp. 24–25.

70. Firmicus Maternus, *De errore profanarum religionum*, 12.8 (Edelstein, *Asclepius*, 1:T.114).

71. See *Contra Galilaeos*, 200 A–B, Julian (Loeb), 3:374, where Julian outlines a theology regarding Asklepeios which is patterned on the Christian doctrine of the Trinity. Julian assigns Asklepios the position of the Son.

72. Edelstein, *Asclepius*, 2:132–38.

73. In the East, Jerome still found the Asklepios cult active among the pagans. See *In Isaiam commentaria*, 18, PG, 24:657, and *De vita Hilarionis*, 2, PG, 23:39.

74. Origen, *Homilia I in psalmam XXXVII*, PG, 12:1369.

75. Greg. Naz., *In laudem Basilii*, chaps. 40, 63.6, and 81 (PG, 36:549, 580, 604).

76. Isidore, *Ep.* 165, PG, 78:1424.

77. *Vita Ioannis* (Leontios), chap. 16, pp. 33–34.

78. Isidore of Seville, *De officiis ecclesiasticis*, 2.5.12, PL, 83:783–84.

79. *Ignatii deaconi vita S. Nicephori*, ed. Charles de Boor, in *Nicephori archiepiscopi Constantinopolitani opuscula historica* (Leipzig, 1880), p. 156.

80. Edelstein, *Asclepius*, 2:228–29.

81. *Vita Euthymii*, p. 17.

82. *Vie de Théodore de Sykéôn*, 146, p. 115.

83. John Klimax, *Liber ad pastorem*, PG, 88:1168–69.

84. *Theodori epistolae, ep.* 45, p. 61. Regarding Blemmydes' medical career see Blemmydes, *Curriculum*, pp. 2–3.

85. Ἑλληνικῶν θεραπευτικὴ παθημάτων.

86. *Nicholas I Patriarch of Constantinople: Miscellaneous Writings*, ed. Leendert G. Westerink (Washington, D.C.: Dumbarton Oaks, 1981), opus 199, p. 46.

87. Ibid., opus 200.B, p. 60.

88. See Chap. 5.

89. Mirjana Živojinović, "L'hôpital du roi Milutin à Constantinople" (Serbian with French resumé), *Zbornik Radova*, 1975, *16*: 105–15; for summary, 116–17.

90. Greg. Naz., *In laudem Basilii*, chap. 63.1 (PG, 36:577).

91. *Palladii dialogus*, p. 32.

92. *Vita Sampsonis*, PG, 115:281.

93. PG, 99:1509.
94. *PantTyp*, 129.1628–51.
95. *PantTyp*, 87.985–89.995.
96. *PantTyp*, 29.33–31.44.
97. Chortasmenos, ep. 8, pp. 157–58.
98. Ibid., p. 158, lines 59–60; cf. Greg. Naz., *In laudem Basilii*, chap. 63.1 (PG, 36:577).
99. Barsanouphios, *questiones* 327, 313, 314, and 316.
100. For the hospital of St. Athanasios see *Vita Athanasii Athonitae B*, chap. 25, lines 26–27, and chap. 41, lines 1–5. Stoudite monasticism is discussed in Chap. 7 below.
101. *Actes de Lavra*, no. 123.
102. For example, *Kosmas und Damianos*, mir. 16, pp. 138–39; mir. 23, pp. 160–61.
103. *Vita Sampsonis*, PG, 115:281.
104. Ibid., 284–88.
105. *Miracula Artemii*, mir. 36, pp. 57–58.
106. Ibid., mir. 24, p. 34.
107. See Chap. 5 below.
108. *Anargyroi* was the epithet applied to the most famous of doctor saints, Cosmas and Damian, and to all the lesser physician saints. See *RAC* 1:725 and Kötting, pp. 202–22. For the Kosmidion shrine to Cosmas and Damian in Constantinople see Janin, *Églises*, pp. 286–89. The cult of Saint Artemios was centered at the Church of St. John Prodromos in Oxeia, overlooking the Golden Horn (ibid., pp. 419–20). Saint Sampson's cult had two centers: the xenon which bore his name, located close to Hagia Sophia, and the Church of St. Mokios, where his relics rested (ibid., pp. 354–58 and 561–62; see also Chap. 5 below).
109. Hunger, *Reich*, p. 177; Ernst Lucius, *Die Anfänge des Heiligenkults in der christlichen Kirche* (Tübingen: Mohr, 1904), pp. 252–56.
110. *Vita Sampsonis*, PG, 115:281–92, recounts the founding of the hospital; ibid., 292–307, describes Sampson's posthumous miracles, most of which involve his xenon in some way.
111. *Kosmas und Damianos*, mir. 30, pp. 173–76.
112. *Miracula Artemii*, mir. 3, p. 4.
113. The church and adjoining hospital were founded by the *magister militum per Orientem* under Maurice, a man named Narses (Zonaras, 3:199, lines 8–10). The Panteleemon Xenon was still functioning in 1204 and was refurbished during the fourteenth century (see Chap. 10 below).
114. *Scriptores originum*, p. 255.
115. *Vita Theophylacti*, p. 75.
116. *PantTyp*, 95.1097 and 105.1297.
117. *Kosmas und Damianos*, mir. 17, pp. 142–43.
118. *Miracula Artemii*, mir. 6, p. 7.
119. Ibid., mir. 24, p. 34.
120. See Harry J. Magoulias, "The lives of the saints as sources of data for the history of Byzantine medicine in the sixth and seventh centuries," *BZ*, 1964, 57: 127–50, who emphasizes that the anargyroi often used medical remedies to cure their suppliants.
121. *Vie et miracles de Saint Thècle*, ed. Gilbert Dagron, Subhag, 62 (Brussels, 1978).
122. *Miracula Artemii*, mir. 21, pp. 25–28.
123. Ibid., mir. 22, pp. 28–31.
124. Ibid., mir. 1, p. 2.
125. See *kantakia* 31 and 33 in *Sancti Romani Melodi cantica: Cantica genuina*, ed. Paul Maas and Constantine Trypanis (Oxford: Clarendon Press, 1963); see also Eva Topping, "The apostle Peter, Justinian, and Romanos the Melodos," *Byzantine and Modern Greek Studies*, 1976, 2: 12–15.
126. John of Ephesus, *Fragmenta*, in "Histoire ecclésiastique de Jean d'Asie," ed. François Nau, *Revue de l'Orient Chrétien*, 1897, 2: 481–82.
127. See *Vita S. Thallelaei*, acta recentiora, *ActaSS*, Maii V, 15–16; *Vita Sampsonis*, PG, 115:281–92.

128. Prodromos, *Gedichte*, poem 46, p. 432, line 45.
129. *Vita Sampsonis* (antiquior), p. 14.
130. See Chap. 9 below.

CHAPTER FIVE: THE FOURTH CENTURY

1. See Chap. 2 at nn. 46–50.
2. Neilos of Ankyra, *Ep.* 110, PG, 79:248: Πολλοὶ ἐν τῷ νοσοκομείῳ τοῦ παρόντος αἰῶνος ὑπάρχουσιν ἄρρωστοι καὶ παραλυτικοί. οὐ πᾶσι δὲ ἡ αὐτὴ ἁρμόζει φαρμακία, οὐ δὲ πᾶσιν ἡ αὐτὴ συμβάλλεται τράπεζα. ἄλλῳ γὰρ ἄλλως τὴν περιωδίαν καὶ τὴν διαίτην προσφέρει ὁ ἰατρός.
3. Brown, *Antiquity*, pp. 34–111. Arnaldo Momigliano, "Das Christentum und der Niedergang des römischen Reiches," in *Der Untergang des römischen Reiches*, WF, 269 (Darmstadt, 1970), pp. 404–24, emphasizes the role Christianity played in destroying the Greco-Roman city. Momigliano does not consider the new city institutions which the church developed.
4. The political history of Arianism suggests that Arian sects were concerned primarily with controlling the episcopal centers of the church. Moreover, Kazhdan and Constable, *People and Power*, p. 85, present some prosopographical evidence that Arianism drew its support from urban areas.
5. For a description of the differing conditions in East and West by the end of the century see E. Demougeot, *De l'unité à la division de l'empire romain, 395–410* (Paris: Adrien-Maisonneuve, 1951), pp. 530–32.
6. For a short discussion of this difference see Arnold H. M. Jones, "The social background of the struggle between paganism and Christianity," in *Paganism and Christianity in the Fourth Century*, ed. Arnaldo Momigliano (Oxford: Clarendon Press, 1963), pp. 17–37. See also Kopecek, pp. 293–303. For the strength of paganism in the West among aristocrats see Herbert Bloch, "The pagan revival in the West at the end of the fourth century," in Momigliano, *Paganism and Christianity* (see above), pp. 193–218, and idem, "Ein neues inschriftliches Zeugnis der letzten Erhebung des Heidentums in Westrom, 393–94 n. Chr.," in *Das frühe Christentum im römischen Staat*, WF, 267 (Darmstadt, 1971), pp. 129–86.
7. See the summary by Henri Gregoire, "Die 'Bekehrung' Konstantins des Grossen," in *Konstantin der Grosse*, WF, 131 (Darmstadt, 1974), pp. 175–223. See also Harnack, *Mission*, 529–958, esp. 946–58 and maps.
8. Patlagean, *Pauvreté*, pp. 301–40, presents some of the latest evidence for a population increase in rural areas of Palestine and Syria. She summarizes the evidence by stating that all signs—prosperity in rural areas, expansion of cities, monastic settlements, and an aggressive foreign policy on the part of the government—indicate demographic increase throughout Asia Minor, Syria, and Palestine (ibid., pp. 426–27). Peter Charanis, "Observations on the demography of the Byzantine Empire," *XIII International Congress of Byzantine Studies: Main Papers* (Oxford, 1966), pp. 9–10, reviews the evidence of population growth in the East from the fourth to the sixth century. Brown, *Antiquity*, p. 44, reflects the prosperity of the East, but stops short of asserting that the population was increasing. Jones, *LRE*, 2:1038–45, holds the traditional view of population decline for the empire as a whole, citing the increase in *agri deserti* and the absence of any attempt to import foodstuffs as a reflection of this decline. The overwhelming weight of the archaeological evidence, however, supports the new view that the population was increasing in the East. For Palestine in general, see Michael Avi-Yonah, "The economics of Byzantine Palestine," *Israel Exploration Journal*, 1958, *8:* 39–51; for Caesarea Maritima, see Robert Wiemken and Kenneth Holum, "The joint expedition to Caesarea Maritima: Eighth season, 1979," *Bulletin of the American Schools of Oriental Research*, 1981, *no. 244:* 27–51, esp. the list of coin finds on p. 46. Claudine Dauphin, "Mosaic pavements as an index of prosperity and fashion," *Levant*, 1980, *12:* 112–34, reviews the archaeological remains of an increasingly wealthy population in Cilicia, Syria, and Palestine.

For population decline in the West see Arthur Boak, *Manpower Shortage and the Fall of the Roman Empire in the West* (Ann Arbor: University of Michigan Press, 1955), and the report of Edith M. Wightman, in *Abstracts of Papers: Sixth Annual Byzantine Studies Conference* (Oberlin, Ohio, 1980), pp. 31–32. Wightman's study of archaeological evidence indicates population decline in Gaul and Italy and increase in Britain.

9. For evidence of population increase in Eastern cities see Patlagean, *Pauvreté*, pp. 156–81; Jones, *LRE*, 1:763, admits that archaeological evidence indicates that some Eastern cities flourished in the years after Constantine. Claude, *Stadt*, pp. 162–67, also offers evidence that some Eastern cities had been growing in population before the reign of Justinian.

10. For examples of bishops maintaining the traditions of urban life, see Kopecek, pp. 293–303. Synesius, bishop of Ptolemais, even organized his city's defense against marauders at the beginning of the fifth century. Carl Kraeling, *Ptolemais: City of the Libyan Pentapolis* (Chicago: University of Chicago Press, 1962), p . 24. Bishop Theodoretos of Kyrrhos took over maintenance of public buildings. Theodoretos, *ep.* 81, PG, 83:1261. Under the emperor Anastasios (491–518) a process began by which the bishop with his clergy and a group of local *archontes* assumed control of the cities from the old curial class. See Claude, *Stadt*, pp. 107–44, and Jones, *LRE*, 1:758–60. On the other hand, when Justinian's army invaded Italy, the lay aristocrats still seemed to dominate the *civitates* of the West while the bishops were relatively unimportant. Claude, *Stadt*, pp. 123–26.

11. See *Const. apost.* 4.2–4 (pp. 219–21).

12. Cyprian, *ep.* 41, ed. Guilhelmus Hartel, Corpus scriptorum ecclesiasticorum latinorum, 3 vols. (Vienna, 1868), 3.2:587–88.

13. Uhlhorn, *Liebestätigkeit*, 1:317.

14. Soz. 6.31.7–8.

15. For the growing strength of Christians in cities of the East during the third century see Lukas De Blois, *The Policy of the Emperor Gallienus* (Leiden: Brill, 1976), pp. 175–85. Regarding Christians at Antioch, see John Liebeschuetz, *Antioch: City and Imperial Administration in the Later Roman Empire* (Oxford: Clarendon Press, 1972), p. 224.

16. See the evidence collected by Patlagean, *Pauvreté*, pp. 156–81.

17. Libanios, *or.* 41.11.

18. For special privileges given by Justinian to the Church of Jerusalem so that it could support poor immigrants see *JNov*, 40; with *JNov*, 80, on the other hand, Justinian established a special officer to limit access to the capital.

19. Greg. Nys., *Pauperibus, or.* 1, pp. 6–7; Greg. Naz., *De pauperum amando*, PG, 35:869–73. Basil refers to the desperately poor as δῆμον ὅλον ῥιγῶντα (*Homilia in divites*, PG, 31:292).

20. Uhlhorn, *Liebestätigkeit*, 1:99–109; *RPT*, 21:436–39. One of the older standard works on the Late Roman Empire—Ferdinand Lot, *The End of the Ancient World and the Beginnings of the Middle Ages* (original Fr. ed., 1927; New York: Harper and Row, 1961)—emphasized the economic collapse of late antique society without differentiating between East and West.

21. Brown, *Antiquity*, pp. 43–44. Though he is unaware of population growth in the East, Jones, *LRE*, 2:1064–68, recognizes the prosperity of the Eastern provinces.

22. Patlagean discusses both the rural population growth (*Pauvreté*, pp. 301–40) and the population increases in East Roman cities and the inability of the early Byzantine economy to employ unskilled migrants from the countryside (ibid., pp. 156–81). Urban economies could not absorb large numbers of unskilled workers until the dawn of the industrial revolution. Medieval Western Europe suffered similar population increases on the land, again stimulating migration to the towns; and, like East Roman cities, the towns of twelfth-century Europe were unable to employ the large numbers of unskilled newcomers, a situation which resulted in a growing class of urban poor. Here, as in the Eastern provinces of the Late Roman Empire, the church was forced to develop new caritative services. See Miller, "Knights," pp. 712–13.

23. For the economic health of the cities see Roger Remondon, *La crise de l'empire romain de Marc-Aurèle à Anastase*, Nouvelle Clio (Paris: Presses Universitaires de France, 1964), pp. 89–90, and Jones, *LRE*, 1:11–14; see also the documents and commentary in *Roman Civilization,*

II: The Empire, ed. Naphtali Lewis and Meyer Reinhold (New York: Harper and Row, 1955), pp. 341–43. For the *curiales,* see Jones, *LRE,* 1:748–50.

24. Jones, *LRE,* 1:740–50. See also the letter of Gregory of Nazianz (*ep.* 41, pp. 36–37), where Gregory, as bishop, is helping a friend to enter the clergy and thus to be free of civic duties on the curial council.

25. See the short description of the classical polis of the fifth and fourth centuries in M. I. Finley, *The Ancient Greeks* (New York: Viking Press, 1963), pp. 37–43. For the growth of a wealthy ruling class in Hellenistic poleis see Arnold H. M. Jones, *The Greek City from Alexander to Justinian* (Oxford: Clarendon Press, 1940), pp. 157–69.

26. Glen W. Bowersock, *Augustus and the Greek World* (Oxford: Clarendon Press, 1965), pp. 85–100; C. P. Jones, *Plutarch and Rome* (Oxford: Clarendon Press, 1971), pp. 3, 45–47.

27. Jones, *LRE,* 1:16–18.

28. Patlagean, *Pauvreté,* pp. 1–17; see esp. John Chrysostom, *De eleemosyna sermo,* PG, 51:269–70, who describes the many strangers and fugitives from the countryside streaming into Antioch.

29. Patlagean, *Pauvreté,* pp. 11–35. Thus, Basil (*Homilia in divites,* PG, 31:292) uses *demos* to refer to the poor.

30. John Chrysostom, *De eleemosyna sermo,* PG, 51:261: Πρεσβείαν τινὰ δικαίαν καὶ λυσιτελῆ καὶ πρέπουσαν ὑμῖν ἀνέστην ποιησόμενος τήμερον πρὸς ὑμᾶς. ἑτέρου μὲν οὐδένος, τῶν δὲ τὴν πόλιν οἰκούντων ἡμῖν πτωχῶν ἐπὶ ταύτην με χειροτονησάντων, οὐ ῥήμασι καὶ ψηφίσμασι καὶ κοινῆς γνώμῃ βουλῆς, ἀλλὰ διὰ τῶν θεαμάτων τῶν ἐλεεινῶν καὶ πικροτάτων. In the same sermon (cols. 269–70) Chrysostom accuses the older citizenry of refusing to help the newcomers. His accusations are confirmed by Libanios, a representative of the pagan curial class at Antioch, who compared the migrants to an urban disease (*or.* 41.11).

31. Basil, *ep.* 28 (Loeb, 1:166).

32. Kopecek, pp. 296–98.

33. Greg. Naz., *In laudem Basilii,* chap. 80.3 (PG, 36:601–5).

34. Kopecek, pp. 293–98.

35. Theodoretos, *ep.* 81, PG, 83:1261.

36. In *De eleemosyna sermo* (PG, 51:269–70) Chrysostom urges the Antiochenes to give to the poor on the basis of their need, rather than excluding them because they lacked skills or local citizenship. In *De perfecta caritate* (PG, 56:279), he emphasizes the need for sharing skills and talents to create the Christian society.

37. Patlagean, *Pauvreté,* pp. 181–96; Kopecek, pp. 293–303.

38. *Theophanis chronographia,* p. 29 describes *xenodocheia* serving the poor under the emperor Constantine. Gerhard Uhlhorn, in *RPT* (2d ed.), 17:301, states that permanent charitable institutions first opened during the reign of the first Christian emperor. Albert Hauck, in *RPT* (3d ed.), 21:436–37, revises Uhlhorn's statement. Hauck sees the charitable foundation of Eustathios in Sebasteia (in the 350s) as the first permanent philanthropic institution. See also Patlagean, *Pauvreté,* pp. 188–95, who believes that the new institutions sprang up sometime before the end of the fourth century.

39. Greg. Naz., *Contra Julianum* 1, PG, 35:648, accused Julian of constructing καταγωγία and ξενῶνες in imitation of Christian institutions. Julian himself mentions his pagan ξενοδοκεῖα (Julian [Loeb], 3:68). See also Soz. 5.16.1–5.

40. *Epit. Theo. Ana.,* p. 59, lines 4–6: Ἰουλιανὸς ἀπατᾶν τοὺς δήμους οἰόμενος τὰς Χριστιανῶν εὐποιίας μιμεῖσθαι καθυπεκρίνατο. διὸ ξένοισι καὶ πτωχείοις χορηγεῖσθαι προσέταττε. . . .

41. Greg. Naz., *In laudem Basilii,* chaps. 34–37 (PG, 36:541–45).

42. Gregory of Nazianz (ibid., chap. 57) states that the whole population was angry, but especially the workers in the imperial factories.

43. Soz. 8.18.1–8.

44. Greg. Naz., *In laudem Basilii,* chap. 28 (PG, 36:533–36). At the time of this struggle

Basil did not hold the office of oikonomos, though he was closely associated with the Cappadocian monks who were active supporters of charity.

45. Greg. Naz., *epp.* 219 and 220, pp. 157–59.

46. *Palladii dialogus,* pp. 35–36.

47. See also the dispute between Eustathios, bishop of Sebasteia, and Areios, his assistant in charge of the ptochotropheion, in Epiphanios, *Panarion,* 75.1–2 (3:333–34).

48. *Iohannis Ephesini . . . pars tertia,* 2.15 (pp. 55–56).

49. Janin, *Eglises,* pp. 551–52; Patlagean, *Pauvreté,* p. 192.

50. See the summary in Stein, *Le bas-empire,* 1:108–10 and 134–36; see also Brown, *Antiquity,* pp. 86–90. For a thorough treatment of the history of Arianism, see Jean Palanque, *De la paix constantinienne à la morte de Théodose,* in *Histoire de l'église depuis les origines jusqu'à nos jours,* ed. Augustin Fliche and Victor Martin (Paris: Bloud and Gay, 1936), vol. 3.

51. Dagron, *Naissance,* pp. 422–25; William Telfer, "Paul of Constantinople," *Harvard Theological Review,* 1950, *43:* 45–53.

52. Dagron, *Naissance,* pp. 425–53, traces the intricacies of Constantinopolitan church politics during the Arian controversy.

53. Albertz, "Jung-arianischen Kirchengemeinschaft," p. 230. Albertz (pp. 205–10 and 276) maintains that the Anomoian party alone among the Arian factions was committed in conscience to its creed.

54. Dagron, *Naissance,* pp. 447–49; Albertz, "Jung-arianischen Kirchengemeinschaft," pp. 230–32. Gregory of Nazianz, *In pentecosten,* PG, 36:440–41, ridiculed the many divisions among the Arians.

55. Epiphanios, *Panarion,* 76.1 (3:341).

56. *Iohannis Ephesini . . . pars tertia,* 2.15 (pp. 55–56).

57. Julian (Loeb), *ep.* 22, 3:68–70, and his *fragmentum epistolae,* Julian (Loeb), 2:298–304, where he fails to include the sick among those whom he urged pious pagans to assist.

58. For Aetios' early years see Philostorgios, 3.14–20 (pp. 44–48). His account is confirmed for the most part by a harsh critic of Aetios, Gregory of Nyssa. *Contra Eunomium,* 1.36–48, in *Opera* (Jaeger), 1:34–40 (PG, 45:260–64). Gregory's account indicates that Arianism was strong among medical students (Ibid., p. 38).

59. Philostorgios, 3.17 (pp. 47–48); *Histoire de Barhadbešabba Arabaia,* 14, ed. François Nau, PO, 23:279.

60. Philostorgios, 3.15 (p. 47), mentions that Aetios studied medicine under Sopolis in Alexandria, before he was ordained a deacon by Leontios (after 344). Barhadbešabba, *Histoire* (see above), p. 279, states clearly that Aetios practiced medicine in Antioch after he was ordained a deacon. Barhadbešabba wrote his history at the School of Nisibis in the sixth century, but he drew on earlier works, perhaps a lost *Contra Eunomium* by Theodore of Mopsuestia. See Ortiz de Urbina, p. 132. For the supposition regarding the lost work of Theodore Mopsuestia see Richard P. Vaggione, "Some neglected fragments of Theodore of Mopsuestia's *contra Eunomium,*" *Journal of Theological Studies,* 1980, *31:* 403–70.

61. *Chronicon pascale,* 1:535.

62. The famous mosaic of Yakto, unearthed in Daphne, presents a strip of buildings and famous places in the city. One of those buildings pictured is labeled τὸ Λεοντίου. Jean Lassus, "La mosaique de Yakto," in *Antioch-on-the Orontes, I: The Excavations of 1932,* ed. George Elderkin (Princeton: Department of Art and Archaeology, 1934), 1:128–56. Devreesse, p. 111 and note 11, identifies the *to Leontiou* of the mosaic with one of Bishop Leontios' xenodocheia.

63. *Contra Eunomium,* 1.42, in *Opera* (Jaeger), 1:36–37 (PG, 45:261).

64. *Ad Stagirium a daemone vexatum,* 3, PG, 47:490.

65. For a summary of Anomoian maneuvers see Albertz, "Jung-arianischen Kirchengemeinschaft," pp. 210–46. Philostorgios, 3.17 (pp. 47–48), recounts Aetios' meeting with Theophilos and Eunomios; Gregory of Nyssa, *Contra Eunomium,* 1.47, in *Opera* (Jaeger), 1:38, mentions Aetios' meeting with Theophilos. The latest work on the Anomoians is Thomas Kopecek, *A History of Neo-Arianism,* 2 vols. (Cambridge, Mass.: Philadelphia Patristic Foundation, 1979).

66. Philostorgios, 9.6 (p. 118).
67. Philostorgios, 3.20 (p. 48).
68. Philostorgios, 4.7 (p. 61).
69. Philostorgios, 9.1 (p. 116), claims that Aetios, Eunomios, and other Anomoian leaders performed miracles of healing. Photios unfortunately did not include the miracle accounts in his epitome of Philostorgios' history.
70. Philostorgios, 3.16 (p. 47) and 4.8 (pp. 61–62). For Basil of Ancyra see Johannes Schladebach, *Basilius von Ancyra* (Leipzig, 1898).
71. Schladebach, *Basilius von Ancyra* (see above), p. 8, advises caution here.
72. Philostorgios, 3.16, 27 (pp. 47, 52) and 4.8 (p. 62). See the account of Basil's activity in Schladebach, *Basilius von Ancyra*, pp. 5–22.
73. Jaakke Gummerus, *Die homöusianische Partei bis zum Tode des Konstantius* (Leipzig, 1900), pp. 36–89.
74. Soz. 6.34.8; Dagron, "Les moines," pp. 249–53. See also Basil of Caesarea's elegant apology for Eustathian monasticism over Egyptian anchoritism, in *Regulae fusius tractatae, quaest.* 7, PG, 31:928–29.
75. Epiphanios, *Panarion,* 75.1 (3:333).
76. Ibid.: τοιαῦτα γάρ τινα κατασκευάζουσι κατὰ φιλοξενίαν καὶ τοὺς λελωβημένους καὶ ἀδυνάτους ἐκεῖσε ποιοῦντες καταλύειν . . . οἱ τῶν ἐκκλησιῶν προστάται.
77. Basil, *ep.* 94 (Loeb, 2:150). The passage is quoted below, n. 132.
78. Philostorgios, 9.1 (p. 116), discusses the miracle-working Anomoians. See Albertz, "Jung-arianischen Kirchengemeinschaft," pp. 231–36, for a description of the Anomoian party's field of action. Philostorgios, 5.2 (pp. 67–68), mentions Aetios' miracles in Amblada, just north of the Taurus Mountains.
79. Dagron, "Les moines," pp. 246–53; idem, *Naissance,* pp. 436–42.
80. Soz. 4.27.4.
81. Soz. 4.20.2 and 27.4; Socrat. 2.38 (PG, 67:324).
82. Socrat. 2.38 (PG, 67:324); Soz. 4.2.3 and 20.2.
83. Soz. 4.27.2–5.
84. *Vie des saints Notaires,* in *AnalBoll,* 1946, *64*: 170, lines 21–23. This is the capstone of Dagron's account regarding Makedonios (*Naissance,* p. 440).
85. Greg. Naz., *In Pentecosten,* PG, 36:440.
86. Soz. 4.27.4: συνοικίας νοσούντων καὶ πτωχῶν ἐπεμελεῖτο. . . .
87. *Vita Sampsonis,* PG, 115:284–88; *Vita Sampsonis* (antiquior), pp. 10–12.
88. Sampson is included in a list of leading Romans who were summoned to Constantinople by Constantine (*Synaxarion,* p. 359, line 44). The short vita of Sampson himself (*Synaxarion,* p. 773), on the other hand, says only that Sampson was of Constantine's family.
89. *JNov,* 59.3; Prokopios, *De aedif.* 1.2.15: τούτον [xenon] ἀνήρ τις θεοσεβὴς ἐν τοῖς ἄνω χρόνοις ἐδείματο, Σαμψὼν ὄνομα.
90. *JNov,* 59.3.
91. *JNov,* 131.15.
92. Dagron, *Naissance,* pp. 511–12 and p. 512, n. 1.
93. *De cerimoniis,* 1.32 (1:173; Vogt, 1:161–62). This section of the *Book of Ceremonies* derives from a description of court ceremonial drawn up under the emperor Michael III (842–67). See John B. Bury, "The Ceremonial Book of Constantine Porphyrogennitos," *English Historical Review,* 1907, *22*: 417–27. Vogt's commentary (2:168–69) says nothing about the order in which the xenodochoi appear.
94. *Scriptores originum,* p. 246.
95. Zonaras, 3:199, *Scriptores originum,* p. 249.
96. *Vita Marciani* (antiquior), pp. 265–67; *Scriptores originum,* p. 234.
97. *Vita Sampsonis,* PG, 115:281. See also Chap. 3 above.
98. *Palladii dialogus,* p. 32.
99. *Vita Sampsonis,* PG, 115:292. Ibid., col. 304, demonstrates that the staff of the Sampson

xenon left their hospital wards to celebrate the founder's feast at the distant church of St. Mokios. See also *Vita Sampsonis* (antiquior), 15.

100. *Vita Sampsonis* (antiquior), pp. 8–9. For the relics of Sampson at St. Mokios, see Janin, *Eglises,* p. 356.

101. See map 1 accompanying Janin, *Eglises.*

102. Socrat. 5.7 (PG, 67:573–76); Soz. 7.5.5–7.

103. *Scriptores originum,* p. 209.

104. Ibid., pp. 198–99.

105. *Vita Sampsonis* (antiquior), pp. 9–10.

106. Ibid., pp. 12–13.

107. Ibid., p. 8. In New Testament Greek μοναί means mansions or dwellings, but during the Patristic period it was most often used to refer to monasteries.

108. Ibid., p. 10.

109. *Passio Artemii,* PG, 96:1256–60. The *Passio* was written during the sixth century by John, a monk from the island of Rhodes. John, however, took much of his information regarding Artemios from the Anomoian historian Philostorgios (Philostorgios, intro., pp. xliv–xlv).

110. *Passio Artemii,* PG, 96:1268 (Constantius appoints Artemios *dux* of Egypt); 1284 (Artemios assumes special military command for Julian's Persian campaign); 1316 (Artemios' body is sent to Constantinople).

111. For Artemios dressed as a physician see *Miracula Artemii,* mir. 1, p. 2, and mir. 40, p. 66; for Artemios with his bag of medical instruments, ibid., mir. 42, p. 71.

112. In a similar manner the *gesta* of the Arian bishop of Alexandria, George of Cappadocia, were woven into the legend of Saint George the Dragon Slayer. See Hippolyte Delehaye, *Les légendes grecques des saints militaires* (Paris: Librairie A. Picard, 1909), pp. 68–73.

113. *Theodoreti haereticarum fabularum compendium,* PG, 83:418.

114. See Quasten, 3:204–7.

115. Greg. Naz., *In laudem Basilii,* chap. 63.1 (PG, 36:577): καὶ θέασαι τὴν καινὴν πόλιν, τὸ τῆς εὐσεβείας ταμεῖον....

116. Friedrich Loofs, *Eustathios von Sebaste und die Chronologie der Basilius-Briefe* (Halle, 1898), pp. 53–97; Amand de Mendieta, "Système," pp. 72–76.

117. Basil, *ep.* 223 (Loeb, 3:292–98).

118. Amand de Mendieta, "Système," pp. 74–76 compares Basil's *regulae* with the decrees of the Council of Gangres, a synod which condemned some practices of the monks in Asia Minor shortly before 341.

119. Soz. 3.14.31.

120. Amand de Mendieta, "Système," pp. 42–43.

121. Ibid., pp. 43–46.

122. Ibid., pp. 64–68. For Basil's monastery in Caesarea see Greg. Naz., *In laudem Basilii,* chap. 62 (PG, 36:577); see also his letters 211 and 219 (Greg. Naz., *Ep.,* pp. 153 and 158), which state that the priest Sakerdos was the head of the monastery associated with the ptocheion after Basil's death. See also the introduction to these letters, in Greg. Naz., *Ep.,* p. xxxvi. No source explains in detail the relationship between the monastery and the ptocheion, though Basil's *Interogatio* 155 (*Regulae brevius tractatae,* PG, 31:1184) indicates that the brothers of the monastery served the sick in the house of charity.

123. Soz. 6.34.8: the monks of Galatia and Cappadocia κατὰ συνοικίας δὲ ἐν πόλεσιν ἢ κώμαις οἱ πλείους ᾤκουν. Soz. (6.34.9) follows this description of Cappadocian monasticism with a short statement concerning Basil's ptocheion in Caesarea.

124. Epiphanios, *Panarion,* 75.1 (3:333): τό τε ξενοδοχεῖον... ὅπερ ἐν τῷ Πόντῳ καλεῖται πτωχοτροφεῖον. Basil himself calls his institution a *ptochotropheion.* Basil, *ep.* 150 (Loeb, 2:366).

125. Greg. Naz., *In laudem Basilii,* chaps. 63 and 82.3 (PG, 36:577–80, 600–605).

126. Ibid., chap. 63.1.

127. *Basilii regulae fusius tractatae, interogatio* 35, PG, 31:1004–8, provides some details indicating the size of Basil's community; William K. Clarke, *Saint Basil the Great: A Study in*

Monasticism (Cambridge: Cambridge University Press, 1913), p. 117, estimates 30 to 40 members.

128. Greg. Naz., *In laudem Basilii,* chap. 63.1 (PG, 36:577).

129. Basil, *ep.* 94 (Loeb, 2:150).

130. Greg. Naz., *In laudem Basilii,* chap. 63.5–6 (PG, 36:580).

131. Ibid., chap. 23.6.

132. Basil, *ep.* 94 (Loeb, 2:150): τίνα δὲ ἀδικοῦμεν καταγώγια τοῖς ξένοις οἰκοδομοῦντες, τοῖς τε κατὰ πάροδον ἐφοιτῶσι καὶ τοῖς θεραπείας τινὸς διὰ τὴν ἀσθένειαν δεομένοις, καὶ τὴν ἀναγκαίαν τούτοις παραμυθίαν ἐγκαθιστῶντες, τοὺς νοσοκομοῦντας, τοὺς ἰατρεύοντας, τὰ νωτοφόρα, τοὺς παραπέμποντας;

133. See Chap. 2 above.

134. See Philipsborn, "Krankenhauswesen," p. 347; Constantelos, *Philanthropy,* p. 154. Hunger, *Reich,* p. 174, on the other hand, mentions two distinct philanthropic agencies, one of which he describes as a hospital.

135. Cf. Gregory's description (*In laudem Basilii,* chap. 63.1) and Basil's letter (*ep.* 94[Loeb, 2:150]) with the summary of the Pantokrator complex (see Chap. 2 above).

136. On Basil's interest in and study of medicine, Greg. Naz., *In laudem Basilii,* chap. 23.6 (PG, 36:528); on references to medicine in his sermons and writings, Chap. 4 above, at nn. 33–36; on his medical treatment of his patients, *In laudem Basilii,* chap. 63.5–6 (PG, 36:580).

137. Basil, *ep.* 94 (Loeb, 2:150).

138. Gregory of Nazianz (*In laudem Basilii,* chap. 63.5–6) implies that Basil was in competition with the heretical bishops of the East.

139. Socrat. 5.13 (PG, 67:600); Soz. 7.14.5.

CHAPTER SIX: CITY, CHURCH, AND STATE

1. See Chap. 4 above.

2. See Chap. 5 above.

3. Soz. 2.3.6–7.

4. *Palladii dialogus,* p. 32.

5. See the text of Chap. 5, above, at n. 93 regarding the chronological list (*De cerimoniis,* 1.32[1:173]).

6. External sources confirm that four of the institutions in the list were hospitals during the ninth and tenth centuries. The Metaphrast's version of the *Vita Sampsonis* includes a later collection of miracle tales. One from the reign of Romanos I (920–44) describes the Sampson Xenon as a hospital with a staff of physicians and *hyperetai* (servants). PG, 115:304 and 308. The Euboulos is surely a hospital in the tenth-century (*Vita Lucae Stylitae,* p. 218). So, too, the empress Irene (797–802) founded her xenon as a hospital, as did Theophilos (829–42). *Scriptores originum,* p. 246; *Theo. Cont.,* p. 95. Clearly, the xenones in this list were all hospitals by the mid-Byzantine period.

7. *Vita Sampsonis* (antiquior), p. 10; Prokopios, *De aedif.* 1.2.14; *JNov,* 59.3.

8. *Chronicon paschale,* 1:622; *Theophanis chronographia,* p. 184; Kedrenos, 1:647.

9. *Vita Sampsonis* (antiquior), p. 14; *Miracula Artemii,* mir. 21, pp. 25–26.

10. Kedrenos, 1:647, mentions the patients of both the Sampson and the Euboulos who died in the Nika fire.

11. *Scriptores originum,* p. 255.

12. *Iohannis Ephesini . . . pars tertia,* 2.4–6 (pp. 41–46).

13. Kedrenos, 1:647; *Scriptores originum,* p. 254.

14. *Scriptores originum,* p. 234.

15. *Vita Marciani* (antiquior), pp. 267–68.

16. For *oikos* as a term used to describe a hospital see *Vita Theodosii* (Theodore), p. 40. For *oikos* used in reference to a church see *Kosmas und Damianos,* mir. 1, p. 98; mir. 2, p. 101; mir. 6, p. 110; and passim.

17. Prokopios, *Anecdota*, 26.5. See Chap. 3 above.
18. *Kosmas und Damianos*, mir. 30, pp. 174–75; mir. 14, pp. 135–136.
19. See Chap. 7 below.
20. *Miracula Artemii*, mir. 22, pp. 28–31.
21. *De cerimoniis*,1.32 (1:173; Vogt, 1:161–62); Zonaras, 3:199; *Scriptores originum*, p. 249.
22. *Palladii dialogus*, p. 32.
23. Soz. 9.1.10.
24. *Epit. Theo. Ana.*, p. 91, lines 11–13.
25. Kallistos, PG, 146:1240, probably drawing on Theodore Anagnostes (cf. *Epit. Theo. Ana.*, p. 95) and perhaps the *Vita Euthymii*, p. 53. See also Chap. 7 below.
26. *Vita Theodosii* (Theodore), p. 40.
27. *Vita Sabae* (Cyril), pp. 175–77.
28. Epiphanios, *Panarion*, 76.1 (3:341).
29. Ibid.
30. *ACO*, 2.1.2:214–15.
31. *Vita SS. Cyri et Ioannis*, PG, 114:1232–33.
32. *Vita Ioannis* (Leontios), chap. 7, pp. 13–14.
33. *Papyrus* (Maspero), vol. 2, no. 67151.
34. *London Papyrus*, no. 1028, pp. 276–77, presents a list of professional guilds which have contributed to a festival of some sort. One contribution was made διὰ τῶν ὑπούργων τῶν νοσοκομείων.
35. For example, *Sammelbuch griechischer Urkunden aus Ägypten*, ed. Friedrich Preisigke, 3 vols. (Strassburg: K. J. Trübner, 1915), vol. 1, nos. 4668, 4869, 4903, and 4904; *OxPap*, no. 1898; *Studien zur Palaeographie und Papyruskunde*, ed. Carl Wessely, 21 vols. (Leipzig: Haessel, 1901–24), vol. 3 and 8, p. 157 (no. 875); *The Amherst Papyri*, ed. Bernard Grenfell and Arthur Hunt, 2 vols. (London: H. Frowde, 1901), vol. 2, no. 154.
36. Prokopios, *De aedif.* 2.10.2–25; section 25 describes the hospital.
37. Evagrios, *Hist. eccl.* 4.35 (pp. 184–85).
38. See Chap. 5 above.
39. *Les saints stylites*, ed. Hippolyte Delehaye, Subhag, 14 (Brussels, 1923), chap. 87, pp. 81–82. The text does not use the word *iatros* (physician). Rather it says that the injured traveller was carefully treated (περιοδευθείς). This verb was commonly used to describe a physician's careful observations and treatment. See Alexander Tralleis, 11.4, ed. Theodor Puschmann, 2 vols. (Vienna, 1879), 2:489. *JDigest*, 27.1.6.1, refers to physicians as περιοδευταί. Indeed, the passage of the vita leaves no doubt that here physicians carried out the medical treatment. When the Metaphrast recast the story in the tenth century, he simply stated that physicians attempted to cure the patient. *Les saints stylites*, p. 143.
40. *CIG*, no. 9256.
41. See the study of George Ostrogorsky, "Byzantine cities in the Early Middle Ages," *DOP*, 1959, *13*: 47–66, and Browning, *Empire*, pp. 62–65.
42. *De cerimoniis*, 1.32 (1:173; Vogt, 1:161–62).
43. For the Sampson Xenon see the violation of the hospital described in the tract *Graeci in Latinos*, in *Ecclesiae graecae monumenta*, 3:512. For the Panteleemon, see the comment in *Actes de Lavra*, no. 123, p. 23.
44. In *Vita Lucae Stylitae*, pp. 217–20.
45. *Scriptores originum*, p. 246.
46. *Theo. Cont.*, p. 95.
47. Ibid., p. 339.
48. Skylitzes, p. 231, mentions that Romanos founded a new monastery at the Myrelaion. The xenon is attested in the introduction to the tenth-century medical treatise by the physician Romanos, published by Kouses, "Contribution," pp. 83–84. See also Symeon Magister, p. 733; *Theo. Cont.*, pp. 402, 473. See also Janin, *Eglises*, pp. 351–52.
49. Skylitzes, pp. 476–77.

50. Niketas Choniates, p. 445.
51. *Vita Andreae*, p. 176.
52. *Vita Theophylacti*, p. 75.
53. Eustathios, *Espugnazione*, p. 146.
54. *Typikon Kosmosoteiras*, 70 (p. 53).
55. Theodore Metochites, *Nikaeus*, p. 145.
56. See Chap. 5 above.
57. *DACL*, 1:1109.
58. Malalas, p. 344; Carl Watzinger and Karl Wulzinger, *Damaskus: Die antike Stadt* (Berlin and Leipzig: Vereinigung wissenschaftlicher Verleger, 1921), pp. 77–97.
59. Denis Zakythinos, "La grande brèche dans la tradition historique de l'hellénisme du septième au neuvième siècle," in *Charisterion eis Anastasion K. Orlandon*, 4 vols. (Athens: Bibliothekē tēs en Athenais archaiologikēs hetaireias, 1965), 3:305–6.
60. Greg. Naz., *De se ipso*, PG, 36:280.
61. John Chrysostom, *In acta apost. homilia XI*, PG, 60:96–98.
62. Greg. Naz., *In laudem Basilii*, chap. 63.1–2 (PG, 36:577–80).
63. See Chap. 7 below.
64. The Euboulos Xenon, second after the Sampson in the procession described by Constantine VII (*De cerimoniis*, 1.32 [1:173]. See n. 5 above.
65. See the *Vita Marciani* (antiquior), pp. 264–65, 269.
66. *ACO*, 2.1.3:405.
67. *JNov*, 120 and *JNov*, 131.
68. Prokopios, *De aedif.* 2.10.2–25.
69. Ibid. 5.4.15–16.
70. Ibid., 4.10.20–21.
71. *JCod*. 1.3.45.
72. The history of the burial association is not clear. *JNov*, 43, *proem.*, and *JNov*, 59, *proem.*, provide information on the history of the institution. See also Rasi, "Spese funeralizie," pp. 269–89. Still, I have not been able to determine the relative roles of the church, the state, and the urban monastic movement of the late fourth and fifth century in developing these burial groups. See Chap. 7 below for a discussion of the urban, or Anatolian, monastic movement and its relationship to the *asketriai* and *dekanoi* appointed by Justinian to perform the free burials.
73. *JNov*, 59.1–3.
74. The staff of the xenodocheion at Edessa buried plague victims in 500–501. These victims died, not in the xenodocheion (in Syriac this term can designate a hospital), but in the streets of the town. See the *Chronicle of Joshua the Stylite, Composed in Syriac*, ed. and trans. William Wright (Cambridge, 1882), pp. 32–33.
75. *Nov*. 12 (Leo VI), *Jus*, 1:70.
76. *PantTyp*, 107.1324–109.1344, and for the pallbearers, 89.1005.
77. *Theodori Epistulae*, ep. 118, pp. 164–65.
78. *De cerimoniis*, 1.32 (1:171–73; Vogt, 1:161–62). See also the *Kletorologion of Philotheos*, p. 197.
79. *De cerimoniis*, 1.19 (1:115), and *Kletorologion of Philotheos*, p. 216.
80. *Kletorologion of Philotheos*, p. 183. For the duties of the Count of the Walls see Oikonomides' commentary in *Préséance*, pp. 336–37; for those of the Domestic of the Noumera see Rodolphe Guilland, *Etudes de topographie de Constantinople byzantine*, 2 vols. (Berlin: Akademie-Verlag; Amsterdam: Hakkert, 1969), p. 50.
81. *Sammelbuch*, ed. Preisigke (see n. 35 above), nos. 4668 and 4903, mentions a nosokomeion τῆς Ἀρσινοειτῶν πόλεως.
82. See Chap. 5.
83. *Panegyrica Rabulae*, pp. 202–3 (Bickell, pp. 205–6).
84. Waddington, *Inscriptions*, no. 2327.
85. *Vita SS. Cyri et Ioannis*, PG, 114:1233.

86. Arabic Canons of Nicaea, canon 70, Mansi, 2:976. For the date and provenance of these rules see Georg Graf, *Geschichte der christlichen arabischen Literatur*, 2 vols., Studi e Testi, 118 (Rome: Biblioteca apostolica vaticana, 1944), 1:586–89.

87. Canons 8 and 10, *ACO*, 2.1.2:355–56.

88. See esp. *JNov*, 131.1.

89. *JNov*, 7, *proem.*: πᾶσι τοῖς τῶν ἁγιωτάτων ἐκκλησιῶν καὶ ξενώνων καὶ νοσοκομείων καὶ πτωχείων . . . κτλ . . . *JNov*, 120.6: ἐκκλησίαις καὶ μοναστηρίοις καὶ ξενῶσι καὶ νοσοκομείοις καὶ λοιποῖς εὐαγέσιν οἴκοις. . . . *JCod*, 1.3.48, assigns unconditional bequests for the poor to the local xenon for the sick. *JCod*, 1.3.45, provides an illustration of a private philanthropic institution by referring to a xenon and its beds for the sick.

90. *JNov*, 120.6.

91. *JNov*, 131.10.

92. Ibid.

93. *In Matthaeum homilia*, 66, PG, 58:630–31.

94. Arabic Canons of Nicaea, canon 70, Mansi, 2:976.

95. *JNov*, 131.9.

96. *JCod*, 1.3.45.

97. Canons 8 and 10, *ACO*, 2.1.2:355–56.

98. *Palladii dialogus*, p. 32.

99. *JNov*, 120.1, lists the property of the Great Church (that of the patriarch) first, followed by that of the Orphanotropheion and then of the other philanthropic houses. *JNov*, 131.15, grants the rights which the property of the Great Church enjoys also to the property of the Orphanotropheion and to that of the Sampson Xenon and its dependent houses. Both these novels demonstrate that the leading philanthropic institutions of Constantinople were distinct legal entities, not branches of the patriarchal (episcopal) church.

100. *JNov*, 59.1–4.

101. *Iohannis Ephesini . . . pars tertia*, 2.4 (p. 41).

102. *Miracula Artemii*, mir. 22, p. 28.

103. *The Stoa of Attalos II in Athens* (Princeton: American School of Classical Studies at Athens, 1959).

104. Pausanias I (Attica), 18.6.

105. Jones, *LRE*, 1:89–91.

106. Herbert Hunger, "Philanthropia: Eine griechische Wortprägung auf ihrem Wege von Aeschylos bis Theodoros Metochites," *Anzeiger phil.-hist. Klasse, Österreichische Akademie der Wissenschaft*, 1963, *100:* 2–12.

107. Themistios, *or.* 1 (*De philanthropia*).8a.

108. *Theophanis chronographia*, p. 29.

109. Aristides (Keil) 39.11 (2:322).

110. Theodoretos, *Hist. eccl.* 4.19.13.

111. For Pulcheria's benefactions see Soz. 9.1.10 and *Epit. Theo. Ana.*, p. 91, lines 11–13. For Eudocia's benefactions see Kallistos, PG, 146:1240, probably drawing on Theodore Anagnostes (cf. *Epit. Theo. Ana.*, p. 95) and the *Vita Euthymii*, p. 53.

112. In Zacos and Veglery, no. 129, τοῦ εὐαγοῦς δεσποτικοῦ ξενῶνος above the bust of Justin II and perhaps his empress Sophia. The authors interpret *despotikos* to mean "belonging to the emperor."

113. *Theophanis chronographia*, p. 29.

114. *Vita Sabae* (Cyril), pp. 175–77.

115. *Vita Sampsonis* (antiquior), p. 14: Justinian ἀπέδοτο εἰς πλούτου πολλοῦ διαμονὴν ἐν ἐπαρκείᾳ καὶ περισσείᾳ ὄντα συμπροαστείων πλείστων καὶ μεγίστων σὺν εἰσφοραῖς κρατύνας ὁσήμεραι.

116. Patrick W. Duff, *Personality in Roman Private Law* (Cambridge: University Press, 1938), pp. 168–205.

117. *JNov*, 131.5-6, summarizes the privileges of ecclesiastical land.

118. *JNov*, 7, *proem.*, provides a sketch of the history of the rules against alienation. *JNov*, 120, is the fullest summary of the rules regarding alienation of ecclesiastical property.

119. Prokopios, *Anecdota*, 26.5-6, refers to Justinian's cancellation of the annona payments made from the public treasury (the *arca* of the praetorian prefect) to both the city archiatroi and the teachers of the liberal arts. Nutton, "Archiatroi," p. 211, supposes that Justinian made some change in financing the public physicians. See also the text at note 162.

120. *JNov*, 59.1-3.

121. See Paul Gautier's table listing the staff members and their salaries for the various institutions which made up the Pantokrator complex (*PantTyp*, intro., pp. 12-17). According to Gautier's calculations, the staff of the xenon numbered 103, that of the gerokomeion, 8.

122. *JNov*, 131.15, gave the property of the Sampson Xenon and that of the Orphanotropheion the same status as that of the Great Church.

123. *JCod*, 1.3.48, demonstrates that Justinian considered the city xenon for the sick as the philanthropy which should be given first place in the plans of any polis. According to the provision of this constitution, if a benefactor leaves his estate simply to the poor of a given city, the xenodochos of the xenon for the sick should obtain the estate for the benefit of the patients in his hospital.

124. For the cities of Asia Minor see Clive Foss, "Archaeology and the 'Twenty Cities' of Byzantine Asia," *AJA*, 1977, *81:* 469-86. For Constantinople see Mango, pp. 77-81.

125. *PantTyp*, 127.1613ff.

126. *Typikon Kosmosoteiras*, chap. 4, p. 21, and chap. 12, p. 26.

127. RP, 2:236.

128. RP, 2:234-35.

129. *PantTyp*, 89.1002-5.

130. *OxPap*, no. 1898.

131. *Papyri* (Maspero), no. 67151.

132. *JCod*, 1.3.45, and *JNov*, 131.7 and 10. Regarding the legal personality of philanthropic houses see Duff, *Personality in Roman Private Law*, (see n. 116 above), pp. 168-203.

133. *JNov*, 131.11.

134. In the twelfth century legal fights over charitable bequests still raged. See Manuel I's novel in RP, 1:84-85.

135. *Synopsis major*, E.10.4 (*Jus*, 5:262).

136. *Peira*, 15.4 (*Jus*, 4:49-50).

137. "Diataxis Attaleiate," pp. 41-43; see also the commentary in Lemerle, *Cinq études*, p. 103.

138. "Diataxis Attaleiate," p. 35.

139. *JNov*, 120 and 131, are incorporated into *Basilika*, 5.2 and 5.3.

140. "Diataxis Attaleiate," pp. 41-43; concerning the eparch, ibid., p. 69.

141. *Typikon Kosmosoteiras*, chap. 12, p. 26.

142. For Attaleiates' biography see Paul Gautier's introduction in "Diataxis Attaleiate," pp. 11-16; see also Lemerle, *Cinq études*, pp. 99-112.

143. *PantTyp*, 127.1613ff.

144. *JCod*, 1.3.45.

145. A detailed study of this process can be found in Walther Schönfeld, "Die Xenodochien in Italien und Frankreich in frühen Mittelalter," *Zeitschrift der Savigny—Stiftung für Rechtsgeschichte* 43, Kan. Abt., 1922, *12:* 1-52. Schönfeld blames this corruption of Justinianic Roman law on the Germanic influence in Lombard Italy. The same process, however, took place in Byzantium, outside the scope of Germanic influence.

146. *MGH Cap*, vol. 2, cap. 15, p. 121.

147. Lemerle, *Cinq études*, pp. 99-112.

148. *Peira*, 15.12 (*Jus*, 4:53).

149. *Typikon Kosmosoteiras*, chap. 61, pp. 48-49, and chap. 70, pp. 53-56. The other private

foundation is the seventh-century nosokomeion of Philentolos at Constantia in Cyprus ("La vision de Kaioumos," ed. François Halkin, *AnalBoll,* 1945, *63:* 62).

150. *Typikon Kosmosoteiras,* chap. 61, p. 48, calls the house a *gerokomeion.* See the discussion of this institution in Chap. 2 above.

151. *Vita Andreae,* p. 176.

152. *Vita Theophilacti,* p. 75.

153. *MGH SSrerMerov,* 5:235: "Xenodochium quoque in propriis rebus, orientalium more secutus, in loco qui Columbarius dicitur, fabricare curavit."

154. *Biography of Ibn Buṭlān,* by Ibn Al-Qifṭī, passage translated and annotated in Joseph Schacht and Max Meyerhof, *The Medico-Philosophical Controversy between Ibn Buṭlān of Baghdad and Ibn Riḍwān of Cairo* (Cairo: Egyptian University, Faculty of Arts, 1937), p. 56.

155. Eustathios, *Espugnazione,* p. 146.

156. *Vita Theophylacti,* p. 75.

157. *Ashburner Traktat,* in Dölger, *Finanzverwaltung,* p. 117, lines 1–8, and commentary, pp. 144–45.

158. Oikonomides, *Préséance,* p. 315. See also Justinian's allotments to the Sampson hospital, in *Vita Sampsonis* (antiquior), p. 14.

159. *Kletorologion of Philotheos,* p. 121. The organization of the middle Byzantine bureaucracy is extremely confusing, and the exact duties and responsibilities which attached to each office are not yet known. John B. Bury, *The Imperial Administrative System in the Ninth Century* (London: H. Frowde, 1911), provides an outline of the whole system as it appears in the *Kletorologion of Philotheos,* composed in the reign of Leo VI (886–912). Dölger, *Finanzverwaltung,* makes the only attempt to understand the maze of imperial treasuries and accounting offices that were concerned with state finances. Oikonomides, *Préséance,* offers some of the latest information on the middle Byzantine bureaucracy.

160. *Kletorologion of Philotheos,* pp. 197 (Palm Sunday) and 217 (Feast of Elijah).

161. *De cerimoniis,* 1.32 (1:173; Vogt, 1:161–62).

162. *Kletorologion of Philotheos,* p. 183.

163. Oikonomides, *Préséance,* p. 315, suspects that the central treasury made some regular payment to the xenodochoi.

164. The laws of Valentinian I regarding the archiatroi are addressed to the urban prefect of Rome, but these archiatroi received annona allotments as pay. *Cod. Theo.* 13.3.8–10. The praetorian prefects were in charge of both collecting and distributing the annona. Jones, *LRE,* 1:448–62. Moreover, we have evidence that professors at Rome collected their annonae from the praetorian prefect. Ibid., 1:707. Since imperial legislation always associated archiatroi and city professors (cf. *Cod. Theo.* 13.3.1–19), we can be sure that the archiatroi were paid in the same fashion. Constantinople was organized in the same way as Rome, so that the archiatroi there must also have been paid from the *arca* of the praetorian prefect.

165. The xenodochoi are listed in the *officium* of the chartoularioi of the sakelle (*Kletorologion of Philotheos,* p. 121), and are described as accompanying the *sakellarios* in two imperial ceremonies (Ibid., pp. 197, 216).

166. *Kletorologion of Philotheos,* p. 155.

167. Oikonomides, *Préséance,* p. 297, and Paul Lemerle, "Roga et rente d'état aux Xe–XIe siècles," *REB,* 1967, *25:* 77–100.

168. Zacos and Veglery, no. 1779.

169. *Kletorologion of Philotheos,* p. 123.

170. Oikonomides, *Préséance,* pp. 315 and 318.

171. Janin, *Eglises,* pp. 555 and 560.

172. Symeon Magister, p. 733, and esp. *Theo. Cont.,* p. 402.

173. *Kletorologion of Philotheos,* p. 123, and Dölger, *Finanzverwaltung,* pp. 39–40. Cf. *Theo. Cont.,* p. 337.

174. It is more likely that these xenodochoi governed xenones, since such institutions were expensive and probably required imperial support to sustain their activities. Simple xenodocheia

were far less expensive and could be supported by aristocrats or ecclesiastical figures—bishops or monastic superiors.

175. *Peira*, 15.12 (*Jus*, 4:53).

176. RP, 5:364. See also Nicolas Oikonomides, "L'evolution de l'organisation administrative de l'empire byzantine au XI siècle," *Travaux et Mémoires*, 1976, *6*: 138–40.

177. Dölger, *Finanzverwaltung*, pp. 40–42.

178. *Vita S. Nicephori, episcopi Milesii, AnalBoll*, 1895, *14*: 143–44; *Vita S. Lazari, ActaSS*, Nov., vol. 3:540 A.

179. *Theo. Cont.*, p. 458 (the Petrion); "Diataxis Attaleiate," p. 121 (the chrysobull). Cf. the earlier chrysobull of March 1075, where the Petrion still seems to be subject to the *oikonomos evagōn oikōn* (manager of the pious houses). Ibid., pp. 101, 107. For a discussion of the various changes in the management of imperial estates see Dölger, *Finanzverwaltung*, pp. 40–47.

180. *PantTyp*, 127.1613ff. The officials managing imperial properties are the ἀνακτορικὴν ἐξουσίαν; the regular officials of the state are the ἀρχοντικὴν ἐξουσίαν.

181. *PantTyp*, 113.1414–115.1445.

182. Regarding the nosokomos, see *PantTyp*, 93.1074–97.1119.

183. See *JNov*, 120.5, 6. See also *Vita Sampsonis*, PG, 115:301, which pictures the xenodochos Leo drawing up a contract.

184. E.g., the xenodochos and deacon Eugenios (*JNov*, 59.3) and the xenodochos of the Christodotes (*Miracula Artemii*, mir. 22, p. 28).

185. The nosokomos of the Pantokrator Xenon is described as an eminent physician in Tzetzes, *ep.* 81, p. 121; the nosokomos of an unknown twelfth-century xenon as a practicing surgeon in Prodromos, *Gedichte*, poem 46, pp. 432–33.

186. *JNov*, 120. These chartoularioi were still important in the independent xenones of Constantinople at the end of the ninth century, when they appear with the xenodochoi and archiatroi at the Christmas banquet. *Kletorologion of Philotheos*, p. 183. See also *Vita Sampsonis*, PG, 115:304.

187. *Theo. Cont.*, pp. 94–95.

188. Romanos was buried there (Skylitzes, p. 237); so too was his wife Theodora (Symeon Magister, p. 733), his daughter Helena (*Theo. Cont.*, p. 473), and his son Christophoros (*Leonis grammatici chronographia*, CSHB [1848], p. 321).

189. Skylitzes, pp. 477–78.

190. See Delehaye, *Deux typica byzantins*, p. 175; see also Janin, *Eglises*, pp. 307–10.

191. *Vat. gr.*, 292, fol. 200: προσταγαὶ καὶ τύποι τῶν μεγάλων ξενώνων. . . .

CHAPTER SEVEN: MONASTICISM

1. Greg. Naz., *In laudem Basilii*, chaps. 62–63 (PG, 36:576–77); Greg. Naz., *ep.* 219, pp. 157–58.

2. Epiphanios, *Panarion*, 75.1–3 (3:333–34).

3. Socrat. 2.38; Soz. 4.27.4.

4. The Anomoians were indifferent or even hostile to the monastic movement, whose leaders in Anatolia—Eustathios of Sebasteia and Basil of Cappadocia—were among their chief opponents. Philostorgios, intro., pp. cxii–cxiii.

5. *Vita Antonii*, 2–3, PG, 26:841–44.

6. *NCE*, 10:853. See the account in the *Historia lausiaca*, 32.1, where an angel tells Pachomios to organize a monastic community.

7. Philipsborn, "Krankenhauswesen," p. 341; see the *Praecepta Pachomii*, nos. 50 and 51, in *Pachomiana*, pp. 26–27, which mention the xenodocheion or xenodocheia.

8. *Praecepta Pachomii*, nos. 50 and 51, *Pachomiana*, pp. 26–27; Amand de Mendieta, "Système," p. 35; Paulin Ladeuve, *Études sur le cénobitisme Pakhomien* (Louvain and Paris, 1898), pp. 292–93. See also Henry Chadwick, "Pachomios and the idea of sanctity," in *The Byzantine*

Saint: University of Birmingham Fourteenth Spring Symposium of Byzantine Studies, ed. Sergei Hackel (London: Fellowship of St. Alban and St. Sergius, 1981), pp. 11–24.

9. Amand de Mendieta, "Système," p. 35; Ladeuve, *Cénobitisme Pakhomien* (see above), p. 292.

10. Basil, *ep.* 223 (Loeb, 3:292–94).

11. Basil, *Regulae fusius tractatae, interogatio* 7, PG, 31:928–33.

12. Basil, *ep.* 223 (Loeb, 3:292–94); for the urban orientation of Anatolian monasticism see Soz. 6.34.8.

13. Dagron, "Les moines," p. 252; see also Chap. 5 above.

14. Greg. Naz., *Synkrisis biōn,* ed. Heinrich M. Werhahn (Wiesbaden: In Kommission bei O. Harrassowitz, 1953), lines 245–55.

15. Basil, *Regulae fusius tractatae, interogatio* 37, PG, 31:1009.

16. Greg. Naz., *In laudem Basilii,* chap. 62.4–5 (PG, 36:577).

17. See n. 1 above.

18. *Palladii dialogus,* p. 32.

19. *Panegyrica Rabulae,* pp. 202–3 (Ger. trans. [Bickell], p. 206).

20. Arabic Canons of Nicaea, canon 70, Mansi, 2:976. For a discussion of the Arabic Canons and their dating see Georg Graf, *Geschichte der christlichen arabischen Literatur,* 2 vols., Studi e Testi, 118 (Rome: Biblioteca apostolica vaticana, 1944), 1:586–89.

21. Dagron, "Les moines," pp. 250–53.

22. Epiphanios, *Panarion,* 75.2 (3:333).

23. Greg. Naz., *In laudem Basilii,* chap. 28 (PG, 36:533–36).

24. Greg. Naz., *Epp.* 219 and 220, pp. 157–59.

25. Dagron, "Les moines," pp. 250–52.

26. Soz. 8.9.4–6; John Chrysostom, *De lazaro concio,* 3, PG, 48:992.

27. Jean Chrysostome, *Les cohabitations suspectes,* ed. Jean Dumortier (Paris: "Les Belles Lettres," 1955) (also PG, 47:495–532); *Palladii dialogus,* p. 31.

28. Certainly, his organization of nosokomeia emphasized episcopal leadership, although he allowed monks to serve in his hospitals. *Palladii dialogus,* p. 32.

29. *Palladii dialogus,* p. 34.

30. Dagron, "Les moines," p. 260.

31. Marcel Viller and Karl Rahner, *Aszese und Mystik in der Väterzeit* (Freiburg: Herder, 1939), pp. 100–107; *Dict. Spirit,* 4.2:1731–44.

32. Quasten, 3:496–502.

33. Neilos of Ankyra, *De monachorum praestantia,* PG, 79:1061–93 passim.; for the passage regarding the dangers of assisting others, see col. 1077.

34. Ibid., col. 1077: τί οὖν βέλτιον ἑαυτὸν ἐλεεῖν καὶ περιΐστασθαι τὰ σκάνδαλα ἢ τὸ δῆθεν ἄλλους ἐλεεῖν, βρόχοις δυσεκλύτοις ἐμπλέκεσθαι τῷ βοηθεῖν ἐθέλειν ἑτέροις. . . .

35. Dagron, "Les moines," pp. 261–75, recounts the struggle in Constantinople between the urban monastic party, or *tagma,* and the episcopal leadership.

36. *ACO,* 2.1.2:355.

37. Dagron, "Les moines," p. 252; Soz. 4.27.4.

38. Soz. 4.27.4.

39. For the dating of Sampson's foundation see Chap. 5 above. For Sampson as an urban monk see *Vita Sampsonis* (antiquior), pp. 8, 10.

40. *Palladii dialogus,* p. 32.

41. Dagron, "Les moines," p. 264.

42. Soz. 9.1.10; *Epit. Theo. Ana.,* p. 91, lines 11–13. For Pulcheria's support of other forms of monasticism see Callinicos, *Vie d'Hypatios,* 42.14, ed. J. B. Bartelink, SC, 117 (Paris, 1971), p. 246.

43. *Scriptores originum,* p. 234; cf. *De cerimoniis,* 1.32 (1, 73; Vogt, 1:161).

44. Soz. 7.21.6–8.

45. *Vita Auxentii,* PG, 114;1380. *Spoudaios* first seems to have been used in connection with

the monastic movement throughout the East by Epiphanios, *De fide*, 22.11, in Epiphanios, *Panarion*, 3:523. The *spoudaioi* of fifth-century Jerusalem, however, were clearly urban monks; see *Vita Theodosii* (Cyril), pp. 105–6).

46. Several of the older *synaxaria* of Constantinople refer to Anthimos as one of the spoudaioi. S. Petrides, "Le monastère des spoudaei de Jérusalem et les spoudaei de Constantinople," *EO*, 1900–1901, 4: 228. For services with both men and women—a practice promoted by the urban ascetics—see Dagron, "Les moines," p. 251. Basil, *ep.* 207 (Loeb, 3:186), mentions that his ascetic communities conducted night vigil services during which both men and women sang.

47. *Vita Auxentii*, PG, 114:1380.

48. *Vita Marciani* (antiquior), p. 269; *Vita Marciani*, PG, 114:449–52.

49. *Vita Marciani*, PG, 114:452–53.

50. *Vita Marciani* (antiquior), pp. 269–70.

51. *Scriptores originum*, pp. 261–62; Janin, *Eglises*, pp. 286–87.

52. In 518 an archimandrite of the μονῆς Παυλίνου named Eleutheros signed a letter to the patriarch (*ACO*, 3:70). From this one can deduce the presence of a monastic community attached to Paulinos' church. Miracle 30 (*Kosmas und Damianos*, p. 174) describes a xenon next to the church.

53. *Kosmas und Damianos*, mir. 30, pp. 174–75; mir. 14, pp. 135–36.

54. Greg. Naz., *In laudem Basilii*, chap. 63.1 (PG, 36:577).

55. For the location of the Paulinos complex see Janin, *Eglises*, pp. 286, 289.

56. See Chap. 4 above.

57. *ACO*, 3:70.

58. See below.

59. Mango, *Byzantium*, pp. 109–10.

60. *Vita Theodosii* (Cyril), pp. 105–6.

61. Ibid.

62. Evagrios, *Hist. eccl.* 1.21 (pp. 29–31).

63. Evagrios, *Hist. eccl.* 1.21–22 (pp. 31–32), indicates that Eudocia associated especially with the urban monks. Kallistos (PG, 146:1240) describes the many churches, monasteries, and charitable institutions she founded. Although Kallistos was writing much later, in the fourteenth century, his additions to Evagrios' account probably rest on the full account of Theodore Anagnostes; cf. the epitome of Theodore Anagnostes, *Epit. Theo. Ana.* 95.

64. Evagrios, *Hist. eccl.* 1.21 (p. 32), describes their primary activity as σώμασί τε ἄκη προσφέροντες. . . .

65. *Vita Theodosii* (Theodore), p. 40.

66. Canons 8 and 10, *ACO*, 2.1.2:355–56.

67. *JNov*, 120 and 131.

68. *Vita Marciani* (antiquior), pp. 259–60.

69. In Constantinople the xenones, orphanotropheia, and other charitable foundations were distinct legal entities. See Chap. 6 above.

70. *Historia beatorum orientalium*, pp. 668–71 (Isaak).

71. *Miracula Artemii*, mir. 22, p. 31.

72. *Vita Sampsonis*, PG, 115:300–307. Cf. *Palladii dialogus*, p. 32.

73. *Iohannis Ephesini . . . pars tertia*, 2.4–6 (pp. 41–46).

74. See n. 52 above.

75. *Kosmas und Damianos*, mir. 14, pp. 135–36. Cf. the description of urban monks in Evagrios, *Hist. eccl.* 1.21 (p. 31).

76. *Vita Auxentii*, PG, 114:1385–88; for a monastic community see *Vie de Saint Auxence*, ed. Léon Clugnet (Paris: A. Picard and Sons, 1904), pp. 10–11.

77. Dagron, "Les moines," pp. 235–36; Janin, *Eglises*, p. 430.

78. *Vita Marcelli*, *AnalBoll*, 1968, 86: 296–98.

79. *JNov*, 59.4.

80. Basil, *ep.* 207 (Loeb, 3:186).
81. See Soz. 4.27.4.
82. *JNov,* 59.1–3; also *JNov,* 43.1.
83. Callinicos, *Vie d'Hypatios* (see n. 42 above), 41.10, p. 244.
84. *Vie de Saint Auxence* (see n. 76 above), p. 3.
85. *Vita Marciani* (antiquior), p. 269; *Vita Marciani,* PG, 114:449.
86. Evagrios, *Hist. eccl.* 1.21 (pp. 29–32).
87. Neilos of Ankyra, *De monachorum praestantia,* PG, 79:1061–93.
88. *Vita Theodosii* (Cyril), pp. 105–9; *Lex. Theo. Kir.,* 10:48–49.
89. *Vita Sabae* (Cyril), p. 116.
90. *Vita Severi,* p. 24, equates Alexandrian philoponoi with spoudaioi in other cities. Ibid., p. 12, describes their lifestyle.
91. Cf. the description of the early Anatolian monks which Dagron has extracted from the Gangra decrees. Dagron, "Les moines," pp. 250–52.
92. *Miracula Joannis et Cyri,* mir. 35, p. 320.
93. *London Papyrus,* no. 1028, pp. 276–77.
94. *Vita Severi,* pp. 54–55.
95. *Oxford Dictionary of the Christian Church,* 2d ed., ed. Frank L. Cross (London: Oxford University Press, 1977), p. 1266.
96. *Historiae beatorum orientalium,* cols. 671–73 (Paul); cf. *Vita Marciani,* PG, 114: 449–52.
97. *Historiae beatorum orientalium,* col. 673 (Paul).
98. Ibid., cols. 674–75.
99. *Iohannis Ephesini . . . pars tertia,* 2.15 (p. 55).
100. Ibid., p. 56.
101. Ibid., p. 55.
102. See Janin, *Eglises,* pp. 551–52.
103. *Miracula Artemii,* mir. 18, pp. 20–23.
104. See Chap. 4 above.
105. *Dict. Spirit.,* 1:171–75.
106. *Vita Marcelli, AnalBoll,* 1968, *86:* 296–97.
107. Ibid., pp. 297–98.
108. *Vita Theodosii* (Theodore), pp. 34–35, 40–41.
109. For Dorotheos' life and work see *Dict. Spirit.,* 3:1651ff.
110. Dorotheos of Gaza, *Vita Dosithei,* in *Dorothée de Gaza: Oeuvres Spirituelles,* ed. and trans. Lucien Regnault and J. de Préville, SC, 92 (Paris, 1963), p. 123. When Dorotheos tells Dositheos to give his clothes either to a brother—i.e., a monk—or a sick person (ibid., 132), he implies that some of the sick were not monks. Dorotheos' question (Barsanouphios, *questio* 333) makes the same distinction. Ibid., *questio* 313, states explicitly that laymen came to the monastery's nosokomeion as outpatients.
111. Barsanouphios, *questio* 316; *questio* 327 mentions that Dorotheos had to consult physicians in the course of his work as nosokomos.
112. Barsanouphios, *questiones* 313, 316, and 333.
113. Ibid., *questio* 314.
114. Ibid., *questio* 313.
115. Ibid., *questio* 327.
116. Julien Leroy, "La réforme studite," in *Il monachesimo orientale,* Orientalia Christiana Analecta, 153 (Rome: Pont. Institutum Orientalium Studiorum, 1958), pp. 189–91 and 209.
117. Katechesis 1.1: ἐπαρκῶμεν καὶ ἑαυτοῖς, καὶ ἀσθενοῦσι καὶ ξένοις, . . . Cited in Leroy, "La réforme studite" (see above), p. 197, n. 123.
118. *Theodoros Studites: Jamben auf verschiedene Gegenstände,* nos. 17 and 29, ed. Paul Speck (Berlin: De Gruyter, 1968), pp. 148, 173.
119. Much of this biographical information is found in the *Typikon Athanasii* published in

Die Hauptturkunden für die Geschichte der Athosklöster, ed. Philipp Meyer (Leipzig, 1894), pp. 102–10. See also Julien Leroy, "La conversion de Saint Athanase l'Athonite à l'idéal cénobitique et l'influence Studite," in *Le Millénaire du Mont Athos,* 2 vols. (Chevetogne: Éditions de Chevetogne, 1963), 1:101–20.

120. *Vita Athanasii Athonitae B,* chap. 25, pp. 151–52, mentions hospital, bath, and hospice; ibid., chap. 41, p. 173, demonstrates that patients came to the nosokomeion from outside the monastery.

121. *Vita Athanasii Athonitae B,* chap. 41, 173–75.

122. Cf. *Typikon Kosmosoteiras,* no. 61, p. 48.

123. *JNov,* 120. For example, Menas had been xenodochos of the Sampson and a priest when elected patriarch in 536. Malalas, p. 479. According to the Sampson legend (reflecting sixth-century realities), Sampson was xenodochos of the Sampson and at the same time a priest and *skeuophylax* of the Great Church. *Vita Sampsonis* (antiquior), p. 7.

124. For Romanos' monastery see Symeon Magister, p. 733, and *Theo. Cont.,* pp. 402 and 473; also Skylitzes, p. 231.

125. For the Petrion see *Theo. Cont.,* p. 458; for the Mangana, see Skylitzes, pp. 476–77.

126. *PantTyp,* 127.1613–20.

127. *PantTyp,* 113.1414–36.

128. "Diataxis Attaleiate," pp. 73–75; *Typikon Kosmosoteiras,* no. 12, pp. 26–27; no. 31, pp. 37–38; and no. 61, pp. 48–49.

129. *PantTyp,* 99.1176–109.1346, gives absolutely no indication of monastic help in the xenon. All employees are salaried laymen. Moreover, a reading of the whole typikon shows that no monastic office had any relationship with the xenon beyond the fiscal responsibilities for the hospital which the superior and his oikonomoi assumed.

130. *PantTyp,* 53.379–96; cf. *Vita Theodosii* (Theodore), p. 40.

131. *PantTyp,* 99.1164–66.

132. See Ann W. Epstein, "Formulas for salvation: A comparison of two Byzantine monasteries and their founders," *Church History,* 1981, *50:* 385–400, esp. 394.

133. *Typikon Kosmosoteiras,* no. 70, pp. 53–55, provides for the hospital; no. 96, pp. 65–66, warns the superior never to neglect the hospital and its patients; no. 61, p. 48, provides for hiring a physician; no. 94, p. 65, provides evidence that hypourgoi were also hired, not recruited from among the monks; no. 39, pp. 40–41, lists the duties of the monks without once mentioning any work done in or for the hospital.

134. *Typikon Libos,* nos. 50–51, pp. 134–35.

135. Nowhere in the typikon is there any evidence of Christian praxis. The nuns are to be totally free from the cares of the world. *Typikon Libos,* no. 1, p. 106.

136. *Typikon Libos,* nos. 50–51, p. 134.

137. *Vita Athanasii Athonitae A,* chaps. 114–19, pp. 54–57; *Vita Athanasii Athonitae B,* chap. 36, pp. 168–69.

138. *Symeon neos Theologos: Hymnen,* ed. Athanasios Kambylis (Berlin: De Gruyter, 1976), intro., pp. xv–xviii.

139. Ibid., hymn 33, lines 14–17.

140. Walther Völker, *Praxis und Theoria bei Symeon dem neuen Theologen* (Wiesbaden: Steiner, 1974), pp. 87–96.

141. *Syméon le nouveau théologien: Catéchèses,* Kat. IX, ed. Basile Krivochéine and Joseph Paramelle, SC, 104 (Paris, 1964), pp. 106–8.

142. Ibid., pp. 108–10; cf. *Vita Mariae aegyptiacae,* PG, 87.3:3709–16.

143. *Syméon: Catéchèses,* pp. 124–32.

144. Völker, *Praxis und Theoria* (see n. 140 above), pp. 88–96; Kazhdan and Constable, *People and Power,* pp. 159–60.

145. Hunger, *Reich,* pp. 290–91, places Symeon in the tradition of hesychast writers. He did not invent all the techniques of later hesychasts, however.

146. *Typikon Kosmosoteiras,* no. 70, p. 53.

147. *PantTyp,* 113.1414–37; see also Chap. 6 above.
148. *Ms. Scorialensis,* 3.Y.14, described in *Codices hispanienses,* p. 38. Since monks were considered laymen in canon law, the prohibition of Patriarch Lukas Chrysoberges (RP, 3:344) against deacons' or priests' practicing medicine did not apply to them, unless, of course, they had received those orders.
149. Notice in Dioskorides ms. (*Vend. med. gr.* 1), published in *Katalog* (Hunger), p. 40.
150. *Emperios and Margarona,* lines 631–76, in *Collection de romans grecs,* ed. Spyridon Lambros (Paris, 1880), pp. 276–78.
151. Regarding the poem's story and its history, see Hans-Georg Beck, *Geschichte der byzantinischen Volksliteratur,* Handbuch der Altertumswissenschaft (Munich: Beck, 1971), pp. 143–47. Cf. the description of Margarona's xenon (*Emperios and Margarona* [see above], lines 670–76, p. 278) with that of Athanasios' philanthropies (*Vita Athanasii Athonitae B,* chap. 25, pp. 151–52, and chap. 41, pp. 173–74).

CHAPTER EIGHT: THE HOSPITAL IN ACTION

1. Philipsborn, "Krankenhauswesen," p. 355; Schreiber, "Hospital," p. 10, emphasizes the singular quality of the Pantokrator Typikon.
2. *Paris. gr.* 510, fol. 149. For the date of the ms. see Sirarpie Der Nersessian, "The illustrations of the homilies of Gregory of Nazianz Paris G. 510," *DOP,* 1962, *16:* 197; for a description of this particular illumination see ibid., p. 207 and fig. 7.
3. Orlandos, *Monasterike,* pp. 79–83.
4. *Typikon Evergetis,* ed. Paul Gautier, *REB,* 1982, *40:* 87.
5. *Theodori Studitae epistolae,* PG, 99:1509.
6. *Typikon Kosmosoteiras,* no. 70, p. 55.
7. *PantTyp,* 99.1152–54.
8. Anastasios Orlandos, "E anaparastasis tou xenonos tēs en Konstantinoupolei monēs tēs Pantokratoros," *EEBS,* 1941, *17:* 198–207.
9. *Panegyrica Rabulae,* pp. 202–3 (Ger. trans. [Bickell], pp. 205–6); Prokopios, *De aedif.* 2.10.25.
10. *Kosmas und Damianos,* mir. 30, pp. 173–75.
11. *Miracula Artemii,* mir. 21, p. 26.
12. Prodromos, *Gedichte,* poem 46, p. 432.
13. *PantTyp,* 83.907–11 and 85.937–39.
14. *PantTyp,* 99.1152–54.
15. See its use in *Das Strategikon des Maurikios,* ed. George T. Dennis, trans. Ernest Gamillscheg (Vienna: Österreichische Akademie der Wissenschaften, 1981), esp. 12.B.22, lines 15–21.
16. Prokopios, *De aedif.* 1.2.14–16 (Justinian's rebuilding of the Sampson Xenon); *Theodori Studitae epistolae,* PG, 99:1509. One cannot help but contrast the emphasis on proper heating for patients in Byzantine hospitals with the extreme cold in the dormitories of the Parisian Hôtel-Dieu as late as the nineteenth century (see Chap. 1 above).
17. *Kosmas und Damianos,* mir. 14, pp 135–36.
18. *Miracula Artemii,* mir. 11, p. 11.
19. *Vita Athanasii Athonitae B,* chap. 25, pp. 151–52.
20. *PantTyp,* 91.1051–93.1056; regarding the residents of the gerokomeion, ibid., 111.1377–78.
21. *Miracula Artemii,* mir. 11, p. 11.
22. *Typikon Kosmosoteiras,* no. 97, p. 66.
23. *PantTyp,* 85.947–87.954.
24. See the text and a black-and-white reproduction of the miniature in Jeanselme and Oeconomos, "Dispensaire."
25. See Chap. 4.

26. *Manuelis Philae carmina,* vol. 1, no. 98, pp. 280–81.

27. One can assume the presence of such facilities from the description of services in the Pantokrator Typikon and in the *Typikon Libos* (p. 134). For libraries and lecture rooms see below, under "Medical Training."

28. *PantTyp,* 95.1116–97.1119.

29. *PantTyp,* 93.1088–90.

30. For Dioskoros' prison see *ACO,* 2.1.2:214–15; for John of Ephesus' ordeal, see *Iohannis Ephesini . . . pars tertia,* 2.4–6 (pp. 41–46).

31. *Typikon Libos,* no. 11, p. 113.

32. *PantTyp,* 83.907–85.936.

33. *Panegyrica Rabulae,* pp. 202–3 (Ger. trans. [Bickell], pp. 205–6).

34. De Lacy O'Leary, *How Greek Science Passed to the Arabs* (London: Routledge and K. Paul, 1949), pp. 49–50.

35. *Kosmas und Damianos,* mir. 30, pp. 173–75; Prodromos, *Gedichte,* poem 46, pp. 432–33.

36. Jeanselme and Oeconomos, "Dispensaire."

37. See Chap. 5 above.

38. *Vita Sampsonis,* PG, 115:281–84.

39. *Panegyrica Rabulae,* pp. 202–3 (Ger. trans. [Bickell], pp. 205–6).

40. *Vita Theodosii* (Theodore), p. 40.

41. *JNov,* 40.

42. Jerome, *ep,* 108 (5:159–201). Paula was so famous that the proconsul of Palestine offered her rooms in the praetorium for her visit to Jerusalem (ibid, p. 167).

43. *JCod,* 6.4.4.2.

44. *Miracula Artemii,* mir. 21, pp. 25–27.

45. *PantTyp,* 107.1307–8.

46. *Poèmes prodromiques en grec vulgaire,* ed. Dirk-Christiaan Hesseling and H. Pernot (Amsterdam: J. Müller, 1910), poem 3, lines 326–45, esp. line 334a.

47. Ibid., poem 4, lines 79–89. See Hans-Georg Beck, *Geschichte der byzantinischen Volks-literatur,* Handbuch der Altertumswissenschaft (Munich: Beck, 1971), p. 104.

48. *Vie de Théodore de Sykéôn,* chap. 161, pp. 138–45.

49. *Vita S. Theophano,* ed. Eduard Kurtz, *Mémoires de l'academie impériale des sciences de St. Pétersbourg* (in Russian), series 8.3, no. 2 (1898), pp. 1 and 18.

50. *Cecaumeni Strategicon,* chap. 125, ed. Basil Wasseliewsky and Victor Jernstedt (St. Petersburg, 1896), p. 53.

51. *PantTyp,* 107.1305–12.

52. Skylitzes, p. 477; Zonaras, 3:651.

53. Anne Comnène, *Alexiade,* 15.11.9, ed. Bernard Leib, 3 vols (Paris: "Les Belles Lettres," 1945), 3:234–36; Zonaras, 3:759: ἀκεσώδυνα τὴν τῶν Μαγγάνων κατοικίαν ἐξηγοῦντό τε καὶ ὠνόμαζον διὰ τὸ ἰατρεῖον τὸ ἐν αὐτοῖς. . . .

54. *Monodie sur Pantechnès,* in *Italikos,* pp. 113–15.

55. See the commentary by Petrus Possinus in Pachymeres, 1:539–41.

56. *Vat. gr.* 299, fol. 374: τοῦ Σαρακηνοῦ τοῦ Ἀβρὰμ καὶ ἀκτ(ου)αρίου τῶν Μαγγάνων καὶ βασιλικοῦ ἀρχιϊατροῦ. Abram is called *aktouarios* of the Mangana, but this is clearly abbreviated from the xenon of the Mangana, since the preceding remedy comes ἐκ τοῦ ξενῶνος τῶν Μαγγάνων (fol. 374). Indeed, the treatments contained on fols. 368–92ᵛ represent a xenon treatment list from the Mangana Xenon.

57. Anne Comnène, *Alexiade* (see n. 53 above), 15.11.13 (3:236).

58. Ep. 33, in *Italikos,* pp. 209–10.

59. *PantTyp,* 107.1313–23.

60. Laurent, no. 1147.

61. Jones, *LRE,* 1:626.

62. Prokopios, *De aedif.* 2.10.25.

63. Romanos, *De acutis et diurnis morbis*, intro., published in Kouses, "Contribution," p. 84.

64. *Vita Lucae Stylitae*, pp. 217–20.

65. *PantTyp*, 85.925–26 and 107.1324–108.1344.

66. *Passio Thallelaei*, p. 16 (Bröcker, p. 39).

67. See Herbert Hunger's comment in Hunger, *Reich*, p. 181.

68. *Vita Lucae Stylitae*, p. 218.

69. *Miracula Artemii*, mir. 21, pp. 25–26.

70. Richard Shryock, *Medicine and Society in America, 1660–1860* (Ithaca: Cornell University Press, 1972), pp. 22–23.

71. For Basil's hospital see Basil, *ep.* 94 (Loeb, 2:150); for Chrysostom's hospital, see *Palladii dialogus*, p. 32.

72. See Chap. 7 above.

73. Although the *Miracula Artemii* were collected after 650, the elaborate hospitals which two of the tales describe (mir. 21 and mir. 22, pp. 25–31) must have been organized in the sixth century, since the strain of constant warfare between 600 and 650 left the East Roman state few resources for the development of hospitals. The sixth century witnessed the growth in xenon services which the *Miracula Artemii* reflect.

74. *Miracula Artemii*, mir. 21, p. 26.

75. *Miracula Artemii*, mir. 21, p. 26; *PantTyp*, 83.908–10.

76. *Miracula Artemii*, mir. 22, pp. 28–31.

77. Ibid., mir. 22, p. 30; cf. *PantTyp*, 85.939–41.

78. *Miracula Artemii*, mir. 22, p. 28; cf. *PantTyp*, 87.980–84. See also Chap. 6 above.

79. *Miracula Artemii*, mir. 22, pp. 28 and 30; cf. *PantTyp*, 87.955–64.

80. *Miracula Artemii*, mir. 22, p. 30.

81. *PantTyp*, 87.965–79.

82. *Theodori Studitae epistolae*, PG, 99:1509; cf. Chap. 2, above, regarding the Pantokrator organization.

83. *Miracula Artemii*, mir. 22, p. 30.

84. Romanos, *De acutis et diurnis morbis*, in Kouses, "Contribution," p. 84.

85. Ostrogorsky, *History*, pp. 367–69.

86. *Kletorologion of Philotheos*, p. 183.

87. *Vat. gr.* 299, fol. 368ᵛ.

88. *Typikon Libos*, no. 51, p. 134.

89. *Poèmes prodromiques* (see n. 46 above), poem 3, line 334a.

90. Kinnamos, p. 190.

91. Eustathios, *Espugnazione*, p. 146.

92. *PantTyp*, 85.847–87.954.

93. Jeanselme and Oeconomos, "Dispensaire."

94. Again Jeanselme and Oeconomos (ibid.) provide an excellent description of the uniforms pictured.

95. *Kletorologion of Philotheos*, p. 183.

96. Evagrios, *Hist. eccl.* 1.21–22 (pp. 31–32).

97. See Philipsborn, "Parabalani," pp. 185–90.

98. *Passio Thallelaei*, p. 16 (Bröcker, p. 39).

99. Paul the Deacon, *De vita patrum Emeritensium*, PL, 80:139.

100. Romanos, *De acutis et diurnis morbis*, in Kouses, "Contribution," p. 84.

101. *PantTyp*, 107.1313–23.

102. For a discussion of the staff organization at the Pantokrator Xenon see Chap. 2.

103. Philipsborn, "Krankenhauswesen," p. 355.

104. Aeschines, *Contra Timarchum*, 40.

105. Greg. Nys., *Contra Eunomium*, 1.44–46, in *Opera* (Jaeger), 1:37 (PG, 45:261); Philostorgios, 3.15 (p. 47).

106. John Chrysostom, *In acta apostolorum*, 52, PG, 60:365.
107. *Passio Thallelaei*, p. 12 (Bröcker, p. 32); *Vie de Théodore de Sykéôn*, chap. 146, p. 115.
108. *JCod*, 10.53.6, reissued *Theo. Cod*. 13.3.3 (27 Sept. 333).
109. Hunger, *Literatur*, 2:301.
110. The manuscript (*Laurentianus* 74.7) is described in Bandini, *Catalogus*, pp. 53ff. Bandini (p. 55) dates the manuscript to the late eleventh century, but the recent study of Jutta Kollesch and Fridolf Kudlien, *Apollonios von Kition: Kommentar zu Hippokrates über das Einrenken der Gelenke*, CMG, 11.1.1 (Berlin, 1965), p. 5, prefers the tenth century. The epigrams on fol. 7ᵛ indicating that the manuscript was used at a xenon are published in Bandini, *Catalogus*, pp. 80–83.
111. Second epigram, in Bandini, *Catalogus*, p. 82: [this codex] ἄριστον ἔργον εὐφυῶς ἠσκημένον, / διδάσκαλον φέριστον ἐμπράκτῳ λόγῳ.
112. *Georgii Lacapeni, ep.* 19, 21 *scolium* ad lin. 26.
113. Notice in Dioskorides ms. (*Vind. med. gr.* 1) in *Katalog* (Hunger), p. 40.
114. Spyridon Lampros, *Argyropouleia* (Athens: P. D. Sakellarios, 1910), p. 227; Fuchs, *Schulen*, p. 71.
115. Venance Grumel, "La profession medicale à Byzance a l'époque des Comnènes," *REB*, 1949, 7: 42–46, who reproduces the relevant passage; it is also published in Mansi, 21:552, and in RP, 5:76.
116. *PantTyp*, 107.1313–23.
117. See Chap. 2 above.
118. For the monastic infirmary, *PantTyp*, 93.1063–73; for the outpatient clinic, *PantTyp*, 87.948–50.
119. *Liber prefecti*, 1.1–3.
120. Ibid., 1.1.
121. Grumel, "La profession medicale" (see n. 115 above), p. 43; cf. *Liber prefecti*, 1.2–3.
122. Theodore Balsamon's commentary on Canon 16 of the Council of Carthage, RP, 3:344.
123. *Liber prefecti*, 1.4; for the gowns, ibid., 1.3, 26.
124. Grumel, "La profession medicale" (see n. 115 above), p. 45; see also *Italikos*, intro., pp. 46–47.
125. *London Papyri*, no. 1028 (pp. 276–77).
126. At Athens in the fourth century B.C., the *demosieuontes iatroi* made collective offerings at the Temple of Asklepeios (Cohn-Haft, p. 11).
127. *Cod. Theo.* 13.3.8.
128. *Kletorologion of Philotheos*, p. 183.
129. It is even possible that the testing of medical students was carried out by the primmikerioi of the hospital. In the ninth-century xenon which Theodore Stoudites describes (PG, 99:1509), the highest-ranking physician was the *protarchos* (πρώταρχος), an official bearing a title similar to the examiner (προεξάρχων) mentioned by Patriarch Stypes (Grumel, "La profession medicale" [see n. 115 above], p. 43). As I demonstrated above (see the text at n. 82 above), the title *primmikerios* probably replaced *protarchos* in many hospitals sometime between the tenth and the twelfth century. Since a primmikerios supervised the examining of the notarial students, it is a good guess that the hospital primmikerios or protarchos conducted the tests and licensing of physicians in the xenon where he led the medical staff.
130. *PantTyp*, intro., p. 13; for the value of a *modios* of wheat see Ostrogorsky, "Löhne," pp. 319–24.
131. *Typikon Libos*, chap. 51, p. 134. See Chap. 10, n. 78, below, for an explanation of the devaluation of the thirteenth-century Byzantine noumisma.
132. Ostrogorsky, "Löhne," pp. 295–301.
133. Such voluntary hospitals began in eighteenth-century England (Abel-Smith, pp. 5–6) and then spread to the colonies (Starr, pp. 151–52).
134. Abel-Smith, p. 5; Starr, pp. 152 and 162–63.
135. Starr, pp. 162–63.

136. *PantTyp,* 107.1305–12.
137. *PantTyp,* intro., p. 13.
138. *Kletorologion of Philotheos,* p. 155, line 3; Zacos and Veglery, no. 1779.
139. Paul Lemerle, "Roga et rente d'état aux Xe–XIe siècle," *REB,* 1967, *25:* 88 and 95–96.
140. *Palladii dialogus,* p. 32.
141. *Miracula Artemii,* mir. 22, p. 28.
142. Tzetzes, ep. 81, p. 121.
143. Prodromos, *Gedichte,* poem 46, p. 432.
144. See Chap. 6 above.
145. For Aetios see Philostorgios, *Hist. eccl.* 3.15 (p. 47); for Basil, Greg. Naz., *In laudem Basilii,* chaps. 23.6 and 63.5–6 (PG, 36:528, 580).
146. See Chap. 3 above.
147. Neilos of Ankyra, *ep.* 110, PG, 79:248.
148. *Miracula Artemii,* mir. 22, p. 31.
149. See the description of the Nuri Hospital in Damascus in *Encyclopedia of Islam,* 1:1224.
150. Ibid., 2:1119–20; see the recent article by Friedrun R. Hau, "Gondeschapur: Eine Medizinschule aus dem 6 Jahrhundert," *Gesnerus,* 1979, *36:* 98–115.
151. *Paris suppl. gr.* 764, fol. 84: Θεραπευτικαὶ ἰατρεῖαι συντεθεῖσαι παρὰ διαφόρων ἰατρῶν κατὰ τὴν ἐκτεθεῖσαν ἀκολουθίαν τοῦ ξενῶνος. (title published by Jeanselme, "Therapeutique," p. 168).
152. See Jeanselme's explanation of the disorder at the end of the list (Jeanselme, "Therapeutique," pp. 147–48).
153. *Vat. gr.* 292, fol. 200: προσταγαὶ καὶ τύποι τῶν μεγάλων ξενώνων ὅσα ἐκ πείρας ἰατρῶν παῖδες θεραπείας χάριν προσάγουσι καὶ τοῖς ἄλλοις πως πάσχουσιν ἐν τοῖς ξενῶσιν.
154. Kouses, "Contribution," p. 84.
155. *Vat. gr.* 292, fols. 207–207^v.
156. *Laurentianus* 74.7 (Bandini, *Catalogus,* pp. 53–93).
157. Temkin, "Byzantine Medicine," pp. 215–22; Hunger, *Literatur,* 2:287 and 315. See also Gerhard Harig, "Von den arabischen Quellen des Simeon Seth," *Medizin-historisches Journal,* 1967, *2:* 248–68, who emphasizes that nearly 60 percent of the drugs mentioned by Seth cannot be found in Galen's works.
158. Eustathios, *Espugnazione,* p. 146.
159. Prodromos, *Gedichte,* intro., pp. 21–35.
160. Ibid., poem 46, pp. 431–32.
161. Ibid., pp. 432–33.
162. Ibid., intro., pp. 31–32.
163. Kantakouzenos, *Historia,* 3:223.

CHAPTER NINE: HOSPITALS AND MEDICAL LITERATURE

1. Basil, *ep.* 94 (Loeb, 2:150); *Palladii dialogus,* p. 32.
2. *Syriac Chronicle,* 12.7 (pp. 331–32): "Out of kindness towards the captives [East Romans] and the holy men he [the shah] has now by the advice of the Christian physicians attached to him made a hospital, a thing not previously known, and has given 100 mules and 50 camels laden with goods from the royal stores, and 12 physicians and whatever is required is given; and in the king's retinue . . . [manuscript breaks off]."
3. *PantTyp,* intro., p. 13.
4. See Chap. 8 above.
5. See Herbert Hunger's summary of the situation in Hunger, *Literatur,* 2:304, as well as his comments on the poor state of our knowledge regarding the works of Theophilos Protospatharios, ibid., pp. 299–301.
6. Aktouarios, *De urinis, liber IV,* Ideler, 2:95; Hohlweg, "Aktuarios," p. 309.
7. *Oribasii collectionum medicarum reliquiae,* ed. Johannes Raeder, CMG, 6.1–4 (Leipzig,

1928–33). Only about a third of the work survives. See Hunger, *Literatur*, 2:293–94. See also Photios' essay in Photios, *Bibliotheca*, 217 (3:132ff.).

8. Photios, *Bibliotheca*, 220 (3:139–40).

9. Ibid., p. 139, line 25.

10. Ibid., p. 139, lines 30–33, and p. 140, lines 40–45.

11. For Aetios, see the brief sketch with bibliography in Hunger, *Literatur*, 2:294–95; for Alexander of Tralleis, ibid., p. 297, and Bloch, "Byzantinische Medizin," pp. 535–36.

12. Photios, *Bibliotheca*, 221 (3:152). A partial edition of Aetios (first eight books) was prepared by Alessandro Olivieri, 2 vols., CMG, 8.1–2 (Berlin, 1935–50).

13. Hunger, *Literatur*, 2:298.

14. John Scarborough, "Early byzantine pharmacology," in *Byzantine Medicine* (Scarborough).

15. John Duffy, "Byzantine medicine in the sixth and seventh centuries: Aspects of theology and practice," in *Byzantine Medicine* (Scarborough); Hunger, *Literatur*, 2:297.

16. *Vat. gr.* 299, fols. 368–393ᵛ.

17. Marie-Thérèse Fontanille, "Les bains dans la médicine gréco-romaine," *Revue archeologique du centre de la France*, 1982, *21:* 121–30; Hunger, *Literatur*, 2:298.

18. *PantTyp*, 93.1057–60. See also the list of therapies in the Vatican List (*Vat. gr.* 292, fols. 200–210ᵛ).

19. Hunger, *Literatur*, 2:297; edition by Theodor Puschmann, in *Berliner Studien für classische Philologie und Archeologie*, 1886, *5.2:* 134–78.

20. Regarding eye specialists in the Greco-Roman period see Vivian Nutton, "Roman oculists," *Epigraphica* (Milan), 1972, *34:* 16–29.

21. *Miracula Artemii*, mir. 21, p. 26.

22. Hunger, *Literatur*, 2:302.

23. Paul of Aegina, *Epitome*, ed. Johann L. Heiberg, CMG, 9.1 and 2 (Leipzig, 1921–24). See also the English translation by Francis Adams, 3 vols. (London, 1844–47).

24. Hunger, *Literatur*, 2:292 and 302; Bloch, "Byzantinische Medizin," pp. 548–50; Fuat Sezgin, *Geschichte des arabischen Schrifttums*, 3 vols. (Leiden: Brill. 1970), 3:168–70.

25. *Vita Joannis Eleemosynarii*, chap. 7, PG, 114:900; another version is "Une vie inédite de Saint Jean l'Aumônier," ed. Hippolyte Delehaye, *AnalBoll*, 1927, *45:* 22. Hunger, *Literatur*, 2:292, suggests that Paul practiced gynecology in Alexandria. He does not mention Patriarch John's special hospitals, however.

26. Richard Friedländer, *Die wichtigen Leistungen der Chirurgie in der byzantinischen Periode* (Breslau, 1883). For an example see the lithotomy operations discussed by Ernst Gurlt, *Geschichte der Chirurgie und ihrer Ausübung*, 3 vols. (Berlin, 1898), 3:774–79, where Paul's description makes the ancient procedure comprehensible.

27. *Laurentianus* 74.7, fols. 239ᵛ–262, contains sections of Paul's chapter 6; fol. 7ˣ preserves the poems which address Niketas as the executor of the codex and mention that he prepared it primarily to teach the various grades of physicians and interns at a hospital (the poems are published in Bandini, *Catalogus*, pp. 80–83); fol. 349 has the marginal note regarding the Hospital of the Forty Martyrs. See also Jeanselme, "Thérapeutique," p. 168.

28. See the standard account of the seventh century in Ostrogorsky, *History*, pp. 87–146, and some interesting observations in Brown, *Antiquity*, pp. 150–203.

29. Lemerle, *Humanisme*, pp. 74–108.

30. Browning, *Empire*, pp. 69–70; Hunger, *Literatur*, 1:331; Ostrogorsky, *History*, pp. 87–92.

31. Lemerle, *Humanisme*, pp. 74–85.

32. Clive Foss, "Archaeology and the 'Twenty Cities' of Byzantine Asia," *AJA*, 1977, *81:* 469–86, esp. 477–79.

33. Clive Foss, *Ephesus after Antiquity: A Late Antique, Byzantine, and Turkish City* (Cambridge: Cambridge University Press, 1979), pp. 103–15.

34. Lemerle, *Humanisme*, pp. 97–104; Paul Speck, *Die kaiserliche Universität von Konstan-*

tinopel, Byzantinisches Archiv, 14 (Munich: Beck, 1974), pp. 7–22 and 29–35. See also the rules for the guild of notaries in *Liber prefecti,* 1.

35. *De cerimoniis,* 1.32 (1:173; Vogt, 1:161–62). See the chronology established in Chap. 5 above at n. 93.

36. For the teaching role of xenones see Chap. 8.

37. The title of this treatment list in *Laurentianus* 75.19: ἀποθεραπευτικὴ Θεοφίλου συλλέξαντος ταύτην ἐκ διαφόρων ξενωνικῶν βίβλων. See also Hunger, *Literatur,* 2:301.

38. See Chap. 8.

39. Lemerle, *Humanisme,* p. 76. See also Robert Devreesse, *Le fonds coislin* (Paris: Imprimerie nationale, 1945), ms. no. 120, p. 111.

40. Owsei Temkin, "The Byzantine origins of the names for the basilic and cephalic veins," in *Janus,* pp. 198–201.

41. The xenon treatment list of *Vat. gr.* 292, fols. 200–210ᵛ, also provides a good example of the xenon style.

42. *Mercurii monachi doctrina de pulsibus,* Ideler, 2:254–56.

43. *Vat. gr.* 285, fols. 151–152ᵛ (see *Codices vaticani graeci,* 1:396). See also the comments by Fuchs, *Schulen,* p. 72.

44. For an analysis of John's compendium, see Daremberg, *Notices,* pp. 22–30.

45. *Vita Theophanis,* p. 23.

46. For the account of kidney-stone surgery see Gurlt, *Geschichte der Chirurgie* (see n. 26 above), 3:774–82, esp. 780–82.

47. Paul of Aegina, *Epitome,* 6.60.

48. Browning, *Empire,* pp. 96ff.

49. Hunger sketches the problems involved in dating the works of Theophilos Protospatharios. Hunger, *Literatur,* 2:299–301 and 304–5.

50. In his forthcoming edition of the Theophilos *scholia* to the *Aphorisms of Hippocrates,* Professor Leendert Westerink argues that Theophilos Protospatharios wrote no earlier than ca. 850, since one of the mss. gives him the title πρωτοσπαθάριος τοῦ Χρυσοτρικλινίου (protospatharios of the Golden Hall). Such a title cannot be found in the sources before the second half of the ninth century.

51. Hunger, *Literatur,* 2:299.

52. *Kletorologion of Philotheos,* p. 155.

53. Zacos and Veglery, no. 1779.

54. The fourteenth-century ms. (Vat. gr. 299, fol. 374) describes the aktouarios Abram as βασιλικοῦ ἀρχιιατροῦ, clearly one of the emperor's personal physicians.

55. See Chap. 7 above.

56. For the Byzantine use of *philosophos,* see Franz Dölger, "Zur Bedeutung von φιλόσοφος und φιλοσοφία in byzantinischer Zeit," *Byzanz und die europäische Staatenwelt: Ausgewählte Vorträge und Aufsätze* (Ettal: Buch-Kunstverlag, 1953), pp. 197–208.

57. Bandini, *Catalogus,* pp. 166–68.

58. Hunger, *Literatur,* 2:301 and note 54; Bandini, *Catalogus,* pp. 166–68.

59. Theophilos begins his study of urine with the prayer: Οὐκοῦν δέον ἡμῖν ἐστι περὶ οὔρων μέλλουσι διδάξαι ἐπικαλέσασθαι Χριστὸν τὸν ἀληθινὸν θεὸν ἡμῶν ἀρωγὸν καὶ βοηθὸν καὶ ὁδηγὸν γενέσθαι εἰς τὴν τοιαύτην διδασκαλίαν. . . . (Ideler, 1:262).

60. Hunger, *Literatur,* 2:299.

61. *Die Schriften 'Peri Sphygmōn' des Philaretos,* ed. John A. Pithis (Husum: Matthiesen Verlag, 1983), pp. 35 and 193–94.

62. *Theophilii de urinis,* Ideler, 1:261–62. See John Zachariah Aktouarios' criticism of Theophilos for emphasizing experience at the expense of *logos* (*Ioannis Actuarii de urinis,* Ideler, 2:5).

63. *Ioannis Actuarii de urinis,* Ideler, 2:3–192. Regarding his observations in the xenon, see Ideler, 2:95.

64. See the miniature in *Paris. gr.* 2243, published in Jeanselme, "Dispensaire." For the

importance of Byzantine uroscopy see Gerhard Baader and Gundolf Keil, "Mittelalterliche Diagnostik," in *Medizinische Diagnostik in Geschichte und Gegenwart: Festschrift für Heinz Goerke zum sechzigsten Geburtstag,* ed. Christa Habrich et al. (Munich: W. Fritsch, 1978), pp. 120–24.

65. Jerome J. Bylebyl, "The school of Padua: Humanistic medicine in the sixteenth century," in *Health, Medicine, and Mortality in the Sixteenth Century,* ed. Charles Webster (Cambridge: Cambridge University Press, 1979), p. 350.

66. Hunger, *Literatur,* 2:305–6.

67. *Codices vaticani graeci,* no. 292, p. 407.

68. G. A. Costomiris, "Études sur les écrits inédits des anciens médicins grecs," *Revue des études grecques,* 1891, *4:* 100–101; Jeanselme, "Thérapeutique," p. 166.

69. *Paris. gr.* 2091 includes 156 chapters of Theophanes' *Synopsis* (fols. 10–58), followed by the Paris List (fols. 77–98). *Baroc.* 150 has the Paris List first (fols. 29–32ᵛ), followed by a section of the *Synopsis* (fols. 32ᵛ–37).

70. Joseph Sonderkamp, "Theophanes Nonnus: Medicine in the circle of Constantine Porphyrogenitus, in *Byzantine Medicine* (Scarborough).

71. *Baroc.* 150 (15th cent.); *Paris. gr.* 2091 (15th cent.); *Paris. suppl. grec.* 764 (14th cent.).

72. Jeanselme, "Thérapeutique," p. 164.

73. Costomiris, "Ecrits inédits" (see n. 68 above) pp. 100–101.

74. Θεραπευτικαὶ καὶ ἰατρεῖαι συντεθεῖσαι ὑπὸ διαφόρων ἰατρῶν κατὰ τὴν ἐκτεθεῖσαν ἀκολουθίαν τοῦ ξενῶνος. See Jeanselme, "Thérapeutique," p. 168.

75. Jeanselme, "Thérapeutique," pp. 148–63, provides a French translation of the text. A summary of the contents in modern Greek is found in Kouses, "Contribution," pp. 79–82.

76. Jeanselme, "Thérapeutique," pp. 147–48 and 169–70; Temkin, "Byzantine Medicine," p. 220.

77. Προσταγαὶ καὶ τύποι τῶν μεγάλων ξενώνων ὅσα ἐκ πείρας ἰατρῶν παῖδες θεραπείας χάριν προσάγουσι καὶ τοῖς ἄλλοις πως πάσχουσι ἐν τοῖς ξενῶσι (*Vat. gr.* 292, fol. 200).

78. For the Vatican ms. see *Codices vaticani graeci,* no. 292, and for the Vienna ms. see *Med. gr.* 37, in *Katalog* (Hunger), pp. 89–90.

79. See Chap. 10.

80. *Vat. gr.* 292, fols. 207ᵛ and 209.

81. Ibid., fol. 204ᵛ.

82. Ibid., fols. 205–205ᵛ.

83. Ibid., fol. 209.

84. See the instruments discussed by John S. Milne, *Surgical Instruments in Greek and Roman Times* (Aberdeen: Aberdeen University Studies, 1907).

85. For example, *Vat. gr.* 292, fols. 207–207ᵛ, mentions yellow bile in distinguishing treatments for stomach problems.

86. Hunger, *Literatur,* 2:307.

87. Romanos' heading, introduction, and a summary of the contents of the work are published in Kouses, "Contribution," pp. 84ff. Kouses published the text from *Vat. gr.* 280 in *Praktikon Akademias Athenon,* 1944, *19:* 162–70, which I have not been able to obtain.

88. Hunger, *Literatur,* 2:307.

89. The ms. and contents are described in Bandini, *Catalogus,* pp. 53–93. See also Jeanselme, "Thérapeutique," p. 168, and *Apollonii Citiensis in Hippocratis de articulis commentarius,* ed. Jutta Kollesch and Fridolf Kudlien, CMG, 11.1.1 (Berlin, 1965), intro., pp. 5–6.

90. Bandini, *Catalogus,* p. 81, Poem I:

> Ἀλλ’ οὖν ἅπαντες τῶν σοφῶν ἀκεστόρων
> Νέοι, προγηράσαντες, ὑπουργῶν ὅσοι
> Γυμνὰ κρατεῖτε ῥωστικώτατα ξίφη,
> Στέψατε λοιπὸν τῆς γραφῆς τὸν ἐργάτην
> Ἐκ μουσικῶν πλέκοντες ἄνθη τῶν λόγων.

91. Ibid., p. 82, Poem II:

> Καὶ δὴ (Niketas) προσάψας ἁρμογάς, ὡς ἦν φύσει,
> Τῶν εἰκόνων μὲν τῇ καταλλήλῳ φράσει,

Λόγον δὲ μορφαῖς, τεχνικῇ διαπλάσει, . . .

Ὡς εἶχεν ἐξήνεγκεν . . . ,

Διδάσκαλον φέριστον ἐμπράκτῳ λόγῳ.

92. Text of note in Bandini, *Catalogus*, p. 93, and Jeanselme, "Thérapeutique," p. 168.

93. *Apollonii Citiensis . . . commentarius* (see n. 89 above), intro., p. 5. The physicians of the Greek classical age (fifth and fourth centuries B.C.) transmitted their compositions with the same indifference to preserving the integrity of the *Urtext*. Thus, the *Corpus Hippocraticum* contains many works which are composites of originally distinct treatises or show signs of additions by later editors. Regarding this, see Geoffrey Lloyd, "The Hippocratic Question," *Classical Quarterly*, 1975, n.s. *25*: 178–81.

94. Lawrence Bliquez, "Surgical instruments and the state of surgery in Byzantine times," in *Byzantine Medicine* (Scarborough).

95. *PantTyp*, 83.907–8, 99.1152–53, and 101.1185.

96. Both *Vat. gr.* 292 and *Vendob. med.* 37, which contain the Vatican List (see the text at nn. 67 and 78), are from the fourteenth century. All the mss. containing the Dark Age phlebotomy texts which Temkin studied (Temkin, "The Byzantine origins" [see n. 40 above], pp. 198–201) come from the Late Byzantine period. Temkin was able to date the composition of these Greek phlebotomy texts to the Dark Age because paraphrases of them appear in Arabic and Latin medical literature of the ninth and tenth centuries.

97. *Vat. gr.* 292, fol. 209.

98. *PantTyp*, 105.1271–75.

99. See the description of *Laurentianus* 74.2 in Bandini, *Catalogus*, pp. 46ff. The list is published by H. Schoene, "Zwei Listen chirurgischer Instrumente," *Hermes*, 1903, *38*: 280–84. Cf. the instruments described in Milne, *Surgical Instruments* (see n. 84 above). Lawrence Bliquez, "Surgical instruments and the state of surgery in Byzantine times," in *Byzantine Medicine* (Scarborough), discusses this list thoroughly and identifies some of those instruments in it which are not found in ancient surgical texts.

100. For the Vatican List see n. 78 above; for the Paris List see n. 71 above; for Romanos' guidebook, Kouses, "Contribution," pp. 77–80; for Theophilos' list of tonics, see n. 57 and the accompanying text; for Temkin's phlebotomy texts, n. 96 above.

101. See also Joseph Sonderkamp's introduction to the manuscripts in his forthcoming edition of the *Synopsis* of Theophanes Nonnos.

102. *Codices hispanienses*, pp. 39–41.

103. *Paris gr.* 2315. A translation of the dedication on fol. 23ᵛ can be found in Jeanselme, "Thérapeutique," p. 169. A second ms. (*Paris. gr.*, 2510, fols. 137–39) also contains John Staphides' *antidotarium* and a dedication to the xenon (also found in Jeanselme, "Thérapeutique," pp. 168–69).

104. This list is unpublished. The only known extant copy is *Vat. gr.* 299, fols. 368–393.ᵛ

105. Παρὰ Στεφάνου ἀρχιατροῦ τῶν Μαγγάνων (*Vat. gr.* 299, fol. 368ᵛ); τοῦ Σαρακηνοῦ τοῦ Ἀβρὰμ καὶ ἀκτ(ου)αρίου τῶν Μαγγάνων καὶ βασιλικοῦ ἀρχιατροῦ (fol. 374).

106. Περὶ ἡπατικῶν πρόσταξον ἐκ τοῦ ξενῶνος τῶν Μαγγάνων (fol. 374).

107. For example, Ἀλεξάνδρου περὶ ἥπατος φλεγμονῆς (ibid., fol. 369ᵛ).

108. Ibid., fol. 393.

109. Paul of Aegina, *Epitome*, 6.60.

110. Gurlt, *Geschichte der Chirurgie* (see n. 26 above), 3:780–82.

111. See Chap. 8.

112. Hunger, *Literatur*, 2:312–13. Regarding John Zachariah Aktouarios see also Fridolf Kudlien, "Empirie und Theorie in der Harnlehre des Johannes Aktuarios," *Clio Medica*, 1973, *8*: 19–30.

113. *Georgii Acropolitae opera*, ed. August Heisienberg, 2 vols. (Leipzig: Teubner, 1903), 1:63 (lines 12–16).

114. See Chap. 8.

115. *The Fihrist of al-Nadīm*, ed. and trans. Bayard Dodge, 2 vols., Records of Civilization:

Sources and Studies (New York: Columbia University Press, 1970), 2:698; Friedrun Hau, "Gondeschapur: Eine Medizinschule aus dem 6. Jahrhundert nach Chr.," *Gesnerus*, 1979, *36:* 107.

116. All mss. give him the title *aktouarios.* See his published works in Ideler, vols. 1 and 2, and the recent study by Hohlweg, "Actuarios," pp. 302–21.

117. *Vat. gr.* 299, fol. 374.

118. Ideler, 2:95.

119. He was probably influenced by the Paleologan humanistic movement. Browning, *Empire,* pp. 184–201.

120. Ackerknecht, pp. xi–xiv, provides a summary of the Clinical movement; his study as a whole describes the Clinical movement in Paris in great detail. See also Foucault, pp. ix–xiv, 3–199, for what the author calls "an archaeology of medical perception."

121. *Syriac Chronicle,* 12.7 (pp. 331–32).

122. Bylebyl, "The school of Padua" (see n. 65 above), pp. 342–350.

123. Foucault, pp. 64–87, 107–11; Ackerknecht, pp. 15–22.

124. Ackerknecht, pp. 3–22.

125. "Peu lire, beaucoup voir, beaucoup faire." This was the motto coined by Antoine F. Fourcroy, who played a leading role in reforming the French medical schools under the Convention (1792–95). See Foucault, pp. 69–72.

126. E. Coyecque, *L'Hôtel-Dieu de Paris au moyen-âge: Histoire et documents,* 2 vols. (Paris, 1891), 1:75, states that the Hôtel-Dieu housed between 400 and 500 patients during the fifteenth century and even more during the sixteenth century. He bases his statements on records of the Paris Parlément.

127. Foucault, p. 59.

128. Bylebyl, "The school of Padua," p. 350.

129. Foucault, pp. 120–94.

130. Lawrence Bliquez and Alexander Kazhdan, "Four testimonia to human dissection in Byzantine times," *Bull. Hist. Med., 58:*554–57.

131. *Theophanis chronographia,* p. 436.

132. Ethical Tract VI, in *Symeon le nouveau théologien: Traités théologiques et éthiques,* ed. Jean Darrouzès, 2 vols., SC, 122 and 129 (Paris, 1967), 2:138–40.

133. *Éloge d'Anne Comnène,* in *Tornikeś,* p. 225.

134. Foucault, p. 141, stresses that hospitals provided the Paris clinicians the only opportunity to begin autopsies before the effects of decomposition distorted the internal marks of the disease.

135. Ackerknecht, pp. 145 and 177–78.

136. *Vita Theophanis,* p. 23.

CHAPTER TEN: AFTER 1204

1. A full account of the Latin assault is given in Charles Brand, *Byzantium Confronts the West* (Cambridge: Harvard University Press, 1968), pp. 254–69.

2. *Ecclesiae graecae monumenta,* 3:512.

3. *Actes de Lavra,* no. 123, p. 23.

4. The Panteleemon restored by Niphon (ibid.) and the Mangana (*Vat. gr.* 299, fols. 368–393ᵛ).

5. Ostrogorsky, *History,* pp. 418–65.

6. Browning, *Empire,* p. 186.

7. Ostrogorsky, *History,* pp. 427–31.

8. *Anonymi compendium chronicon,* ed. Constantine Sathas, in *Bibliotheca graeca medii aevi,* 7 (Paris, 1894): 507 (Vatatzes) and 535–36 (Theodore II).

9. Browning, *Empire,* p. 184; Herbert Hunger, "Von Wissenschaft und Kunst der frühen Palaiologenzeit," *Jahrbuch der österreichischen byzantinischen Gesellschaft,* 1958–59, 7–8: 126–27.

10. *Nicephori Gregorae byzantina historia*, ed. Ludwig Schopen, 3 vols., CSHB (1830), 1:44–45; Pachymeres, 1:70–71.

11. Theodore Metochites, *Nikaeus*, p. 145.

12. *Theodori Epistulae, ep.* 118, pp. 164–65.

13. Niketas Choniates, p. 445.

14. Blemmydes, *Curriculum*, 2–3.

15. *Theodori Ducae Lascaris imperatoris in laudem Nicaeae urbis oratio*, ed. Ludwig Bachmann (Progr. Rostock, 1847), p. 5; quoted in Hunger, "Von Wissenschaft und Kunst" (see n. 9 above), p. 136.

16. Pachymeres, 1:530.

17. Janin, *Églises*, p. 578.

18. *Historia occidentalis of Jacques de Vitry*, ed. John F. Hinnebusch (Fribourg: University Press, 1972), pp. 149–50.

19. *Actes de Lavra*, no. 123, pp. 23ff.

20. *Georgi Cypri laudatio Michaelis Paleologi*, PG, 142:377.

21. *Typikon Libos*, pp. 106–36; for the xenon, nos. 50–51, p. 134.

22. Mazaris, p. 92.

23. *Andronici Callisti monodia de Constantinopoli capta*, PG, 161:1135.

24. Fuchs, *Schulen*, p. 71; Giuseppe Cammelli, *I dotti bizantini e le origini dell' umanesimo, II: Giovanni Argiropulo* (Florence: Le Monnier, 1941), pp. 29–36.

25. Speros Vryonis, *Byzantium and Europe* (London: Harcourt, Brace, and World, 1967), pp. 153–59.

26. According to Hunger, "Von Wissenschaft und Kunst" (see n. 9 above), p. 145, both Thomas Magister and Demetrios Triklinios taught in Thessalonica.

27. Browning, *Empire*, pp. 187 and 201.

28. Theodore Metochites, *Nikaeus* p. 145.

29. *Matthaios von Ephesos, ep.* 55, p. 177.

30. Ibid., *ep.* 64, pp. 198–99.

31. Kenneth Setton, *Catalan Domination of Athens, 1311–1388* (Cambridge, Mass.: Medieval Academy of America, 1948), p. 224.

32. Cf. Eustathios, *Espugnazione*, p. 146, with *Symeon, Archbishop of Thessalonica: Political-Historical Works*, ed. David Balfour (Vienna: Österreichische Akademie der Wissenschaften, 1979), pp. 42–43, which describes the Turkish conquest of the city in 1387.

33. See Denis Zakythinos, *Le despotat grec de Morée*, with notes by Chryssa Maltézou, 2 vols. (London: Variorum, 1975).

34. *Georgii Gemisti Plethonis de rebus Peloponnesiacis oratio*, ed. Spyridon Lampros, in *Palaiologeia kai Peloponnesiaka*, 4 vols. (Athens: Epitrope ekdoseōs tōn kataloipōn Spyridonos Lamprou, 1912–30), 3:259 (PG, 160:833): [Monks] ἀγαπῶντας τῷ πλείῳ μὲν καρπουμένους, πλείω δὲ καὶ λειτουργοῦντας, μᾶλλόν τι καὶ χρησίμους εἶναι τοῖς κοινοῖς. . . .

35. Zakythinos, *Le despotat grec de Morée*, (see n. 33 above), 1:175–80.

36. *Vat. gr.* 299, fol. 374.

37. *Manuelis Philae carmina*, poem 98, pp. 280–82; Janin, *Églises*, p. 558.

38. *Actes de Lavra*, no. 123, pp. 20–26.

39. Jeanselme, "Thérapeutique," pp. 168–69.

40. Chortasmenos, *ep.* 8, pp. 157–58.

41. *Danilo II: Stefan Uroš II Milutin*, trans. Stanislaus Hafner, in *Serbisches Mittelalter: Altserbische Herrscherbiographien*, vol. 2 (Graz: Styria, 1976), pp. 174–78; Mirjana Živojinović, "L'hôpital du roi Milutin à Constantinople" (in Serbian with Fr. résumé), *Zbornik Radova*, 1975, *16*: 105–17.

42. *Katalog* (Hunger), p. 40; Fuchs, *Schulen*, p. 71.

43. Browning, *Empire*, p. 187.

44. Ševčenko, "Makrembolites," pp. 212–13.

45. *Philothei patriarchae homilia de Heracliā captā*, in *Anecdota graeca e codicibus bib-*

liothecae S. Marci, ed. Costantino Triantafillis and Alberto Grapputo (Venice, 1874), pp. 2 and 12–13.

46. *Symeon, Archbishop of Thessalonica* (see n. 32 above), p. 47.
47. Ševčenko, "Makrembolites," p. 213.
48. *Theodori epistulae, ep.* 118, pp. 164–65.
49. John Barker, *Manuel II Palaeologus, 1391–1425* (New Brunswick, N.J.: Rutgers University Press, 1968), pp. 79–80.
50. Cf. *Typikon Libos,* no. 1, p. 106, and no. 50, p. 134.
51. Živojinović, "L'hôpital du roi Milutin" (see n. 41 above), pp. 116–17.
52. *Vind. med. gr.* no. 1, fol. 1, reproduced in *Katalog* (Hunger), p. 40.
53. *Codices hispanienses,* p. 38.
54. *Actes de Laura,* no. 123, pp. 23–24.
55. John Meyendorff, *St. Grégoire Palamas et la mystique orthodoxe* (Paris: Éditions du Seuil, 1959), pp. 57–74.
56. *Philothei* (see n. 45 above), pp. 1–5; final decision, p. 29.
57. Found in *Cod. Ambrosianus* H. 81 *suppl.,* fols. 152ᵛ–169ᵛ.
58. Ibid., fols. 154ᵛ–155.
59. See the version in *Vita Sampsonis* (antiquior) and the tenth-century redaction of Symeon Metaphrastes, PG, 115:277–308.
60. Cf. the account in *Actes de Laura,* no. 123, p. 25, with *Vita Athanasii Athonitae B,* chap. 25, pp. 151–52, and chap. 41, p. 173.
61. *Georgii Gemisti Plethonis* (see n. 34 above), 3:257 (PG, 160:832–33): [Hesychasts] τούτους δ᾽ ἀποστάντας, ὥς φασι, πάντων, ἰδίᾳ θεοκλητεῖν τε καὶ τῆς σφετέρας αὐτῶν φάσκειν ἐπιμελεῖσθαι ψυχῆς.
62. *Danilo* (see n. 41 above), p. 177.
63. Mazaris, p. 92.
64. A miniature with inscription in *Baroccianus* 87, fol. 35; text reproduced in Fuchs, *Schulen,* p. 71.
65. *Michaelis Acominati (Choniatis) opera,* ed. Spyridon Lampros, 2 vols. (Athens, 1879), *ep.* 131, 2:263–67.
66. Mazaris, pp. 2–4.
67. Chortasmenos, *ep.* 28, pp. 177–79.
68. Theodore Metochites, *Nikaeus,* p. 145.
69. Chortasmenos, *ep.* 8, pp. 157–58.
70. *Manuelis Philae carmina,* poem 98, p. 282.
71. All the following information on the Lips Xenon can be found in *Typikon Libos,* nos. 50–51, p. 134.
72. See Chap. 8 above.
73. Cf. *PantTyp,* 85.914–16.
74. *PantTyp,* 85.941–43; cf. *PantTyp,* 103.1223, which suggests that three female servants worked in the women's ward.
75. The *optiones* (accountants) are mentioned at *PantTyp,* 85.947 and 101.1200–1201.
76. *PantTyp,* 113.1414–115.1445.
77. See Paul Gautier's chart in *PantTyp,* p. 14, for all of these auxiliary positions.
78. *PantTyp,* 101.1188–89, gives the salary for the male physicians in the women's ward. Ostrogorsky, "Löhne," pp. 319–23, reviews the sources which mention the price of wheat from the fourth to the thirteenth century. They all suggest that one noumisma (hyperperon) bought twelve modioi of wheat. S. Bendall and P. J. Donald, *The Later Palaeologan Coinage, 1282–1453* (London: A. H. Baldwin and Sons, 1979), p. 11, set the hyperperon of 1281 at 14 carats gold, while Michael Hendy, *Coinage and Money in the Byzantine Empire, 1081–1261* (Washington, D.C.: Dumbarton Oaks, 1969), pp. 14–17, sets the Comnenian hyperperon at 20.5 carats. Moreover, the hyperperon of 1281 was somewhat lighter than the Comnenian gold coin—4.42 grams to 4.55 grams; see Tommaso Bertelè, *Numismatique byzantine,* trans. Cécile Morrisson (Wetteren, Belgium: NR, 1978), p. 36.

79. *Vind. med. gr.* 1, fol. 1, *Katalog* (Hunger), p. 40.

80. *Typikon Libos,* no. 50, p. 134, gives the wheat allotments in modioi, but the wine, oil, vegetable, wood, and barley allotments in hyperpera. The sums for these expenditures seem high for one patient's allotment, but too low for that of all twelve patients.

81. Cf. *PantTyp,* pp. 18–19.

82. *Manualis Philae carmina,* no. 98, 1: 281:

Σκοπεῖν γὰρ εἰκὸς τὸν βραβευτὴν τὸν μέγαν,
Μὴ πού τις ἢ ῥάθυμος ἢ κλῶψ ἐνθάδε,
Μηδ᾽ αὐθάδης ἄνθρωπος ἐξ ἀσπλαγχνίας
Πρὸς τοὺς ταπεινοὺς καὶ παραλελυμένους ·
Ἄλλως δ᾽ ἂν οὐκ ἄμισθος ἡ πρᾶξις μένοι,
Καὶ τῇ σχέσει πρέπουσα τῶν δειμαμένων.

83. *PantTyp,* 87.985–89.995.

84. *PantTyp,* 107.1307–8.

85. Mazaris, p. 92: [Malakes] καὶ ἀμνημονήσεις οὐ μόνον πατρίδος . . . , ἀλλὰ δὴ καὶ τῶν συνεισφορῶν τῶν ξενώνων καὶ λημμάτων τῶν ἀρχόντων τοῦ Γαλατᾶ.

86. *PantTyp,* 87.955–64.

87. Chortasmenos, p. 190; see also Hunger's comments (ibid., p. 48).

88. *Ioannis Actuarii de urinis,* Ideler, 2:3–4.

89. *Ioseph Monachou tou Bryenniou ta heurethenta . . . di' epimeleias Eugeniou tou Boulgareos,* 3 vols. (Leipzig, 1784), *ep.* 47, 3:120.

90. *Vat. gr.* 299, fol. 374.

91. Mazaris, pp. 10–12.

92. Hunger, *Literatur,* 2:313–14.

93. Browning, *Empire,* p. 197.

94. Cammelli, *I dotti bizantini* (see n. 24 above), pp. 30–33; a plate (ibid., pp. 30–31) reproduces the drawing from *Baroccianus* 87, fol. 35.

CHAPTER ELEVEN: EPILOGUE

1. John H. Knowles, "The teaching hospital: Historical perspective and contemporary view," in *Hospitals, Doctors, and the Public Interest,* ed. John H. Knowles (Cambridge: Harvard University Press, 1965), pp. 1–2; *Encyclopedia of Bioethics,* s.v. "Hospitals"; Starr, pp. 177–79.

2. Hospices in Norman England supplemented their original endowment by receiving small gifts. See Edward Kealey, *Medieval Medicus: A Social History of Anglo-Norman Medicine* (Baltimore: Johns Hopkins University Press, 1981), pp. 96–97.

3. Starr, pp. 169 and 176.

4. *Vita Sampsonis* (antiquior), p. 14.

5. Darrel Amundsen, "Images of physicians in classical times," *Journal of Popular Culture,* 1977, *11:* 647.

6. For the political influence of Byzantine physicians in the fourteenth century see Mazaris.

7. *JCod,* 1.27.41, established the salaries for five physicians in the African prefecture. There is in this *constitutio* no statement that these were the municipal archiatroi; moreover, the section concerning their salaries appears in a list of salaries paid imperial bureaucrats, not city appointees such as the archiatroi. On the other hand, the number of physicians (five) corresponds to the number of archiatroi in a city established by Antoninus Pius (*JDigest,* 27.1.6.2; Nutton, "Archiatri," pp. 198–204). Moreover, the physicians of Africa are associated with grammarians and rhetors, as the archiatroi of Pius' legislation were (*JDigest,* 27.1.6.2).

8. *PantTyp,* 85.919–20 (beds); 105.1276–77 (hand-washing); 99.1152–55 (heating).

9. Ackerknecht, pp. 16–17.

10. *Theodori epistulae, ep.* 118, pp. 164–65.

11. See the comments by Professor Lawrence Bliquez, "Surgical instruments and the state of surgery in Byzantine times," in *Byzantine Medicine* (Scarborough).

12. Ackerknecht, pp. 15–22.

13. *PantTyp,* 99.1164–65, indicates that the superior performed the washing of feet on Holy Thursday in the xenon chapel.

14. Starr, p. 179: "Within the hospital, there continue to be three separate centers of authority—trustees, physicians, and administrators, posing a great puzzle to students of formal organizations."

15. The Hippocratic tradition is explained by Ludwig Edelstein, "Greek Medicine in its Relation to Religion and Magic," in *Ancient Medicine: Selected Papers of Ludwig Edelstein,* ed. Owsei Temkin and C. Lilian Temkin (Baltimore: Johns Hopkins University Press, 1967), p. 229.

16. See Gautier's chart of xenon staff in *PantTyp,* p. 13.

17. Cf. *PantTyp,* 85.942–43, and *Typikon Libos,* no. 51, p. 134.

18. Lemerle, *Humanisme,* pp. 82–83.

19. *Vita S. Nicephori episcopi Mileti, AnalBoll,* 1895, *14:* 137–39, and commentary, 161–65.

20. Kazhdan and Constable, *People and Power,* esp. pp. 19–58.

Abbreviations and Bibliography

Abel-Smith
> Brian Abel-Smith, *The Hospitals (1800–1948): A Study in Social Administration in England and Wales* (Cambridge: Harvard University Press, 1964).

Ackerknecht
> Erwin H. Ackerknecht, *Medicine at the Paris Hospital, 1794–1848* (Baltimore: Johns Hopkins Press, 1967).

ACO
> *Acta conciliorum oecumenicorum,* ed. Eduard Schwartz, 4 vols. (Berlin and Leipzig: De Gruyter, 1922–74).

ActaSS
> *Acta Sanctorum* (Antwerp, 1643–), 3d ed., 71 vols. (Paris, 1863–1940).

Actes de Lavra
> *Actes de Lavra, III: De 1329 à 1500,* ed. Paul Lemerle et al., Archives de l'Athos, 10 (Paris: P. Lethielleux, 1979).

AJA
> *American Journal of Archaeology*

Albertz, "Jung-arianischen Kirchengemeinschaft"
> Martin Albertz, "Zur Geschichte der jung-arianischen Kirchengemeinschaft," *Studien und Kritiken,* 1909, *82:* 205–78.

Amand de Mendieta, "Système"
> Emmanuel Amand de Mendieta, "Le système cénobitique basilien comparé au système cénobitique pachômien," *Revue de l'histoire des religions,* 1957, *152:* 31–80.

Amundsen and Ferngren
> Darrel Amundsen and Gary Ferngren, "Medicine and religion: Pre-Christian antiquity," in *Health/Medicine and the Faith Traditions,* ed. Martin Marty and Kenneth Vaux (Philadelphia: The Fortress Press, 1982), pp. 53–92.

AnalBoll
> *Analecta Bollandiana*

Aristides, *Opera* (Keil)
> *Aelii Aristidis Smyrnaei quae supersunt omnia,* ed. Bruno Keil, vol. 2 (Berlin, 1898).

Bandini, *Catalogus*
> Angelo M. Bandini, *Catalogus codicum graecorum Bibliothecae Lauren-tianae,* vol. 3 (Florence, 1770).

Barsanouphios
> *Nikodemou Agioreitou Biblos Barsanouphiou kai Ioannou,* ed. Soterios Schoinas (Bolos: Hagioretike Bibliotheke, 1960).

Basil, *ep.* (Loeb)
> *Saint Basil: Letters,* trans. Roy J. Deferrari and Martin R. McGuire, 4 vols., Loeb Classical Library (Cambridge: Harvard University Press, 1961).

Behr
> Charles A. Behr, *Aelius Aristides and the Sacred Tales* (Amsterdam: Hakkert, 1968).

Bildlexikon
> Wolfgang Müller-Wiener, *Bildlexikon zur Topographie Istanbuls* (Tübingen: E. Wasmuth, 1977).

Blemmydes, *Curriculum*
> *Nicephori Blemmydae curriculum vitae et carmina,* ed. August Heisenberg (Leipzig, 1896).

Bloch, "Byzantinische Medizin"
> Iwan Bloch, "Byzantinische Medizin," in *Handbuch der Geschichte der Medizin,* ed. Max Neuburger and Julius Pagel, 2 vols. (Jena: G. Fischer, 1902), 1:492–588.

BNJ
> *Byzantinisch-neugriechische Jahrbücher*

Brown, *Antiquity*
> Peter Brown, *The World of Late Antiquity, A.D. 150–750* (New York: Harcourt Brace Jovanovich, 1971).

Browning, *Empire*
> Robert Browning, *The Byzantine Empire* (London: Weidenfeld and Nicolson, 1980).

Bull. Hist. Med.
> *Bulletin of the History of Medicine*

***Byzantine Medicine* (Scarborough)**
> *Byzantine Medicine,* ed. John Scarborough, *DOP,* 1984, *38* forthcoming.

BZ
> *Byzantinische Zeitschrift*

Chortasmenos
> *Johannes Chortasmenos: Briefe, Gedichte, und kleine Schriften,* ed. Herbert Hunger (Vienna: Österreichische Akademie der Wissenschaften, 1969).

Chronicon paschale
> *Chronicon paschale,* ed. Ludwig Dindorf, CSHB (1832).

CIG

Corpus inscriptionum graecorum, ed. August Boeckh, 4 vols. and index (Berlin, 1828–77)

Claude, *Stadt*

Dietrich Claude, *Die byzantinische Stadt im sechsten Jahrhundert,* Byzantinisches Archiv, 13 (Munich: Beck, 1969).

CMG

Corpus medicorum graecorum (Leipzig and Berlin: Akademie-Verlag, 1927–).

Codices hispanienses

Catalogus codicum astrologorum graecorum: Codices hispanienses, ed. Carlo O. Zuretti (Brussels: H. Lamertin, 1932), vol. 11.1.

Codices vaticani graeci

Codices vaticani graeci, vol. 1, ed. Giovanni Mercati and Pio De' Cavalieri (Rome: Vatican, 1929).

Cod. Theo.

Theodosiani libri XVI cum constitutionibus Sirmondianis, ed. Theodor Mommsen and Paul Meyer, 2 vols. (Berlin: Weidmann, 1905).

Cohn-Haft

Louis Cohn-Haft, *The Public Physicians of Ancient Greece,* Smith College Studies in History, 42 (Northampton, Mass.: Department of History, Smith College, 1956).

Constantelos, *Philanthropy*

Demetrios Constantelos, *Byzantine Philanthropy and Social Welfare* (New Brunswick, N.J.: Rutgers University Press, 1968).

Const. Apost.

Didascalia et constitutiones apostolorum, ed. Francis X. Funk (Paderborn: F. Schoeningh, 1905).

CSHB

Corpus scriptorum historiae byzantinae, 50 vols. (Bonn: W. Weber, 1828–97).

DACL

Dictionnaire d'archéologie chrétienne et de liturgie, ed. Fernand Cabrol et al., 15 vols. (Paris: Letouzey et Ané, 1907–53).

Dagron, "Les moines"

Gilbert Dagron, "Les moines et la ville: Le monachisme à Constantinople jusqu'au concile de Chalcédoine (451)," *Travaux et Mémoires,* 1970: *4:* 229–76.

Dagron, *Naissance*

Gilbert Dagron, *Naissance d'une capitale* (Paris: Presses universitaires de France, 1974).

Daremberg, *Notices*

Charles Daremberg, *Notices et extraits des manuscrits médicaux grecs, latins, et français* . . . (Paris, 1853).

De cerimoniis
Constantini Porphyrogeniti de cerimoniis aulae byzantinae, ed. Johann Reiske, CSHB (1828); new ed. of first 92 chapters by Albert Vogt, 2 vols. (Paris: "Les Belles Lettres," 1935–39).

Delehaye, *Deux typica byzantins*
Deux typica byzantins de l'époque des Paléologues, ed. Hippolyte Delehaye (Brussels: M. Lamertin, 1921).

Devreesse
Robert Devreesse, *Le patriarcat d'Antioche depuis la paix de l'église jusqu'à la conquête arabe* (Paris: J. Gabalda and Co., 1945).

"Diataxis Attaliate"
"La diataxis de Michel Attaliate," ed. Paul Gautier, *REB,* 1981, *39:* 5–143.

Dict. CB
A Dictionary of Christian Biography, 4 vols. (Boston, 1877–78).

Dict. Spirit.
Dictionnaire de spiritualité ascétique et mystique, ed. Marcel Villier et al., 8 vols. (Paris: G. Beauchesne and Sons, 1932–).

Dietz, *Scholia*
Scholia in Hippocratem et Galenum, ed. Friedrich Dietz, 2 vols. (Königsberg, 1834).

Dmitrievskij, *Opisanie*
Aleksei Dmitrievskij, *Opisanie liturgičeskih rukopisej hranjaščihsja v bibliotekah pravoslavnago vostoka, I: Typika* (Kiev, 1895).

Dölger, *Finanzverwaltung*
Franz Dölger, *Beiträge zur Geschichte der byzantinischen Finanzverwaltung, besonders des 10 und 11 Jahrhunderts,* Byzantinisches Archiv, 9 (Leipzig and Berlin: Teubner, 1927).

DOP
Dumbarton Oaks Papers

Ecclesiae graecae monumenta
Ecclesiae graecae monumenta, ed. Jean B. Cotelier, 4 vols. (Paris, 1677–92).

Edelstein, *Asclepius*
Emma J. Edelstein and Ludwig Edelstein, *Asclepius: A Collection and Interpretation of the Testimonies,* 2 vols. (Baltimore: Johns Hopkins Press, 1945).

EEBS
Epiteris Hetaireias Byzantinōn Spoudaiōn

Encyclopedia of Bioethics
Encyclopedia of Bioethics, ed. Warren Reich, 4 vols. (New York: Free Press, 1978).

Encyclopedia of Islam
Encyclopedia of Islam, new ed., 4 vols. (Leiden: Brill, 1960–).

EO
  Echos d'Orient
Epiphanios, Panarion
  Epiphanios, *Panarion,* ed. Karl Holl, 3 vols., GCS, 25, 31, and 37 (Leipzig, 1915–33).
Epit. Theo. Ana.
  Theodoros Anagnostes: Kirchengeschichte, ed. Günther C. Hansen, GCS, 54 (Berlin, 1971).
Eusebios, Hist. eccl.
  Eusebios, *Kirchengeschichte,* ed. Eduard Schwartz, 2 vols., GCS, 9.1 and 9.2 (Leipzig, 1903–8).
Eustathios, Espugnazione
  Eustazio di Tessalonica, *La espugnazione di Tessalonica,* ed. Stilpon Kyriakides (Palermo: Istituto siciliano di studi bizantini e neoellinici, 1961).
Evagrios, Hist. eccl.
  Evagrius, *Historia ecclesiastica,* ed. Joseph Bidez and Leon Parmentier (London, 1898).
Foucault
  Michel Foucault, *The Birth of the Clinic: An Archaeology of Medical Perception,* trans. A. M. Sheridan Smith (New York: Random House, 1973).
Fuchs, Schulen
  Friedrich Fuchs, *Die höheren Schulen von Konstantinopel im Mittelalter,* Byzantinisches Archiv, 8 (Leipzig and Berlin: Teubner, 1926).
Gask and Todd
  George Gask and John Todd, "The origins of hospitals," in *Science, Medicine, and History: Essays on the Evolution of Scientific Thought and Medical Practice Written in Honour of Charles Singer,* ed. Edgar E. Underwood, 2 vols. (New York: Oxford University Press, 1953), 1:122–30.
GCS
  Die griechischen christlichen Schriftsteller der ersten Jahrhunderte (Leipzig and Berlin: Akademie-Verlag, 1897–).
Georgii Lacapeni
  Georgii Lacapeni epistulae X priores cum epimerismis editae, ed. Sigfried Lindstram (Upsala: E. Berling, 1910).
Greg. Naz., ep.
  Gregor von Nazianz, Briefe, ed. Paul Gallay, GCS, 53 (Berlin, 1969).
Greg. Naz., In laudem Basilii
  Grégoire de Nazianze: Discours funèbres, ed. Fernand Boulenger (Paris: A. Picard and Sons, 1908), 58–203; PG, 36: 493–605.
Greg. Nys., Pauperibus
  Gregorii Nysseni de pauperibus amandis: Orationes duo, ed. Adrian van Heck (Leiden: Brill, 1964).

Harig, "Krankenhaus"
Gerhard Harig, "Zum Problem 'Krankenhaus' in der Antike," *Klio,* 1971, *53:* 179–95.

Harig and Kollesch, "Krankenpflege"
Gerhard Harig and Jutta Kollesch, "Arzt, Kranker, und Krankenpflege in der griechisch-römischen Antike und im byzantinischen Mittelalter," *Helikon,* 1973–74, *13–14:* 256–92.

Harnack, *Mission*
Adolf von Harnack, *Die Mission und Ausbreitung des Christentums in den ersten drei Jahrhunderten,* 2 vols. (Leipzig: J. C. Hinrichs, 1915).

Historiae beatorum orientalium
Historiae beatorum orientalium, ed. and trans. Ernest W. Brooks, PO, 18:513–698.

Historia lausiaca
Palladio, *La storia lausiaco,* ed. Gerhard Bartelink (Rome: Fondazione Lorenzo Valla, A. Mondadori, 1974).

Hohlweg, "Aktuarios"
Armin Hohlweg, "Johannes Aktuarios, Leben—Bildung und Ausbildung—De methodo medendi," *BZ,* 1983, *76,* 302–21.

Hunger, *Literatur*
Herbert Hunger, *Die hochsprachliche profane Literatur der Byzantiner,* 2 vols., Handbuch der Altertumswissenschaft (Munich: Beck, 1978).

Hunger, *Reich*
Herbert Hunger, *Reich der neuen Mitte* (Graz: Styria, 1965).

Ideler
Physici et medici graeci minores, ed. Julius L. Ideler, 2 vols. (Leipzig, 1841–42).

IG
Inscriptiones graecae, 14 vols. (Berlin: Georg Reimer, 1873–).

Iohannis Ephesini . . . pars tertia
Iohannis Ephesini historiae ecclesiasticae pars tertia, trans. Ernest W. Brooks, Corpus scriptorum Christianorum orientalium, 106 (Louvain: L. Durbecq, 1952).

Italikos
Michel Italikos: Lettres et discours, ed. Paul Gautier. Archives de l'orient chrétien, 14 (Paris: Institut français d'études byzantines, 1972).

Iuliani epitome
Iuliani epitome latina Novellarum, ed. Gustav Haenel (Leipzig, 1873).

Janin, *Eglises*
Raymond Janin, *La géographie ecclésiastique de l'empire byzantin, première partie: Le siège de Constantinople et le patriarcat oecuménique,* vol. 3. *Les églises et les monastères,* 2d ed. (Paris: Institut français d'études byzantines, 1969).

Janus
> Owsei Temkin, *The Double Face of Janus and Other Essays in the History of Medicine* (Baltimore: The Johns Hopkins University Press, 1977).

JCod
> *Corpus iuris civilis, II: Codex Justinianus,* ed. Paul Krüger (Berlin: Weidmann, 1929).

JDigest
> *Corpus iuris civilis, I: Digesta,* ed. Theodor Mommsen (Berlin: Weidmann, 1928).

Jeanselme, "Thérapeutique"
> Edouard Jeanselme, "Sur un aide-mémoire de thérapeutique byzantin contenu dans un manuscrit de la Bibliotèque Nationale de Paris (suppl. gr. 764)," in *Mélanges Charles Diehl,* 2 vols. (Paris: E. Leroux, 1930), 1:147–70.

Jeanselme and Oeconomos, "Dispensaire"
> Edouard Jeanselme and Lysimachos Oeconomos, "Un dispensaire medical à Byzance au temps des Paléologues," *Aesculape,* 1925, *15:* 26–30.

Jerome, *De viris inlustribus*
> *Hieronymi de viris inlustribus,* ed. Oskar von Gebhardt, *TU,* 1896, *14:* 1–56.

Jerome, *ep.*
> *Saint Jérôme: Lettres,* ed. Jérôme Labourt, 8 vols. (Paris: "Les Belles Lettres," 1949–63).

JNov
> *Corpus juris civilis, III: Novellae,* ed. Rudolf Schoell and Wilhelm Kroll (Berlin: Weidmann, 1928).

Jones, *LRE*
> Arnold H. M. Jones, *The Later Roman Empire, 284–602,* 2 vols. (Norman: University of Oklahoma Press, 1964).

JTS
> *Journal of Theological Studies*

Julian (Loeb)
> Julian, *Opera,* ed. and trans. Wilmer C. Wright, 3 vols. Loeb Classical Library (London: W. Heinemann, 1928–30).

Jus
> *Jus graeco-romanum,* ed. P. Zepos and I. Zepos, 8 vols. (Athens: G. Phexis and Son, 1930–31).

Kallistos
> *Nicephori Callisti Xanthopuli ecclesiasticae historiae libri XVIII,* PG, 145–47.

Kantakouzenos, *Historia*
> *Ioannis Cantacuzeni eximperatoris historiarum libri IV,* ed. Ludwig Schopen, 3 vols., CSHB (1828–32).

Katalog (Hunger)
Herbert Hunger, *Katalog der griechischen Handschriften der öster-reichischen Nationalbibliothek, 2: Codices medici et juridici* (Vienna: G. Prachner, 1969).

Kazhdan and Constable, *People and Power*
Alexander Kazhdan and Giles Constable, *People and Power in By-zantium* (Washington, D.C.: Dumbarton Oaks, 1982).

Kedrenos
Georgii Cedreni historiarum compendium, ed. Immanuel Bekker, 2 vols., CSHB (1838–39).

Kinnamos
Ioannis Cinnami epitome rerum ab Ioanne et Alexio Comnenis gest-arum, ed. August Meineke, CSHB (1836).

Kletorologion of Philotheos
Le traité de Philothée, ed. Nicolas Oikonomides, in Oikonomides, *Préséance,* pp. 81–235.

Kopecek
Thomas A. Kopecek, "The Cappadocian Fathers and civic patriotism," *Church History,* 1974, *43:* 293–303.

Kosmas und Damianos
Kosmas und Damianos, ed. Ludwig Deubner (Leipzig and Berlin: Teubner, 1907).

Kötting
Bernhard Kötting, *Peregrinatio religiosa,* Forschungen zur Volk-skunde, *33–35* (Münster: Regensberg, 1950).

Kouses, "Contribution"
Aristoteles Kouses, "Contribution à l'étude de la médicine des zénons pendant le XVᵉ siècle," *BNJ,* 1928, *6:* 77–90.

Laurent
Vitalien Laurent, *Le corpus des sceaux de l'empire byzantin, II: L'ad-ministration centrale* (Paris: Éditions du centre national de la re-cherche scientifique, 1981).

Lemerle, *Cinq études*
Paul Lemerle, *Cinq études sur le XIᵉ siècle byzantin* (Paris: Éditions du centre national de la recherche scientifique, 1977).

Lemerle, *Humanisme*
Paul Lemerle, *Le premier humanisme byzantin* (Paris: Presses uni-versitaires de France, 1971).

Lex. Theo. Kir.
Lexikon für Theologie und Kirche, ed. Michael Buchberger; 2d ed., ed. Josef Hofer and Karl Rahner, 10 vols. (Freiburg: Herder, 1957–65).

Liber prefecti
The Book of the Eparch, reprinted with introduction by Ivan Dujčev (London: Variorum Reprints, 1970).

London Papyrus
> *Greek Papyri in the British Museum,* ed. Frederic G. Kenyon and Harold I. Bell, 3 vols. (London: The British Museum, 1907), vol. 3.

Malalas
> *Ioannis Malalae chronographia,* ed. Ludwig Dindorf, CSHB (1831).

Mango
> Cyril Mango, *Byzantium: The Empire of New Rome* (New York: Scribner's Sons, 1980).

Mansi
> *Sacrorum conciliorum nova et amplissima collectio,* ed. Joannes D. Mansi, 31 vols. (Florence, 1759–98).

Manuelis Philae carmina
> *Manuelis Philae carmina,* ed. E. Miller, 2 vols. (Paris, 1855–57).

Matthaios von Ephesos
> *Die Briefe des Matthaios von Ephesos im Codex Vindobonensis Theo. Gr. 174,* ed. Diether Reinsch (Berlin: N. Mielke, 1974).

Mazaris
> *Mazaris' Journey to Hades,* ed. Seminar Classics 609, Arethusa Monographs, 5 (Buffalo: Department of Classics, State University of New York at Buffalo, 1975).

Meyer-Steineg
> Theodor Meyer-Steineg, *Kranken-Anstalten im griechisch-römischen Altertum,* in *Jenaer medizin-historische Beiträge,* 3 (Jena: G. Fischer, 1912).

MGH Cap.
> *Monumenta germaniae historica, Legum sectiones quinque, II: Capitularia regum Francorum,* 2 vols. (Hanover and Berlin, 1883–97).

MGH Conc.
> *Monumenta germaniae historica, Legum sectiones quinque, III: Concilia,* 2 vols. (Hanover and Berlin, 1893–).

MGH Poet.
> *Monumenta germaniae historica: Poetae latini medii aevi (Carolini),* 4 vols. (Hanover and Berlin, 1881–).

MGH SSrerMerov.
> *Monumenta germaniae historica: Scriptores rerum Merovingicarum,* 7 vols. (Hanover and Berlin, 1885–1920).

Miller, "Knights"
> Timothy S. Miller, "The Knights of Saint John and the hospitals of the Latin West," *Speculum,* 1978, *53:* 709–33.

Miracula Artemii
> *Miracula S. Artemii,* in Athanasios Papadopoulos-Kerameus, *Varia graeca sacra* (St. Petersburg, 1909), pp. 1–75.

Miracula Joannis et Cyri
> *Los Thaumata de Sofronio,* ed. Natalio Fernandez Marcos (Madrid: Instituto Antonio de Nebrija, 1975); PG, 87.3:3423–3589.

MM
Franz Miklosich and Joseph Müller, *Acta et diplomata graeca medii aevi,* 6 vols. (Vienna, 1860–90).

NCE
New Catholic Encyclopedia, 15 vols. (New York: McGraw Hill, 1967).

Niketas Choniates
Nicetae Choniatae historia, ed. Ioannes A. van Dieten (Berlin: De Gruyter, 1975).

Nutton, "Archiatri"
Vivian Nutton, "Archiatri and the medical profession in antiquity," *Papers of the British School at Rome,* 1977, *45:* 191–226.

Oikonomides, *Préséance*
Nicolas Oikonomides, *Les listes de préséance byzantines des IXe et Xe siècles* (Paris: Editions du centre national de la recherche scientifique, 1972).

***Opera* (Jaeger)**
Gregorii Nysseni opera omnia, ed. Werner Jaeger, 9 vols. (Berlin and Leiden: Weidmann, 1921–72).

***Opera* (Kühn)**
Claudii Galeni opera omnia, ed. Carl G. Kühn, 22 vols. (Leipzig, 1821–33).

Orlandos, *Monasteriake*
Anastasios Orlandos, *Monasteriake architektonike keimenon kai schedia* (Athens: "Hestia," 1927).

Ortiz de Urbina
Ignacio Ortiz de Urbina, *Patrologia Syriaca* (Rome: Pont. Institutum orientalium studiorum, 1958).

Ostrogorsky, *History*
George Ostrogorsky, *History of the Byzantine State* (New Brunswick, N.J.: Rutgers University Press, 1969).

Ostrogorsky, "Löhne"
George Ostrogorsky, "Löhne und Preise in Byzanz," *BZ,* 1932, *32:* 293–333.

OxPap
The Oxyrhynchus Papyri, ed. Bernard Grenfell and Arthur Hunt et al., 51 vols. (London: Egypt Exploration Fund, 1898–).

Pachomiana
Pachomiana latina, ed. Amand Boon (Louvain: Bureaux de la revue, 1932).

Pachymeres
Georgii Pachymeris de Michaele et Andronico Palaeologis libri XIII, ed. Immanuel Bekker, 2 vols., CSHB (1835).

Palladii dialogus
Palladii dialogus de vita S. Joannis Chrysostomi, ed. Paul R. Coleman-Norton (Cambridge: University Press, 1928).

Panegyrica Rabulae
S. Ephraemi syri Rabulae episcopi Edesseni Balaei aliorumque opera selecta, ed. J. Joseph Overbeck (Oxford, 1865); German trans. by Gustav Bickell, in *Bibliothek der Kirchenväter: Ausgewählte Schriften der syrischen Kirchenväter,* ed. Valentin Thalhofer (Kempten, 1874).

PantTyp
"Le typikon du Christ Sauveur Pantocrator," ed. Paul Gautier, *REB,* 1974, *32:* 1–145.

Papyrus (Maspero)
Catalogue général des antiquités égyptiennes du musée du Caire: Papyrus grecs d'époque byzantine, ed. Jean Maspero, 6 vols. (Cairo: Institut français d'archéologie orientale, 1911–16).

Passio Thallelaei
Passio S. Thallelaei, Acta SS, Maii V; new ed. by Heinrich Bröcker, Forschungen zur Volksurkunden, 48 (Münster: Regensburg, 1976).

Patlagean, *Pauvreté*
Evelyne Patlagean, *Pauvreté économique et pauvreté sociale* (Paris: Mouton, 1977).

Paul of Aegina, *Epitome*
Pauli Aeginetae epitome, ed. Johann L. Heiberg, CMG, 9.1 and 9.2 (Leipzig, 1921–24).

PG
Patrologiae cursus completus, Series graeca, ed. Jacques P. Migne, 161 vols. (Paris, 1857–66).

Philipsborn, "Krankenhauswesen"
Alexandre Philipsborn, "Der Fortschritt in der Entwicklung des byzantinischen Krankenhauswesens," *BZ,* 1961, *54:* 338–65.

Philipsborn, "Parabalani"
Alexandre Philipsborn, "La compagnie d'ambulanciers 'parabalani' d'Alexandrie," *Byzantion,* 1950, *20:* 185–90.

Philostorgios
Philostorgios, *Kirchengeschichte,* ed. Joseph Bidez and Friedhelm Winkelmann, 2d ed., GCS, 21 (Berlin, 1972).

Photii epistolae
Photii epistolae, ed. Johannes Valetta (London, 1864).

Photios, *Bibliotheca*
Photios, *Bibliotheca,* ed. René Henry, 8 vols. (Paris: "Les Belles Lettres," 1959–77).

PL
Patrologiae cursus completus, Series latina, ed. Jacques P. Migne, 221 vols. (Paris, 1844–80).

PO
Patrologia orientalis, 39 vols. (Paris: Firmin-Didot, 1907–).

Pohl
Rudolf Pohl, *De graecorum medicis publicis* (Berlin: Georg Reimer, 1905).

Prodromos, *Gedichte*
Theodoros Prodromos, *Historische Gedichte,* ed. Wolfram Hörandner (Vienna: Österreichische Akademie der Wissenschaften, 1974).

Prokopios, *De aedif.*
Procopii Caesariensis opera omnia, ed. Jacob Haury, 4 vols. (Leipzig: Teubner, 1913), vol. 4.

Quasten
Johannes Quasten, *Patrology,* 3 vols. (Westminster, Md.: Newman Press, 1950–60).

RAC
Reallexikon für Antike und Christentum, ed. Theodor Klauser et al., 12 vols. (Stuttgart: Hiersemann, 1950–).

Rasi, "Spese funeralizie"
Piero Rasi, "Donazione di Costantino e di Anastasio alla chiesa di S. Sofia per le spese funeralize a Constantinopoli," *Festschrift für Leopold Wenger zu seinem 70. Geburtstag,* 2 vols. (Munich: Beck, 1944–45), 2:269–82.

RE
Paulys Realencyclopädie der classischen Altertumswissenschaft, rev. ed. Georg Wissowa and Wilhelm Kroll, 24 vols. (Stuttgart: J. B. Metzler, 1893–).

REB
Revue des Études Byzantines

Reicke
Siegfried Reicke, *Das deutsche Spital und sein Recht im Mittelalter,* 2 vols. (Stuttgart: Ferdinand Enke, 1932).

RP
Georgios A. Rhalles and Michael Potles, Syntagma tōn theōn kai hierōn kanonōn, 6 vols. (Athens, 1852–59).

RPT
Realencyclopädie für protestantische Theologie und Kirche, 3d ed., Albert Hauck, 24 vols. (Leipzig: J. A. Hinrichs, 1896–1913).

SC
Sources Chrétiennes, ed. H. de Lubac and J. Danielou (Paris: Éditions du Cerf, 1942–).

Scarborough
John Scarborough, *Roman Medicine* (Ithaca: Cornell University Press, 1969).

Schreiber, "Hospital"
Georg Schreiber, "Byzantinisches und abendländisches Hospital," in

Gemeinschaften des Mittelalters: Recht und Verfassung, Kult und Frömmigkeit (Münster: Regensberg, 1948), pp. 3–80.

Scriptores originum
Scriptores originum Constantinopolitanarum. ed. Theodore Preger (Leipzig: Teubner, 1907).

Ševčenko, "Makrembolites"
Ihor Ševčenko, "Alexios Makrembolites and his dialogue between the rich and the poor," *Zbornik Radova*, 1960, 6:187–228.

Skylitzes
Ioannis Scylitzae synopsis historiarum, ed. Hans Thurn, Corpus fontium historiae byzantinae (Berlin: De Gruyter, 1973).

Socrat.
Socratis scholastici ecclesiastica historia, ed. Robert Hussey, 3 vols. (Oxford, 1853); PG, 67:33–841.

Soz.
Sozomenos, *Kirchengeschichte,* ed. Joseph Bidez, GCS, 50 (Berlin, 1960).

Starr
Paul Starr, *The Social Transformation of American Medicine* (New York: Basic Books, 1982).

Statuts
Statuts d'Hôtels-Dieu et de léproseries, ed. Léon Le Grand (Paris: A. Picard and Sons, 1901).

Stein, *Le bas-empire*
Ernst Stein, *Histoire du bas-empire,* 2 vols. (Paris: Desclée de Brouwer, 1949–59).

Suda
Suidae Lexicon, ed. Ada Adler, 5 vols. (Leipzig: Teubner, 1928–38).

Subhag
Subsidia hagiographica (Brussels: Société des Bollandistes, 1886–).

Symeon Magister
Annales Symeonis Magistri (Pseudo-Symeon), ed. Immanuel Bekker, in *Theo. Cont.,* pp. 601–760.

Synaxarion
Synaxarium ecclesiae Constantinopolitanae e codice Sirmondiano nunc Berolinensi adiectis Synaxariis selectis, ed. Hippolyte Delehaye, *ActaSS, Propylaeum ad acta sanctorum Novembris* (Brussels: Apud socios Bollandianos, 1902).

Syriac Chronicle
The Syriac Chronicle Known as That of Zachariah of Mitylene, trans. Frederick J. Hamilton and Ernest W. Brooks (London: Methuen and Co., 1899).

Temkin, "Byzantine Medicine"
Owsei Temkin, "Byzantine medicine: Tradition and empiricism," in *Janus,* pp. 202–22.

Theo. Cont.
Theophanis Continuati chronographia, ed. Immanuel Bekker, CSHB (1838).

Theodore Metochites, *Nikaeus*
Theodori Metochitis Nikaeus, ed. Constantine Sathas, in *Bibliotheca graeca medii aevi,* 7 vols. (Venice, 1872), 1:139–53.

Theodoretos, *Hist. eccl.*
Theodoret, *Kirchengeschichte,* ed. Léon Parmentier, 2d ed., GCS, 44 (Berlin, 1954).

Theodori Epistulae
Theodori Ducae Lascaris epistulae CCXVII, ed. Nicholas Festa (Florence, 1898).

Theophanis chronographia
Theophanis chronographia, ed. Carolus de Boor, 2 vols. (Leipzig: Teubner, 1883), vol. 1.

Tornikès
Georges et Dèmètrios Tornikès: Lettres et discours, ed Jean Darrouzès (Paris: Éditions du centre national de la recherche scientifique, 1970).

TU
Texte und Untersuchungen zur Geschichte der altchristlichen Literatur.

Typikon Kosmosoteiras
"Typicon du monastère de la Kosmosotira," ed. Louis Petit, *Bulletin de l'institut russe à Constantinople,* 1908, *13:* 19–75.

Typikon Libos
"Le typicon du monastère de Lips," in Delehaye, *Deux typica byzantins,* pp. 106–36.

Tzetzes, *ep.*
Ioannis Tzetzae epistulae, ed. Petrus Leone (Leipzig: Teubner, 1972).

Uhlhorn, *Liebestätigkeit*
Gerhard Uhlhorn, *Die christliche Liebestätigkeit,* 3 vols. (Stuttgart: D. Gundert, 1882–90).

Vie de Théodore de Sykéôn
Vie de Théodore de Sykéôn: Texte grec, ed. André M. J. Festugière, Subhag, 48 (Brussels, 1970).

Vita Andreae
Vita S. Andreae, ed. Athanasios Papadopoulos-Kerameus, in *Analekta hierosolymitikēs stachyologias,* 5 vols. (St. Petersburg, 1891–98), 5: 169–79.

Vita Athanasii Athonitae A
    Vitae duae antiquae sancti Athanasii Athonitae, ed. Jacques Noret,
    Corpus Christianorum: Series graeca, 9 (Turnhout: Brepols University
    Press, 1982), pp. 1–124.
Vita Athanasii Athonitae B
    Vitae duae antiquae sancti Athanasii Athonitae (see above), pp. 125–
    213.
Vita Euthymii
    Vita S. Euthymii, ed. Eduard Schwartz, TU, 1939, *49.2*:3–85.
Vita Ioannis (Leontios)
    *Leontios von Neapolis: Leben des heiligen Johannes des barmherzigen
    Erzbischof von Alexandrien,* ed. Heinrich Gelzer (Freiburg, 1893).
Vita Lucae Stylitae
    Vita S. Lucae Stylitae, in *Les saints stylites* ed. Hippolyte Delehaye,
    Subhag, 14 (Paris and Brussels, 1923).
Vita Marciani (antiquior)
    Vita S. Marciani oeconomi, ed. Athanasios Papadopoulos-Kerameus,
    in *Analekta hierosolymitikēs stachyologias,* 5 vols. (St. Petersburg,
    1891–98), 4:258–70.
Vita Porphyrii
    Marc le Diacre: Vie de Porphyre, évêque de Gaza, ed. Henri Grégoire
    and Marc A. Kugener (Paris: "Les Belles Lettres," 1930).
Vita Sabae (Cyril)
    Cyril of Skythopolis, *Vita S. Sabae,* ed. Eduard Schwartz, *TU,* 1939,
    49.2: 85–200.
Vita Sampsonis (antiquior)
    "Saint Sampson: le xénodoque de Constantinople," ed. François
    Halkin, *Rivista di studi bizantini e neoellenici,* 1977–79, *n.s. 14–16:*
    6–17.
Vita Severi
    Vie de Sévère par Zacharie le Scholastique, ed. and trans. Marc A.
    Kugener, PO, 2:7–115.
Vita Theodosii (Cyril)
    *Lebensnachrichten über den heiligen Theodosios von Kyrillos aus Sky-
    thopolis,* in *Der heilige Theodosios: Schriften des Theodoros und Kyr-
    illos,* ed. Hermann Usener (Leipzig, 1890), pp. 105–13.
Vita Theodosii (Theodore)
    *Lobrede auf den heiligen Theodosios von Theodoros Bischof von Pa-
    trai,* in *Der heilige Theodosios* (see above), pp. 3–101.
Vita Theophanis
    Nicephori Scevophylacis vita S. Theophanis, in *Theophanis chronogra-
    phia,* 2:13–30.

Vita Theophylacti
"Vie de S. Théophylacte de Nicomédie," ed. Albert Vogt, *AnalBoll,* 1932, *50:* 71–82.

Volk, *Klostertypika*
Robert Volk, *Gesundheitswesen und Wohltätigkeit im Spiegel der byzantinischen Klostertypika,* Miscellanea byzantina monacensia, 28 (Munich: Institut für Byzantinistik, neugriechische Philologie, und byzantinische Kunstgeschichte der Universität München, 1983).

Waddington, *Inscriptions*
Inscriptions grecques et latines recueillies en Grèce et en Asie Mineure, ed. William H. Waddington and Philippe Le Bas (Paris, 1870).

WF
Wege der Forschung (Darmstadt: Wissenschaftliche Buchgesellschaft, 1963–).

Zacos and Veglery
George Zacos and Alexander Veglery, *Byzantine Lead Seals,* 1 vol., 4 parts (Basel: J. Augustin, 1972).

Zonaras
Ioannis Zonarae annales, ed. Maurice Pinder and Theodor Büttner-Wobst, 3 vols., CSHB (1841–97).

Index

279

Milton Keynes UK
Ingram Content Group UK Ltd.
UKHW031841280724
446193UK00001B/42

9 780801 856570